ANATOMY & PHYSIOLOGY

AN INTRODUCTION FOR NURSING AND HEALTHCARE

ANATOMY & PHYSIOLOGY

AN INTRODUCTION FOR NURSING AND HEALTHCARE

PAMELA MINETT
LAURA GINESI

Lantern

ISBN: 9781908625731

First published in 2020 by Lantern Publishing Ltd

Lantern Publishing Ltd, The Old Hayloft, Vantage Business Park, Bloxham Rd, Banbury OX16 9UX, UK
www.lanternpublishing.com

British Library Cataloguing in Publication Data
A catalogue record for this book is available from the British Library

The authors and publisher have made every attempt to ensure the content of this book is up to date and accurate. However, healthcare knowledge and information is changing all the time so the reader is advised to double-check any information in this text on drug usage, treatment procedures, the use of equipment, etc. to confirm that it complies with the latest safety recommendations, standards of practice and legislation, as well as local Trust policies and procedures. Students are advised to check with their tutor and/or practice supervisor before carrying out any of the procedures in this textbook.

Illustrations by Matthew McClements at Blink Studio Ltd, www.blink.biz
Cover design by Andrew Magee Design Ltd
Typeset by Medlar Publishing Solutions Pvt Ltd, India
Printed in the UK by Ashford Colour Press Ltd

Last digit is the print number: 10   9   8

CONTENTS

Supplementary chapters to be found online
at www.lanternpublishing.com/AandP:

DETAILED CONTENTS

Chapter 5

The cardiovascular system 65

Chapter 6

The respiratory system. 103

Chapter 7

The digestive system 121

Chapter 8

The urinary system 143

Chapter 9

The nervous system 159

Chapter 10

The sensory system 199

Chapter 11

The endocrine system 221

Supplementary chapters to be found online at www.lanternpublishing.com/AandP:

Chapter 17

Physiological measurements e1

Chapter 18

Principles of drug action e29

Chapter 19

Nutrition e53

Chapter 20

Biochemistry e71

PREFACE

Anatomy and Physiology: an introduction for nursing and healthcare contains the core knowledge of anatomy and physiology and its applications required by a range of health professions. The subject matter is relevant for student nurses, midwives, operating department practitioners, paramedics, physiotherapists, occupational therapists and speech and language therapists.

The healthcare landscape has changed markedly in recent decades because life expectancy has increased dramatically. Healthcare professionals for the 21st century must be able to provide supportive, complex care to people with different chronic conditions (co-morbidities) which may range from hypertension, diabetes, obesity, arthritis and cancers to mental health problems and/or dementia, all depending on self-management.

Based on many years' experience of teaching, we have tried to weave form and function together and we hope that doing this will help our readers to develop an understanding that will prove helpful right through their career.

Pamela Minett
Laura Ginesi

ACKNOWLEDGEMENTS

Many people, drawn from a range of interests and expertise, made a valued contribution to this book by checking drafts, reading proofs, and making suggestions regarding content. The authors would especially like to thank their editor Anna Anderson, and all those listed below:

Karen Blair
Judy Butcher
Clara Crockatt
Patricia Fell
Jane Gall
Kathy Gale
Penny Goacher
Louise Grisedale
Kirsty Henry
Sara Hunt
Madeleine Kerr

Helen Meehan
Dave Morrell
Brian Murray
Rose Niescierowicz
Elizabeth Ramsden
Hannah Schutt
Derek Scott
Jamie Weightman-Murray
Lily White
Alison Wood

They would also like to thank the photographers Andy Tallis, Peter Kaliski and Jack Striker, and also Dr John Greene of Queen Elizabeth University Hospital, Glasgow.

Finally, they would like to express their gratitude to Peter Oates, Jonathan Ray, Clare Boomer and all at Lantern Publishing who have made this book possible.

The publishers would like to thank the following lecturers for their feedback during the development of this book:

Dr Jonny Branney, Department of Nursing Science, Bournemouth University

Tracey Brickell, School of Health and Care Professions, University of Portsmouth

Ruth Broadhead, School of Community Health and Midwifery, University of Central Lancashire

Maggie Bull, Department of Health and Social Care, West Herts College

Dr Steven Crosby, School of Pharmacy and Biomolecular Sciences, Liverpool John Moores University

Richard Hellyar, School of Healthcare Sciences, Cardiff University

Dr Kathryn Jarvis, School of Sport and Health Sciences, University of Central Lancashire

Dorothy Kupara, College of Nursing, Midwifery and Healthcare, University of West London

Kate Morrow, School of Health and Social Work, University of Hertfordshire

Dr Joanne Pike, Faculty of Social and Life Sciences, Wrexham Glyndŵr University

Jay Ragoo, School of Health and Social Work, University of Hertfordshire

Sheila Stott, Department of Nursing, Midwifery and Health, Northumbria University

ABOUT THE AUTHORS

Pamela Minett (BSc (Hons), Biological sciences) is the author of educational textbooks including *Child Care & Development*, now in its 7th edition, and *The Environment Explained* series. She is also co-author, with David Wayne and David Rubenstein, of *Human Form & Function*.

She is also an experienced teacher and publisher, as well as having been an examiner in Human Biology for various awarding bodies. Pamela has also been a director of the Book Trust and was Chair of the former Scientific and Technical Group of the Society of Authors.

Laura Ginesi (PhD; BSc (Hons); PGCE; Cert. HE) is an applied physiologist with more than 30 years' experience of physiological education. Currently working at the University of East Anglia, Laura gained experience across the FE/HE sector teaching a wide range of students who are destined for the healthcare professions. She is also an antenatal educator, life coach and co-author, with Catharine Jenkins and Bernie Keenan, of *Dementia Care at a Glance*. In addition, she is a Fellow of the International Stress Management Association (ISMA) and Fellow of the Higher Education Academy. Her interest in wellbeing, nutrition and stress management first arose through research concerning long-term blood pressure regulation.

ACRONYMS AND ABBREVIATIONS

3D	3-dimensional	C-12	isotope of carbon
A	adenine DNA base	C-13	isotope of carbon
Ab	antibodies	C-14	isotope of carbon
ABCDE	airway; breathing; circulation; disability; exposure	C1–C7	cervical vertebrae or cervical spinal nerves
		cAMP	cyclic AMP
ABG	arterial blood gas	CASH	contraception and sexual health
ABI	acquired brain injury	CBT	cognitive behavioural therapy
ACE	angiotensin-converting enzyme	CCK	cholecystokinin
Ach	acetylcholine	CF	cystic fibrosis
ACTH	adrenocorticotrophic hormone	CFRD	cystic fibrosis-related diabetes
ADH	antidiuretic hormone	CFS	chronic fatigue syndrome
ADHD	attention deficit hyperactivity disorder	CHD	coronary heart disease
ADL	activities of daily living	CKD	chronic kidney disease
AF	atrial fibrillation	CM	cervical mucus
AIDS	acquired immunodeficiency syndrome	CNS	central nervous system
AKI	acute kidney injury	CO	cardiac output
ALA	alpha-linoleic acid	COPD	chronic obstructive pulmonary disorder
ALS	amyotrophic lateral sclerosis	COX	cyclo-oxygenase
AMD	age-related macular degeneration	CP	cerebral palsy
AMH	anti-Müllerian hormone	CPE	chemical permeation enhancer
AMP	adenosine monophosphate	CPR	cardiopulmonary resuscitation
AMR	antimicrobial resistance	CR	cardiac rehabilitation
AN	anorexia nervosa	CRH	corticotrophin-releasing hormone
ANS	autonomic nervous system	CRP	C-reactive protein
APGAR	appearance; pulse; grimace; activity; respiration	CSF	cerebrospinal fluid
		CT	computerised tomograph; calcitonin
ARDS	acute respiratory distress syndrome	CTZ	chemoreceptor trigger zone
ASD	autism spectrum disorder	CVD	cardiovascular disease
ATP	adenosine triphosphate	CYP	cytochrome P450
ATPase	adenosine triphosphatase	DHT	dihydrotestosterone
AV	atrioventricular	DI	diabetes insipidus
AVPU	alert; voice; pain; unresponsive	DIC	disseminated intravascular coagulopathy
BAI	body adiposity index	DKA	diabetic ketoacidosis
BBB	blood–brain barrier	DLB	dementia with Lewy bodies
BIA	bioelectrical impedance analysis	D-MER	dysphoric milk ejection reflex
BMI	body mass index	DNA	deoxyribonucleic acid
BMR	basal metabolic rate	DNAase	deoxyribonuclease
BN	bulimia nervosa	DS	Down syndrome
Botox	*Botulinum* toxin	DVT	deep vein thrombosis
BP	blood pressure	E	effort
BPAD	bipolar affective disorder	EBV	Epstein–Barr virus
BPH	benign prostatic hyperplasia	ECF	extracellular fluid
bpm	beats per minute	ECG	electrocardiogram
BPPV	benign paroxysmal positional vertigo	Echo	echocardiography
BRCA1	breast cancer 1 gene	ED	erectile dysfunction
BRCA2	breast cancer 2 gene	EDD	estimated date of delivery
BUN	blood urea nitrogen	EEG	electroencephalogram
C	cytosine DNA base	EFA	essential fatty acid
C. diff	*Clostridium difficile*	ELISA	enzyme-linked immunosorbent assay

EMG	electromyography
ENS	enteric nervous system
EPO	erythropoietin
ER	endoplasmic reticulum
ERCP	endoscopic retrograde cholangiopancreatography
ERV	expiratory reserve volume
ES	embryonic stem cell
ESR	erythrocyte sedimentation rate
ET	electron transfer
F	fulcrum
FAD	flavin adenine dinucleotide
FAS	foetal alcohol syndrome
FAST	facial weakness; arm weakness; speech problem; time
FBC	full blood count
FOB	faecal occult blood
FRC	functional residual capacity
FSH	follicle-stimulating hormone
FXS	fragile X syndrome
G	guanine DNA base
G1	first growth phase of cell cycle
G2	second growth phase of cell cycle
GA 1	glutaric aciduria type 1
GABA	gamma-amino butyric acid
GAD	generalised anxiety disorder
GCS	Glasgow Coma Scale
GDP	guanosine 5′-diphosphate
gFOBT	guaiac faecal occult blood test
GFR	glomerular filtration rate
GH	growth hormone
GHRH	growth hormone-releasing hormone
GI	gastrointestinal
GnRH	gonadotrophin-releasing hormone
GP	general practitioner
GPCR	G-protein coupled receptor
GTN	glyceryl trinitrate
GTP	guanosine 5′-triphosphate
GUM	genitourinary medicine
GvHD	graft-versus-host disease
H. pylori	Helicobacter pylori
HAI	hospital-acquired infection
HbA1c	glycated haemoglobin
HBV	hepatitis B virus
hCG	human chorionic gonadotrophin
HCU	homocysteinuria
HCV	hepatitis C virus
HD	Huntington's disease
HDL	high density lipoprotein
HGP	Human Genome Project
HHS	hyperosmolar hyperglycaemic state
HIV	human immunodeficiency virus
HLA	human leucocyte antigen
HMG CoA	hydroxy-3-methylglutaryl coenzyme A
HoTN	hypotension
HPV	human papillomavirus
HR	heart rate
HRT	hormone replacement therapy
HTN	hypertension
IBD	inflammatory bowel disease
ICF	intracellular fluid
ICP	intracranial pressure
Ig	immunoglobulins
IgA	immunoglobulin A
IgD	immunoglobulin D
IgE	immunoglobulin E
IgG	immunoglobulin G
IgM	immunoglobulin M
IM	intramuscular
INR	International Normalised Ratio
insP3	inositol-1,4,5 triphosphate
IRV	inspiratory reserve volume
ISF	interstitial fluid
IUD	intrauterine device
IV	intravenous
IVA	isovaleric acidaemia
L	load; litre
L1–L5	lumbar vertebrae or spinal lumbar nerves
LA	linoleic acid
LAM	lactational amenorrhoea method
LDL	low-density lipoprotein
LFT	liver function test
LH	luteinising hormone
LLQ	left lower quadrant
LSD	lysergic acid diethylamide
LUQ	left upper quadrant
M	M (mitosis) phase
MABs	monoclonal antibodies
MAC	membrane attack complex
MALT	mucosa-associated lymphoid tissue
MAOI	monoamine oxidase inhibitor
MAP	mean arterial blood pressure
MCADD	medium-chained acetyl-CoA dehydrogenase deficiency
MCV	meningococcal conjugate vaccine
MDT	multidisciplinary team
ME	myalgic encephalomyelitis
MEC	minimum effective concentration
MFB	median forebrain bundle
MHC	major histocompatibility complex
mHTT	mutant huntingtin
MND	motor neurone disease
MRI	magnetic resonance imaging
mRNA	messenger RNA
MRSA	methicillin-resistant Staphylococcus aureus
MS	multiple sclerosis
MSH	melanocyte-stimulating hormone
MSUD	maple syrup urine disease
MTC	minimum toxic concentration
mtDNA	mitochondrial DNA
MUST	Malnutrition Universal Screening Tool
NAD	nicotinamide adenine dinucleotide
NAFLD	non-alcoholic fatty liver disease
NCV	nerve conduction velocity

NEWS	National Early Warning Score		RR	respiratory rate
NFP	natural family planning; net filtration pressure		rRNA	ribosomal RNA
NHS	National Health Service		RSI	repetitive strain injury
NK	natural killer (cell)		RSV	respiratory syncytial virus
NSAID	non-steroidal anti-inflammatory drug		RTI	respiratory tract infection
NSU	non-specific urethritis		RUQ	right upper quadrant
OCD	obsessive–compulsive disorder		RV	reserve volume
OGTT	oral glucose tolerance test		S	S (synthesis) phase
OM	outer membrane		SA	sinoatrial
OMD	oculomotor dysfunction		SCID	severe combined immunodeficiency disease
OP	osmotic pressure		SEM	scanning electron micrograph
OSA	obstructive sleep apnoea		sER	smooth endoplasmic reticulum
p53	tumour suppressor protein 53		SERMs	selective oestrogen receptor modulator
PAG	periaqueductal grey		SI	international system of units
PC	phosphocreatine		SL	sublingual
P_{CO_2}	partial pressure of carbon dioxide		SLE	systemic lupus erythematosus
PCOS	polycystic ovary syndrome		SPECT	single photon emission computed tomography
PCR	polymerase chain reaction			
PCV	pneumococcal conjugate vaccine		Sp_{O_2}	peripheral capillary oxygen saturation
PEF	peak expiratory flow		SRY	sex-determining region Y
PEFR	peak expiratory flow rate		SSPE	subacute sclerosing panencephalitis
PEG	percutaneous endoscopic gastroscopy		SSRI	selective serotonin reuptake inhibitor
PET	positron emission tomography		STI	sexually transmitted infection
PG	prostaglandins		SV	stroke volume
PGP	pelvic girdle pain		T	thymine DNA base
PID	pelvic inflammatory disease		T1–T12	thoracic vertebrae or thoracic spinal nerves
PKU	phenylketonuria		T3	triiodothyronine
PMDD	premenstrual dysphoric disorder		T4	thyroxine
PMS	premenstrual syndrome		TB	tuberculosis
PNS	peripheral nervous system		TD	topical route
PO	oral route (per os)		TENS	transcutaneous electrical nerve stimulation
P_{O_2}	partial pressure of oxygen		THR	thyroid hormone receptor
POF	premature ovarian failure		TIA	transient ischaemic attack
PPE	personal protective equipment		TLC	total lung capacity
PPH	post-partum haemorrhage		TNF	tumour necrosis factor
PR	rectal route (per rectum)		TORCH	toxoplasmosis; other infections; rubella; cytomegalovirus; herpes virus
pre-D3	precursor to vitamin D			
PT	prothrombin time		TRH	thyrotropin-releasing hormone
PTH	parathyroid hormone		tRNA	transfer RNA
PTSD	post-traumatic stress disorder		TSE	transmissible spongiform encephalopathy
PUFA	polyunsaturated fats		TSH	thyroid-stimulating hormone
PYY	peptide tyrosine tyrosine		TSS	toxic shock syndrome
RA	rheumatoid arthritis		TV	tidal volume
RAAS	renin–angiotensin–aldosterone system		U	uracil
RAS	reticular activating system		UC	ulcerative colitis
RBC	red blood cell count		URTI	upper respiratory tract infection
rER	rough endoplasmic reticulum		UTI	urinary tract infection
Rh	rhesus		UV	ultraviolet
RhD	rhesus factor D		VC	vital capacity
RICE	rest, ice, compression, elevation		VDR	vitamin D receptor
RLQ	right lower quadrant		WHO	World Health Organization
RNA	ribonucleic acid		WHR	waist-to-hip ratio
ROS	reactive oxygen species			

HOW TO USE THIS BOOK

This book has been designed to help you learn quickly and to get the most out of an anatomy and physiology course.

- **Information** is set out clearly and concisely with bullet points to emphasise the structures and functions of the healthy human body.
- **Drawings and flow charts** are included on many pages to illustrate what's been written in the text.
- Each chapter includes examples of **pathophysiology** – which covers the development of disease when homeostasis is disturbed by disordered physiological processes.
- If you are uncertain of the meaning of any word, head to the comprehensive **Glossary** which appears just before the Index.
- **Cross-references in blue introduced by an arrow** (e.g. → Fig. 5.1, → 6.2.1) provide links to other places in the book and in the online chapters which contain more information – think of them as being like hyperlinks on the internet.
- At the end of each chapter you will find **Key points**:

Blue boxes in the margins contain definitions, key ideas and applications of the information in the text and are included to make each topic more interesting and relevant.

Key points

1. These provide a recap of the important aspects of the chapter.
2. Making sure that you have covered everything in the Key points will provide reassurance that your learning is progressing

- Throughout the book you will find **Taking it Further** boxes that guide you to the additional online chapters.
- Once you feel familiar with the material in a chapter, why not test your understanding by trying the **self-assessment questions**, which can be found at www.lanternpublishing.com/AandP? These come in various formats, from multiple choice questions (MCQs) and assertion reasoning questions (ARQs) to test your critical thinking, to free-form questions which may require you to draw a diagram or explain a process. Answers are supplied to most, but not all questions. Some may require you to carry out further research using the book.

Taking it Further
These will guide you towards the material in Chapters 17 to 20 which provides supplementary information. These chapters can be found online at www.lanternpublishing.com/AandP

Test yourself! Go to *www.lanternpublishing.com/AandP* and try the questions to check your understanding.

How to learn anatomy and physiology

1. Make study time a habit

Leaving all your learning until just before your exams is stressful and ineffective. You will be too anxious and worried to learn. Cramming simply doesn't work in the long term. It might mean that you remember some things until your exam is over, but you will probably have forgotten them by the time you go on your next block of practice-based learning.

2. Make the most of your study time

If you start early and schedule your anatomy and physiology study time as part of your regular weekly routine, then studying becomes a habit that enables you to continuously review what you are learning in classrooms, simulation labs and lectures. No cramming therefore means no panic!

3. Make your own clear set of notes

Simply reading a textbook doesn't guarantee that you will remember what you have been reading. Many students find that it helps if they write notes about the topic they are studying in their own words. The combination of seeing the words on a page and then transforming them into your own words helps you to retain the information.

- Read a section of text a couple of times. You might like to write notes in the margin or highlight sentences that are important. Look up key words in the Glossary.
- Then cover up the section of text that you have read, and write it down in your own words, or say it out loud or even sing about it! Try different ways to see what helps the most.
- Read the section again and check what you got right or for any mistakes.
- The next time you sit down to study, review your learning by seeing how much you remember.

4. Get making and creating

Many students like to use their artistic skills to help them learn anatomy and physiology.

- Make large drawings of anatomical structures of the human body and label them; write notes around the drawing to explain its functions and why it is important.
- Make models of anatomical structure using clay, dough or even cake mix!
- You may wish to hang your creations on your wall – or eat it if it's a cake!

5. Make your own flow charts

Think of flow charting as creating your own infographic that describes whichever aspect of human physiology you are learning about.

- Re-draw the illustrations and figures that show how processes in the human body work, by using colours and big sheets of paper or using drawing tools on a tablet device. Don't worry if the result doesn't look like a masterpiece – it's meant to be a learning tool just for you.
- Annotate your flow chart/infographic with facts that describe what could happen if homeostasis is disturbed.

- Follow the blue arrowed links on the pages to find out more, then add any new important items to your flow chart.
- The sections at the end of the chapters introduce pathophysiology. Many students find they help in understanding why basic physiology is important.

6. Practice questions

- When you have finished reviewing and revising a body system, test your knowledge with the online questions that accompany this book. Don't be afraid to have a go without using the book.
- Justify your answers to yourself by trying to work out why you have chosen a particular answer for each question:
- Check what the correct answer is. If you didn't do very well, then go to step 7.

7. Repeat! Repeat! Repeat!

Nobody ever learns their anatomy and physiology in a single sitting.
- You need to keep going over each topic. The more times you go over each body system or topic, the better your chances of remembering it.
- Make use of all the resources your lecturers and tutors provide, including the lecture slides, handouts and online links to videos or physiology websites.

8. Check your understanding with a buddy group

For some students, studying in a team can maximise everyone's learning. In education studies, peer-to-peer teaching is found to be a very effective way of helping people to retain information. It provides the opportunity to:
- practise explaining how body processes work – explaining something to someone else helps you to understand it yourself
- bounce ideas around
- identify areas of weakness that you need to focus on
- quiz each other and work out the answers together
- have a baking/clay modelling competition to use your creative skills to show the structure of body organs.

9. Mix up and mash up

There are lots of different study tactics including those mentioned above. You can help yourself to remember things by making flashcards, writing poetry or haiku, singing out loud, making your own podcasts and being creative in various ways. You won't know what helps you to learn best unless you try out the suggestions.

10. If you're not enjoying studying, take a break

Often people need space to spread out when they are studying or revising, with room for books, laptop or tablet. Feeling cramped and restricted can be stressful, affect your ability to learn and result in feeling worried that you aren't learning much. So if you feel the stress levels rising, stop studying. Go outdoors for a walk or spend some time on a hobby. Many people find that they come back to their studies feeling refreshed and raring to go again.

CHAPTER 1
INTRODUCTION

This chapter introduces the reader to the basic structure of the human body and the anatomical terms in common use by health professionals. It also discusses homeostasis, which is the way the conditions inside the body are maintained in a relatively stable state despite the continuously changing external environment in which we all live. When homeostasis is disturbed, disease may occur.

1.1 The human body

Knowledge of the human body required by health professionals involves the study of:

- **anatomy** – the structure of the human body (→ Fig. 1.1)
- **physiology** – how the body works
- **homeostasis** – a self-regulating process that enables conditions inside the body to remain in a steady state for optimal health (→ 1.3)
- **pathology** – the nature and causes of disease
- **integrated healthcare** – a person-centred approach to health and illness that encompasses physical, emotional, mental and spiritual aspects.

1.2 Structure of the body

Each human, like all other animals, begins life as a single cell which multiplies to produce trillions of cells organised into tissues, organs and systems that are inter-related and interdependent so that they function as a complete individual.

A **cell** is a tiny unit of living matter; there are many types of cells, e.g. red cells, muscle cells and nerve cells. Every cell has a life cycle (→ 13.3).

A **tissue** is a group of cells specialised to perform a particular function, e.g. muscle tissue and nervous tissue.

An **organ** is a part of the body with a special function or functions, e.g. heart, skin and stomach.

A **system** is a group of organs working together to carry out one or more functions, e.g. cardiovascular system and nervous system.

1.2.1 Cavities in the body

A body cavity is a space which contains organs (→ Fig. 1.2). The **cranial cavity** encloses the brain, the **spinal cavity** encloses the spinal cord and the **thoracic cavity** encloses the heart and lungs. The **abdominopelvic cavity** is a large cavity containing the **viscera** (soft internal organs), with the upper part known as the **abdominal cavity** and the lower part as the **pelvic cavity**.

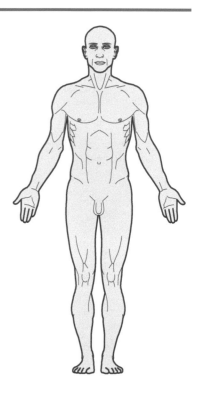

Fig. 1.1 Anterior view of the male body.

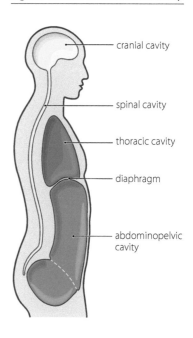

cranial cavity

spinal cavity

thoracic cavity

diaphragm

abdominopelvic cavity

Fig. 1.2 Cavities in the mid-sagittal plane.

1.2.2 Organs

An organ is a structure within the body that comprises two or more tissues and performs one or more specific functions (→ Fig. 1.3). The human body contains 79 organs and each contributes to homeostasis (→ 1.3) in a different way. Five major organs are known as **vital organs** – heart, brain, lungs, liver and kidneys.

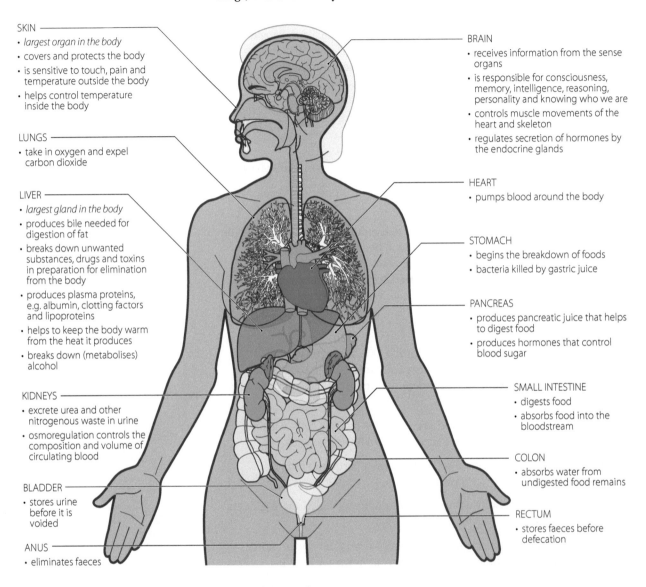

SKIN
- *largest organ in the body*
- covers and protects the body
- is sensitive to touch, pain and temperature outside the body
- helps control temperature inside the body

LUNGS
- take in oxygen and expel carbon dioxide

LIVER
- *largest gland in the body*
- produces bile needed for digestion of fat
- breaks down unwanted substances, drugs and toxins in preparation for elimination from the body
- produces plasma proteins, e.g. albumin, clotting factors and lipoproteins
- helps to keep the body warm from the heat it produces
- breaks down (metabolises) alcohol

KIDNEYS
- excrete urea and other nitrogenous waste in urine
- osmoregulation controls the composition and volume of circulating blood

BLADDER
- stores urine before it is voided

ANUS
- eliminates faeces

BRAIN
- receives information from the sense organs
- is responsible for consciousness, memory, intelligence, reasoning, personality and knowing who we are
- controls muscle movements of the heart and skeleton
- regulates secretion of hormones by the endocrine glands

HEART
- pumps blood around the body

STOMACH
- begins the breakdown of foods
- bacteria killed by gastric juice

PANCREAS
- produces pancreatic juice that helps to digest food
- produces hormones that control blood sugar

SMALL INTESTINE
- digests food
- absorbs food into the bloodstream

COLON
- absorbs water from undigested food remains

RECTUM
- stores faeces before defecation

Fig. 1.3 Some of the organs in the human body and their main functions.

1.2.3 Systems

The systems in the body work together and enable it to function as a whole. Being inter-related, the malfunctioning of one of them can affect the health of the whole body. Nine of the eleven main systems and their funtions are shown below (→ Fig. 1.4). The missing two are the **integumentary system** (skin) and the **immune system**. The skin provides the outer covering that protects the body from the external environment and the immune system protects against disease in all parts of the body.

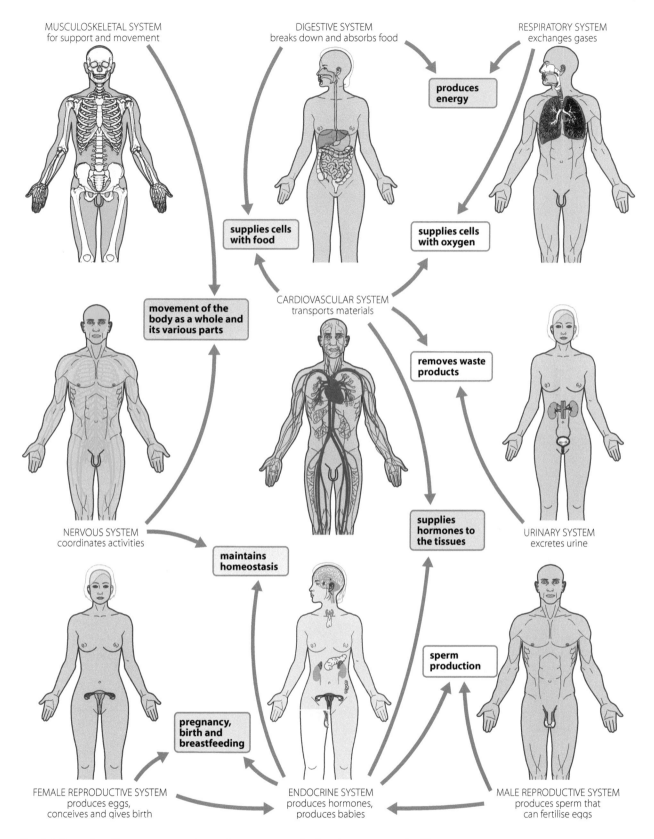

MUSCULOSKELETAL SYSTEM
for support and movement

DIGESTIVE SYSTEM
breaks down and absorbs food

RESPIRATORY SYSTEM
exchanges gases

**produces
energy**

**supplies cells
with food**

**supplies cells
with oxygen**

**movement of the
body as a whole and
its various parts**

CARDIOVASCULAR SYSTEM
transports materials

**removes waste
products**

NERVOUS SYSTEM
coordinates activities

**maintains
homeostasis**

**supplies
hormones to
the tissues**

URINARY SYSTEM
excretes urine

**sperm
production**

**pregnancy,
birth and
breastfeeding**

FEMALE REPRODUCTIVE SYSTEM
produces eggs,
conceives and gives birth

ENDOCRINE SYSTEM
produces hormones,
produces babies

MALE REPRODUCTIVE SYSTEM
produces sperm that
can fertilise eggs

Fig. 1.4 Examples of how systems work together to carry out the functions necessary for life.

3

1.2.4 Anatomical nomenclature

A standard method of naming the position of anatomical structures has been developed to assist in communication of information for diagnosis and therapy. It assumes that the human figure is standing, facing towards the observer, with the arms at the sides of the body and the palms of the hands facing the observer:

- **planes** divide the body into portions (→ Fig. 1.5)
- **quadrants** of the trunk and the **regions** of the abdomen allow the position of pain, tenderness, scars, lumps, etc. to be identified, and the organs and tissues which may be involved (→ Fig. 1.6).

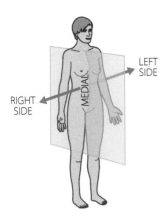

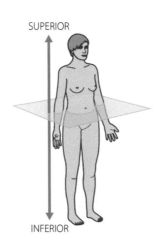

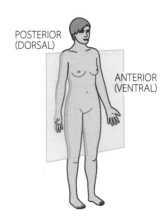

sagittal plane runs through the centre of the body, dividing it into left and right portions

horizontal plane, also called a **cross-section**, divides the body into superior (upper) and inferior (lower) portions

coronal (frontal) plane runs perpendicular to the sagittal plane and divides the body into front and back portions. The front is known as anterior or ventral and the back as posterior or dorsal

Fig. 1.5 The planes of the body.

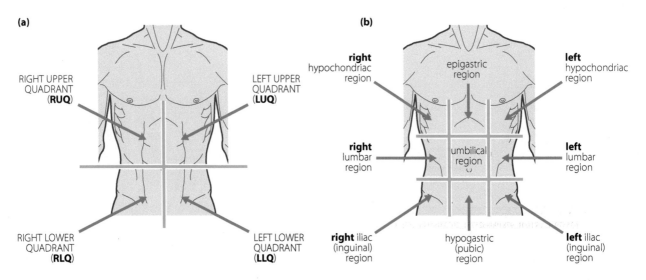

Fig. 1.6 (**a**) The quadrants of the body; (**b**) the regions of the body.

1.3 Homeostasis

The key to health and wellbeing is the maintenance of a steady state within the body called **homeostasis** (*homeo* = same; *stasis* = state). Although the conditions outside the body – the **external environment** – are continually varying, the conditions within the body (**internal environment**) must be kept more or less constant by homeostatic processes for optimal health (→ Box 1.1). Each of the physiological conditions that contribute to the internal environment can vary within a limited range – its **set point**. Too great a variation in any one of them can lead to disease unless corrected by a feedback system to restore the body's natural set point.

1.3.1 The internal environment

Human life and survival depend on the continuous flow of fluids through the tissues carrying substances to the cells for the **metabolic (chemical) processes** that keep the body alive. **Homeostasis of the internal environment** is maintained by the continuous movement of substances between the interstitial fluid, plasma, and intracellular fluid (tissue fluid) (→ Fig. 1.7).

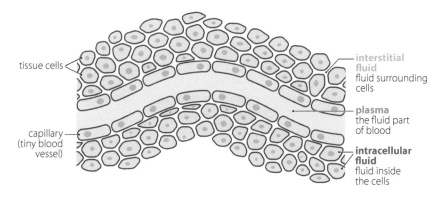

tissue cells

interstitial fluid
fluid surrounding cells

plasma
the fluid part of blood

capillary (tiny blood vessel)

intracellular fluid
fluid inside the cells

Fig. 1.7 Fluids in the internal environment.

1.3.2 Homeostatic regulation

When the composition of interstitial fluid (ISF) is kept more or less constant, the cells can function efficiently and support the body to remain healthy. The many physiological parameters under homeostatic control include:

- blood pressure
- body temperature
- blood pH level (→ Box 1.2)
- blood glucose levels
- levels of circulating hormones
- oxygen and carbon dioxide levels.

Homeostasis is a dynamic process

A small area in the brain called the hypothalamus is responsible for some important homeostatic control mechanisms that are **effected** (carried out) by the endocrine and nervous systems (→ Table 1.1).

Box 1.1 Homeostasis is the self-regulating property by which the human body, like all living systems, uses energy to maintain equilibrium (stability) in response to activity or changing conditions.

The ability of the human body to adapt and maintain stability makes it possible for people to adjust to variations in the internal state such as exercise, stress and pregnancy, and to changes in the external environment.

Box 1.2 The pH scale of 1–14 is used to express the degree of acidity or alkalinity of a solution. pH 7 is neutral, less than 7 is acid, more than 7 is alkaline.

Blood pH is tightly regulated within a narrow range of 7.35–7.45. An incorrect pH alters activity of physiological proteins and enzymes and hence the function of living cells, resulting in health problems known as acid–base disturbances.

Table 1.1 Differences in homeostatic control between the nervous and endocrine systems

Nervous system	Endocrine system
• controls short-term processes by rapid adjustments • signals are sent as electrical impulses along nerves • nerve impulses travel rapidly along nerve pathways • controls the activity of muscle and gland cells	• regulates the body's activities • signals are sent as hormones (chemical messengers) • hormones travel more slowly in the bloodstream • different hormones affect different types of cell

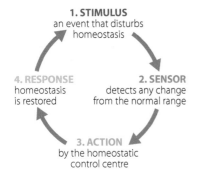

Fig. 1.8 The principle of negative feedback.

1.4 Feedback systems

A feedback system is a homeostatic process that takes very different forms:
- negative feedback – a self-correcting process that results in physiological stability
- positive feedback – amplifies the response that feeds forward to a new physiological state.

1.4.1 Negative feedback

Negative feedback is a self-correcting process to maintain stability. It is necessary when a change in direction away from the set point brings about a change in the opposite direction in order to minimise the change and restore the set point. Key stages in the process are (→ Fig. 1.8):
- **stimulus** – an event that disturbs homeostasis
- **sensor** – the organs or tissues that detect the change from the normal range
- **action** – by the **homeostatic control centre**: the organs or tissues that respond to the stimulus and activate the response
- **response** – the restoration of the set point by the **effector** organs and tissues.

Example of homeostasis

Despite the daily variation in the amount of carbohydrate in the diet (→ Box 1.3), the amount of glucose in the blood (blood sugar) is maintained at a more or less constant level (set point) to prevent disease (→ Box 1.4).

Box 1.3 Carbohydrate in the diet is mainly sugar and starch. Simple sugars, e.g. glucose, do not need to be digested (broken down) before being absorbed into the blood. Starch has first to be converted into sugar by digestion.

Box 1.4 Hyperglycaemia develops when the glucose content in the blood is abnormally high. **Hypoglycaemia** develops when the glucose content in the blood is abnormally low.

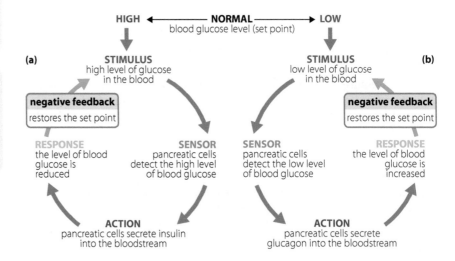

Fig. 1.9 The homeostatic control of blood glucose: (**a**) insulin lowers blood glucose level; (**b**) glucagon raises blood glucose level.

Homeostasis of blood glucose depends on negative feedback, the pancreas as a control centre, an effector pathway and the activity of two hormones:

- **insulin** which lowers the blood glucose level by stimulating liver cells – the effectors of the response – to take up the extra glucose and convert it into glycogen for storage in the liver (→ Fig. 1.9a)
- **glucagon** which raises the blood glucose level by stimulating the conversion of glycogen to glucose (→ Fig. 1.9b).

1.4.2 Positive feedback

Positive feedback occurs when the input of a system is used to increase the output and amplify the response (→ Fig. 1.10). Positive feedback processes usually involve:

1. **input** – the stimulus that initiates the process
2. **output** – amplification of the process, which may take place in stages
3. **outcome** – the end result of the process and restoration that feeds forward to a new steady state (→ Fig. 1.11).

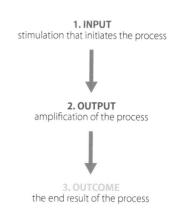

1. INPUT
stimulation that initiates the process

2. OUTPUT
amplification of the process

3. OUTCOME
the end result of the process

Fig. 1.10 The principle of positive feedback.

Example 1

The release of increased amounts of oxytocin from the posterior pituitary gland during labour stimulates the muscles to contract more strongly to push an unborn baby through the birth canal.

Example 2

A cascade of biochemical events leads to clotting and sealing of an injury.

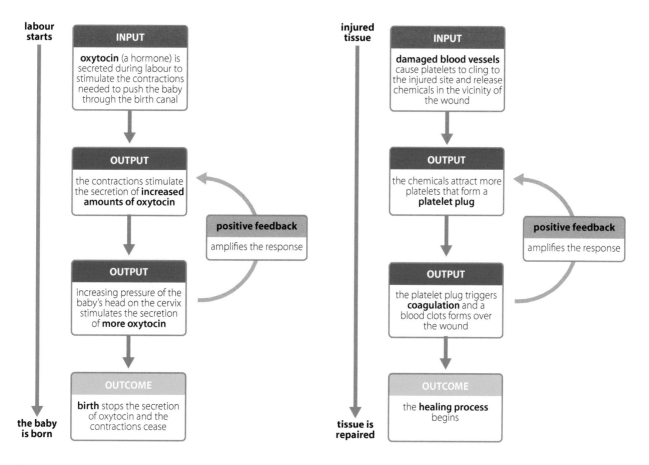

Fig. 1.11 Examples of positive feedback.

1.5 Disturbed homeostasis

Physiological parameters should remain within the normal homeostatic range for survival and wellbeing and, when homeostasis is **temporarily disturbed** by changes, internal or external, feedback mechanisms respond promptly to compensate and **restore** the internal balance of the body, e.g.:

- heat loss and heat gain feedback mechanisms ensure that body temperature remains within normal range despite wide changes in environmental temperature
- when an injury occurs, the damaged tissue triggers both clotting and inflammation which start the process of wound healing and repair
- the immune system responds to each different pathogen – virus, bacterium, fungus or parasite – in a very specific way that leads to its destruction, elimination or tolerance
- disturbances in fluid balance are compensated through coordinated action of the nervous system, endocrine system, cardiovascular system and kidneys.

In the various chapters of the book, readers will be introduced to, and become familiar with, the different types of normal **physiological responses** of each body system. This helps healthcare professionals to understand the basis for the physiological ranges and the ways in which they oscillate around the set point(s). The normal limits for the myriad of different observations, measurements, changing parameters and markers therefore serve as guidelines for physiological observations and clinical assessments.

Homeostasis is a very delicate balancing system and if it becomes disturbed (altered), the internal environment is disrupted, with results that can sometimes destabilise physical health, psychological wellbeing or both. At cell level, altered homeostasis can disturb the way a tissue behaves or an organ performs its function. Many disease processes therefore illustrate what happens in the body when the internal environment is disrupted.

The later section of each chapter includes examples of **pathophysiology** – the study of the processes that lead to disease – that may require healthcare interventions, e.g.:

- blood glucose levels that are outside the expected normal range could indicate diabetes mellitus
- blood pressure outside the normal range is known as **hypertension** when too high or **hypotension** when too low
- low levels of oxygen in blood is termed **hypoxia**
- high body temperature is called **hyperthermia**, and **hypothermia** when it falls below the normal range.

Key points

1. The cell is the basic structural unit of living matter in the human body.
2. The organs of the body are organised into systems each of which contributes to normal, physiological function in a unique way.
3. The systems of the human body work together to maintain an optimal steady state known as homeostasis.
4. Negative feedback is a dynamic, self-correcting process that maintains homeostasis.
5. When homeostasis is disturbed, the internal environment of the human body may be disrupted, leading to pathophysiology.

CHAPTER 2
HISTOLOGY

Histology is the study of the microscopic structure of the cells and tissues of living organisms. The human body contains many different types of cell, each with its own shape, size and function. They are grouped together to form tissues, and the type of cell that a tissue contains is related to its function.

2.1 Cells

Cells are the basic structural units of the body. Although the different types of cell show a remarkable range of shapes, sizes, activities and functions, they all have a complex and highly organised structure (→ Fig. 2.1) with:

- **plasma membrane** (**cell membrane**) – the thin layer around the outside of the cell which separates it from its surroundings
- **nucleus**, often placed near the centre of the cell and which controls its activities
- **cytoplasm**, the semi-liquid material which fills the cell and contains many organelles – an **organelle** being a specialised part of the cytoplasm with its own particular function and, sometimes, enclosed in its own membrane (→ Box 2.1).

Box 2.1 There are more than 250 different types of human cell. The smallest are the sperm, being 0.003 mm at the widest part – the part that contains the genes. Red blood cells are 0.004–0.008 mm in diameter, but as they have lost their nucleus they are no longer complete cells. The ovum (egg cell) is the largest, being 0.15–0.2 mm in diameter, and is just visible to the naked eye.

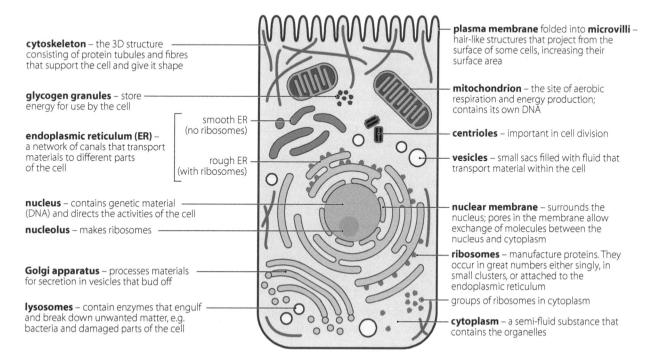

cytoskeleton – the 3D structure consisting of protein tubules and fibres that support the cell and give it shape

glycogen granules – store energy for use by the cell

endoplasmic reticulum (ER) – a network of canals that transport materials to different parts of the cell

smooth ER (no ribosomes)

rough ER (with ribosomes)

nucleus – contains genetic material (DNA) and directs the activities of the cell

nucleolus – makes ribosomes

Golgi apparatus – processes materials for secretion in vesicles that bud off

lysosomes – contain enzymes that engulf and break down unwanted matter, e.g. bacteria and damaged parts of the cell

plasma membrane folded into **microvilli** – hair-like structures that project from the surface of some cells, increasing their surface area

mitochondrion – the site of aerobic respiration and energy production; contains its own DNA

centrioles – important in cell division

vesicles – small sacs filled with fluid that transport material within the cell

nuclear membrane – surrounds the nucleus; pores in the membrane allow exchange of molecules between the nucleus and cytoplasm

ribosomes – manufacture proteins. They occur in great numbers either singly, in small clusters, or attached to the endoplasmic reticulum

groups of ribosomes in cytoplasm

cytoplasm – a semi-fluid substance that contains the organelles

Fig. 2.1 A generalised cell showing the major organelles.

2.2 Plasma membrane

Each cell is bounded by a plasma membrane that forms a flexible, semi-permeable barrier between the interior of the cell and the surrounding environment; similar membranes also form the outer layer of the nucleus and some of the organelles inside the cell.

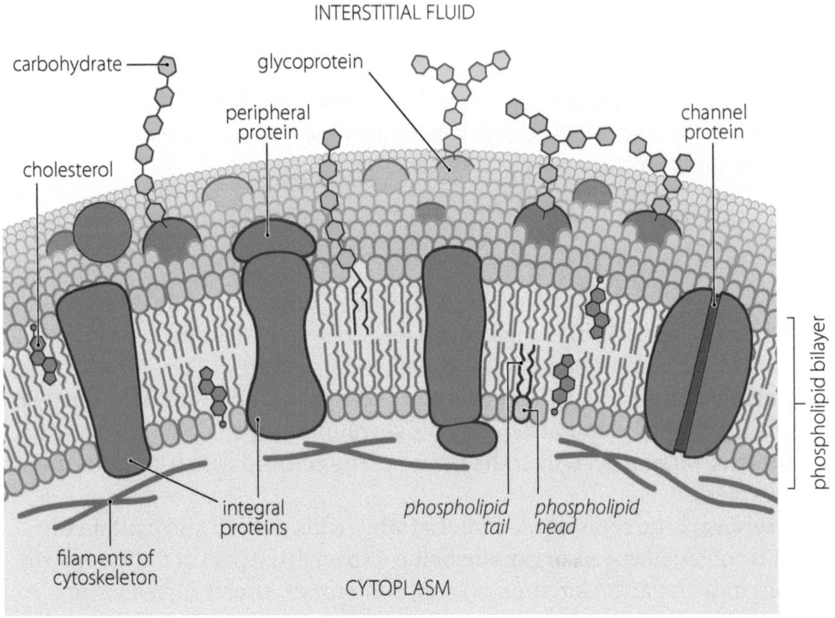

Fig. 2.2 Molecular structure of the plasma membrane.

2.2.1 Molecular structure of the plasma membrane

The plasma membrane is composed of many different types of molecule, each with its own function (→ Fig. 2.2).

The **phospholipid bilayer** forms the basic structure of the plasma membrane. It is composed of **phospholipid molecules** arranged in two layers with the phospholipid heads aligned facing outwards and the phospholipid tails oriented inwards, an arrangement that helps to give flexibility to the membrane (→ Box 2.2).

Peripheral proteins are attached to the outer part of the lipid bilayer or to integral proteins.

Integral proteins span across both lipid layers and are permanently attached to the membrane (→ Box 2.3). Some integral proteins are **receptor proteins** – those that relay signals between the cell's internal environment (cytoplasm) and external environment (interstitial fluid) in response to hormones, neurotransmitters and other signalling molecules.

Transport proteins allow substances to move through specific channels or they transport them across cell membranes by facilitated diffusion or active transport (→ 2.2.2).

Glycoproteins have a carbohydrate chain attached to them and are involved in **cell-to-cell recognition** – the ability to distinguish one type of neighbouring cell from another.

Cholesterol molecules scattered in the membrane help to give it stability (→ Box 2.4).

Box 2.2 The lipid bilayer forms a thin, flexible sheet that encloses the cell and forms a continuous barrier. It is selectively impermeable to water-soluble molecules and ions (charged particles), allowing the cell to regulate the concentrations of salt and acids within.

Box 2.3 Some of the proteins on the surface of the plasma membrane identify the cell as belonging to a particular individual. Before an organ is transplanted, a procedure called **tissue typing** is carried out to ensure that the donor and recipient proteins are compatible (→ 14.8).

Box 2.4 A certain amount of fat is essential in the diet to provide the lipids and cholesterol necessary for the construction of cell membranes.

2.2.2 Crossing the plasma membrane

The plasma membrane is semipermeable and plays an active part in regulating the movement of substances into and out of the cell by allowing some molecules to pass through while preventing larger particles and organelles within the cell from escaping (→ Box 2.5). There is continuous movement in both directions and the processes by which various molecules are transported fall into three general categories – passive, active and vesicle-mediated (→ Fig. 2.3).

Box 2.5 The movement of molecules across the plasma membrane is closely regulated to maintain a balanced internal environment (homeostasis) within the cell.

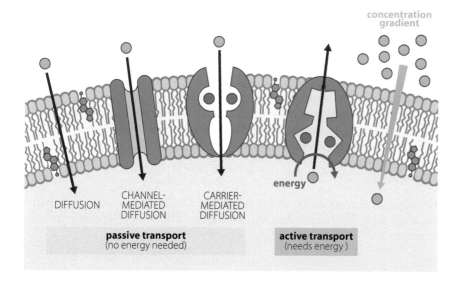

Fig. 2.3 Crossing the plasma membrane.

Taking it Further
See online Chapter 20 to find out more about the ways in which substances are transported across cell membranes.

Passive transport

Passive transport is the movement of substances across the plasma membrane without expenditure of energy. It occurs by means of channel-mediated diffusion, facilitated diffusion or osmosis (→ Box 2.6).

Diffusion is the net movement of molecules from an area of higher concentration to an area of lower concentration along a **concentration gradient**. This process allows small molecules to diffuse across the plasma membrane relatively easily, e.g. oxygen diffuses rapidly from air in the alveolar spaces into the bloodstream (→ Box 2.7).

Channel-mediated diffusion occurs when protein molecules have a pore or channel that allows a specific substance to enter, e.g. water crosses the plasma membrane in this way.

Facilitated diffusion means that a transport protein acts rather like a shuttle through the membrane, e.g. glucose molecules enter the cell in this way.

Osmosis is the movement of water from a high water concentration to a low water concentration through a semipermeable membrane that tends to equalise the concentrations of solutes on the two sides.

Active transport

Active transport requires energy to move substances across the plasma membrane in the opposite direction to their concentration gradient, a process that uses transport proteins or vesicles.

Box 2.6 The difference between passive and active transport is that in passive transport, substances move down a concentration gradient, whereas in active transport they are moved against a concentration gradient which requires energy (→ 20.7.3).

Box 2.7 Concentration gradient
Most transport of materials into and out of cells occurs along concentration gradients from areas of high concentration to areas of low concentration; when the concentration reaches equilibrium, **net** movement of the molecules ceases (→ 20.7.2).

Carrier-assisted active transport uses carrier proteins in the plasma membrane to move molecules against the concentration gradient, e.g. the sodium-potassium 'pump' which uses carrier proteins and energy (ATP) to eject sodium ions (Na^+) from cells and bring in potassium ions (K^+) (→ Fig. 9.11).

Vesicle-mediated transport uses vesicle to transport materials such as protein molecules around the cell or across the plasma membrane. A vesicle is a structure inside or outside a cell that consists of cytoplasm or liquid enclosed by a lipid bilayer. Vesicles form during the process of secretion (exocytosis) or uptake (endocytosis) (→ Fig. 2.4).

Exocytosis

Exocytosis is the movement of substances out of a cell in vesicles. It is used to move substances that are too large to diffuse through the plasma membrane, e.g. hormones and neurotransmitters. These are stored until required in vesicles which have budded off from the Golgi apparatus (→ Fig. 2.1). When the cell is stimulated to release its contents, the vesicle moves to the plasma membrane and fuses with it before releasing its contents into the extracellular space (→ Box 2.8).

Endocytosis

Endocytosis is a process by which cells take in substances by engulfing them, e.g. large molecules such as proteins. **Phagocytosis** is a type of endocytosis where an entire cell is engulfed, e.g. a bacterial cell.

Box 2.8 Secretion of the hormone insulin is an example of exocytosis. Insulin is produced by ribosomes in special cells in the pancreas before being moved in vesicles to the Golgi apparatus where it is prepared for secretion. It is then enclosed in a vesicle and is released from the cell by exocytosis.

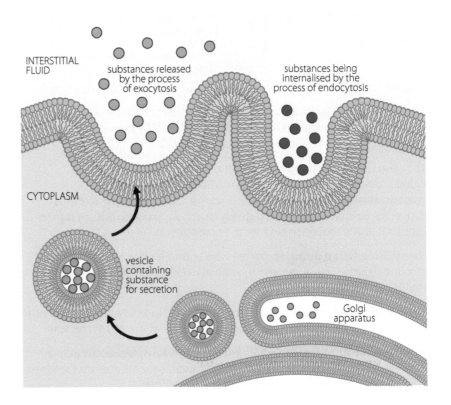

Fig. 2.4 Exocytosis and endocytosis.

2.3 Cytoplasm

Cytoplasm is the gel-like substance between the plasma membrane and the nucleus. A network of protein filaments and microtubules forms the **cytoskeleton** that supports and gives shape to the cell (→ Fig. 2.5).

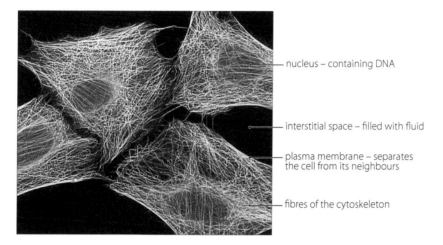

nucleus – containing DNA

interstitial space – filled with fluid

plasma membrane – separates the cell from its neighbours

fibres of the cytoskeleton

Fig. 2.5 Fluorescence micrograph showing cytoskeleton of immortal, cultured cells (known as HeLa cells) used in research; magnification × 670.

2.3.1 Organelles

The cytoplasm contains many **organelles** – specialised parts of the cytoplasm with particular functions. Each is surrounded by a membrane which, in some cases, is similar to the plasma membrane, e.g. mitochondria.

Mitochondria

A mitochondrion (→ Fig. 2.6) has the shape of a tiny sausage with an outer membrane and an inner membrane (crista), the latter being folded into compartments that provide a large surface area on which chemical reactions can occur (→ Fig. 2.6). Mitochondria generate most of the energy needed for the cell's activities in the form of adenosine triphosphate (ATP). The number of mitochondria present in a cell is related to the amount of energy the cell needs; for example, liver cells have high numbers and adipose cells have fewer.

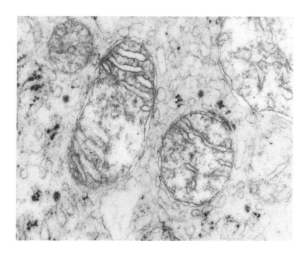

Fig. 2.6 A mitochondrion showing its sausage shape and the folded crista.

Endoplasmic reticulum

The endoplasmic reticulum is an interconnected system of canals and flat curving sacs arranged in parallel rows (→ Fig. 2.7). It exists in two types:

- **rough endoplasmic reticulum** (rER) has ribosomes attached to it which manufacture proteins (e.g. insulin) that move through the canals to the Golgi apparatus
- **smooth endoplasmic reticulum** (sER) does not have ribosomes but is important for the manufacture of lipid-based products, e.g. fats, steroids, cholesterol.

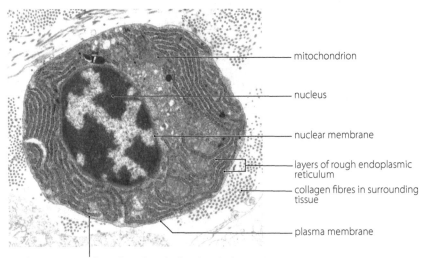

mitochondrion

nucleus

nuclear membrane

layers of rough endoplasmic reticulum

collagen fibres in surrounding tissue

plasma membrane

ribosomes on surface of rough endoplasmic reticulum

Fig. 2.7 Coloured electron micrograph of a plasma cell (mature B-lymphocyte) showing abundant rough endoplasmic reticulum producing antibodies during an immune response; magnification × 400.

Ribosomes

Ribosomes are particles consisting of protein and RNA (→ 13.5.3). Thousands are present in the cytoplasm and their function is the synthesis of the many different proteins used to form the structure of the cell, or for use inside the cell as enzymes, or exported as hormones, antibodies, clotting factors or other products (→ Box 2.9).

Box 2.9 Synthesis is a process of uniting simpler chemical substances to form a complex chemical compound.

Golgi apparatus

The Golgi apparatus is found near the nucleus and consists of flattened vesicles (sacs) stacked one on top of the other. It modifies and sorts the proteins made by the endoplasmic reticulum and loads them into vesicles which bud off from the Golgi apparatus ready for transport to various destinations within or outside the cell (→ Fig. 2.8).

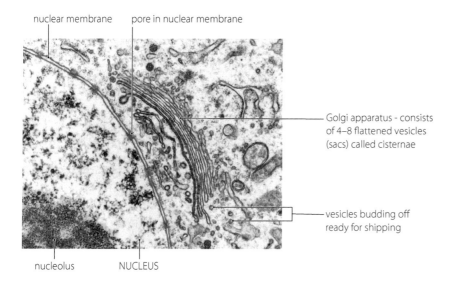

nuclear membrane   pore in nuclear membrane

Golgi apparatus - consists of 4–8 flattened vesicles (sacs) called cisternae

vesicles budding off ready for shipping

nucleolus   NUCLEUS

Fig. 2.8 The Golgi apparatus modifies, sorts and packages macromolecules for transport in vesicles; magnification × 9500.

Vesicles

Some vesicles transport materials within the cytoplasm, others store substances to be secreted (→ Fig. 2.4) or to act as phagosomes. A **phagosome** is a vesicle in which worn-out parts of the cell or pathogenic microorganisms can be digested by phagocytosis (→ Fig. 5.6).

Lysosomes

Lysosomes vary in shape and size from granules to small vesicles. They are filled with fluid containing enzymes that break down (digest) unwanted substances in the cell into simpler substances which can then be reused. When a cell dies the enzymes are released from the lysosomes and break down the cell itself (**autolysis**).

2.4 Stem cells

A **stem cell** is an unspecialised cell that can give rise to one or more different types of specialised cell, e.g. blood cells, nerve cells.

The trillions of cells in the human body all originate from one stem cell – the fertilised egg (→ Box 2.10). After being fertilised, the egg starts to divide to become a tiny, solid ball of cells called, the **morula**. About five days after fertilisation, the morula becomes a fluid-filled ball, the **blastocyst**, containing a small cluster of cells – **embryonic stem cells** (→ Box 2.11). The cells of the outer layer of the blastocyst eventually form part of the placenta; the embryonic stem cells will form all the tissues in the body.

Embryonic stem cells can be:
- **undifferentiated**; they are able to divide by **mitosis** (→ 13.4.2) to produce identical copies of themselves, a process called self-renewal
- **pluripotent**; that is, they have the potential to differentiate into specialised stem cells that mature into more than 200 different types of cells that make up every type of tissue and organ in the body, e.g. muscle cells, nerve cells and blood cells
- **multipotent**; these stem cells are only found in some tissues and organs and they develop into a limited number of cell types, e.g. stem cells in red bone marrow that only give rise to blood cells (haemocystoblasts) (→ Fig. 2.9).

Box 2.10 The unfertillised human egg, also known as an ovum, has half the normal complement of chromosomes. Fertilisation is the process of uniting the chromosomes from a sperm and the egg to generate a unique cell – called the zygote – which has the potential to divide and replicate (→ 12.6).

Box 2.11 When isolated from blastocysts and grown in a laboratory, embryonic stem cells (ES cells) can continue dividing indefinitely.

- **tissue-specific stem cells**; specialised stem cells thought to exist in most of the body's tissues and organs, e.g. those in:
  - cardiac muscle tissue mature into cardiac muscle cells
  - germinal epithelium of testis gives rise to sperm (→ Box 2.12).

2.4.1 Haematopoiesis

Haematopoiesis (also known as haemopoiesis) is the process of producing blood cells and platelets that continues throughout life (→ Box 2.13). The two types of blood cell – red cells (erythrocytes) and white cells (leucocytes) – originate from stem cells in red bone marrow (**myeloid tissue**). As they develop, the blood cells seep into the blood that passes through the bones and travel on into the bloodstream (→ Fig. 2.9).

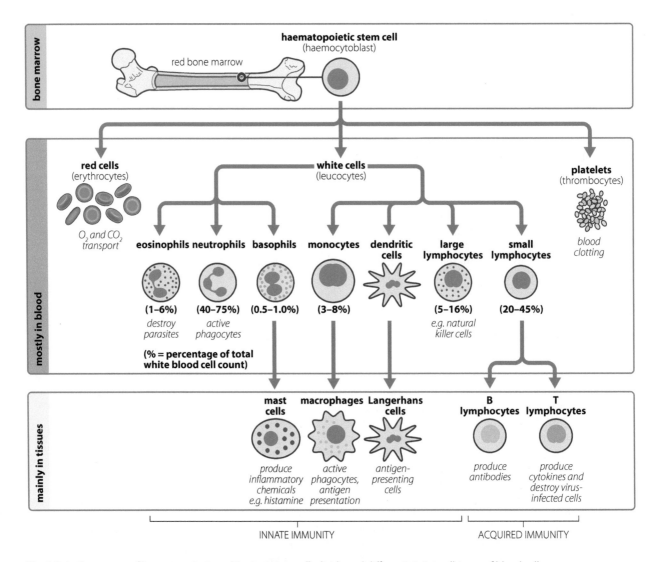

Fig. 2.9 In the process of haematopoiesis, multipotent stem cells divide and differentiate into all types of blood cells.

2.5 Tissues

A **tissue** is a group of cells specialised to perform a particular function. There is usually one main type of cell, and a matrix is often present. The **matrix** (material between the cells) can be hard, soft or liquid depending on the type of tissue. Generally, the matrix aids the movement of nutrients, gases and hormones throughout the tissue and acts as a barrier against pathogens.

2.5.1 Epithelial tissues

Sheets of epithelial tissue cover the outside and inside surfaces of the body and form many glands. The cells are closely packed together in one or more layers on a basal membrane attached to the underlying connective tissue.

Simple epithelium consists of a single layer of thin, flat cells that line blood vessels and form the air sacs in the lungs (→ Fig. 2.10a).

Cuboidal epithelium consists of cube-shaped cells that line the kidney tubules and also form the **germinal epithelium** – the tissue that produces the egg and sperm (→ Fig. 2.10b).

Stratified epithelium consists of several layers (strata) of cells and occurs in places where the surfaces have to withstand the stress of abrasion, e.g. the epidermis of the skin and the lining of the gut and vagina (→ Fig. 2.10c).

Glandular epithelium lines the surfaces and cavities of the glands and consists of cells that produce secretions in both exocrine and endocrine glands (→ Fig. 2.10d). **Exocrine glands** have ducts through which the secretions are removed, e.g. sweat glands and salivary glands. **Endocrine glands** (ductless glands) manufacture one or more hormones and secrete them directly into the bloodstream, e.g. pituitary, thyroid, parathyroid and adrenal glands.

Mucosa (**mucous membrane**) is the moist, mucus-secreting tissue lining the cavities and canals in the body which link to the external environment, chiefly the respiratory, digestive and urogenital tracts. The membranes vary in structure but all have a surface layer of epithelium over a layer of the connective tissue.

Mucus is the viscous fluid, usually colourless, that covers the surface of mucous membranes and protects them from damage and infection. It is secreted by glands called goblet cells which together, on average, produce 1 litre of mucus per day (→ 6.4).

Ciliated mucous membrane. Some mucous membranes have cilia (tiny hairs) on their surface that beat regularly in the same direction to produce wave-like movements that move the mucus over the surface. Such membranes move, for example, mucus out of the lungs and the egg along the Fallopian tube to the uterus (→ Fig. 2.10e).

Serosa (**serous membrane**) is a thin layer of epithelium that covers the walls and organs within the thoracic and abdominal cavities. It secretes **serous fluid**, which is the thin watery fluid found in many body cavities. Serous membranes include the:
- **pericardium** – the membrane covering the heart which secretes pericardial fluid
- **pleura** – line the thoracic cavity and surround the lungs; they secrete pleural fluid
- **peritoneum** – lines the abdominopelvic cavity and covers the viscera (→ Box 2.14); and secretes **peritoneal fluid**

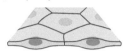

(a) simple epithelium

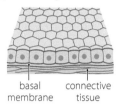

(b) cuboidal epithelium

basal membrane   connective tissue

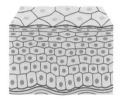

(c) stratified epithelium

(d) glandular epithelium

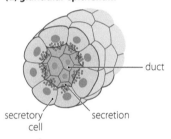

duct

secretory cell   secretion

(e) ciliated mucous epithelium

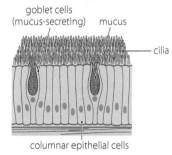

goblet cells (mucus-secreting)   mucus

cilia

columnar epithelial cells

Fig. 2.10 Epithelia. (**a**) Simple epithelium; (**b**) Cuboidal epithelium; (**c**) Stratified epithelium; (**d**) Glandular epithelium; (**e**) Ciliated mucous epithelium.

Box 2.14 Viscera – the soft internal organs of the body, especially those contained within the abdominopelvic and thoracic cavities.

(a) loose areolar tissue

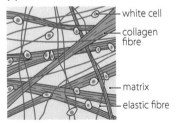

- white cell
- collagen fibre
- matrix
- elastic fibre

(b) adipose tissue

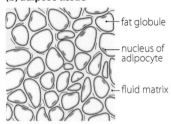

- fat globule
- nucleus of adipocyte
- fluid matrix

(c) dense fibrous tissue

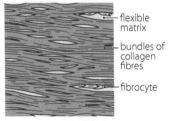

- flexible matrix
- bundles of collagen fibres
- fibrocyte

(d) hyaline cartilage

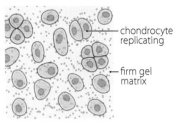

- chondrocyte replicating
- firm gel matrix

(e) elastic cartilage

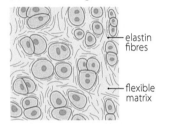

- elastin fibres
- flexible matrix

Fig. 2.11 Microscopic structure of connective tissues: (**a**) Areolar tissue; (**b**) Adipose tissue; (**c**) Fibrous tissue; (**d**) Hyaline cartilage; (**e**) Elastic cartilage.

- **endothelium** – lines the heart, blood vessels and lymphatic vessels and forms a very smooth lining that allows blood to keep flowing. It is a special form of epithelium as it does not secrete fluid.

2.5.2 Connective tissue

Connective tissue is the most abundant tissue in the body and is sometimes described as 'the body's glue and filling material' because its function is to hold the other tissues together (→ Box 2.15). It has three components – cells, fibres and matrix:

Many different types of cell are found in connective tissue including:
- **fibrocytes** – the cells that synthesise the fibres and the gel-like matrix in which the fibres are embedded (→ Fig. 2.11c)
- **white cells** (**leucocytes**) that have migrated from the blood
- **adipocytes** – cells which store fat (→ Fig. 2.11b)
- **chondrocytes** – produce the cartilage matrix (→ Fig. 2.11d).

Fibres found in connective tissue include:
- **collagen fibres** (white fibres) are the tough fibres that often occur in bundles, which confers great tensile strength (→ Fig. 2.11a)
- **elastin fibres**, which as their name implies, are stretchable (→ Fig. 2.11e).

Matrix is the ground substance in which the cells and fibres are embedded. Depending on its function, the matrix varies widely from a fluid, e.g. blood plasma, to a slippery gel, e.g. in fibro-cartilage. Alternatively it can be hardened by crystals of calcium and phosphate, as happens in teeth.

Some types of connective tissue

Areolar tissue is the loose, thin, filmy tissue that holds organs together. The matrix is a soft, viscous gel containing a meshwork of fibres and several types of cell, e.g. the mesentery between the parts of the intestine (→ Fig. 2.11a).

Adipose tissue is connective tissue packed with adipose (fat) cells that acts as a food reserve (→ Fig. 2.11b).

Fibrous tissue consists mainly of dense bundles of collagen fibres arranged in parallel rows, which gives the tissue strength, e.g. ligaments and tendons (→ Fig. 2.11c).

Hyaline cartilage is bluish-white in colour and forms a smooth surface on bones at places where they meet at a joint. It also joins the ribs to the sternum, which allows the ribcage to move during breathing, and is found in the larynx and the rings of cartilage of the airways (→ Fig. 2.11d).

Elastic cartilage contains elastic fibres scattered throughout the solid but flexible matrix, e.g. earlobes and epiglottis (→ Fig. 2.11e).

2.5.3 Bone tissue

Bone tissue forms the skeleton and strengthens it. The hard matrix takes up much more space than the **osteocytes** (bone cells) and is built from a framework of collagen fibres embedded in a cement-like substance containing calcium. **Compact bone** forms the outer shell of a bone and is thickest in places which receive the greatest stress. **Spongy** (cancellous) **bone** consists of a meshwork of **trabeculae** (bony bars) with many interconnecting spaces that are filled with marrow. Continuous activity takes place inside bones as they grow, repair and remodel (→ 4.5), store and release calcium, and make blood cells (→ 2.4.1).

Osteons (**Haversian systems**) are the basic units of compact bone. They are more or less cylindrical and each consists of concentric layers (**lamellae**) surrounding a **central canal**. Osteocytes are embedded in small spaces (**lacunae**) in the lamellae and they communicate with neighbouring osteocytes and the central canal via a network of **canaliculi** (tiny channels). Extracellular fluid fills the canals and canaliculi that permeate bone tissue and enables the exchange of nutrients and waste materials that keeps the cells alive (→ Fig. 2.12).

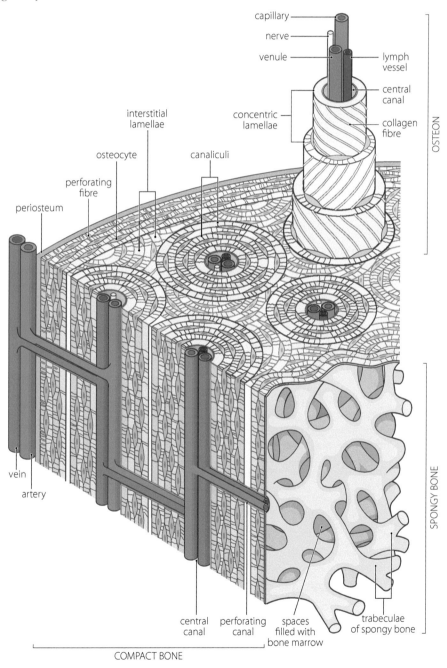

Fig. 2.12 Microscopic structure of bone tissues.

2.5.4 Nerve tissue

Nerve tissue forms a network throughout the body and is composed of two types of cell – **neurons** (nerve cells) and **glia** (supporting cells).

Neurons

Box 2.16 Neurons are unusual cells in that they can be extremely long, e.g. those that connect the toes to the spinal cord may have axons one metre or more in length.

The function of neurons is to transmit information in the form of nerve impulses from one part of the body to another (➔ Box 2.16). A typical neuron consists of:
- a cell body
- one or more **dendrites** – short, branching nerve fibres that carry impulses into the cell body
- an **axon** – a single nerve fibre that carries impulses away from the cell body
- **axon terminals** – the axon ends by dividing into several branches which make contact with other neurons or with muscle or gland cells.

Myelin sheath

Some long nerve fibres are surrounded by a myelin sheath which insulates the nerve fibre and also give the nerves a white colour due to the presence of a fatty substance – **myelin**. The myelin sheath is in sections, each section having been formed by a **Schwann cell** which wraps itself around the axon; the gap between two sections is called a **node of Ranvier** and helps in the conduction of impulses.

Types of neuron

There are an enormous number of different shapes and sizes of neurons, but they can be classified into three groups according to their function:
- **sensory neurons** transmit impulses from the sense organs towards the central nervous system (CNS; brain and spinal cord) (➔ Fig. 2.13a)
- **motor neurons** transmit impulses away from the CNS to the muscles and glands – parts of the body that can respond by taking action (➔ Fig. 2.13b)

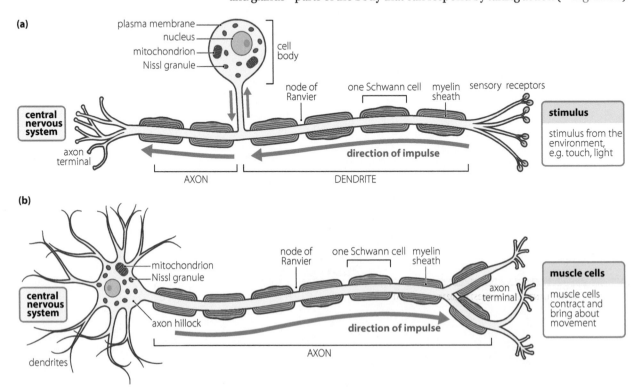

Fig. 2.13 Neurons: (**a**) Sensory neuron; (**b**) Motor neuron.

- **interneurons** (**association neurons**) are found only in the brain and spinal cord; they allow communication between sensory and motor neuron. They usually have numerous branching dendrites, which enables them to form many networks within the CNS, e.g. reflex arc (→ Fig. 9.6.1).

2.5.5 Glia

Glia (**neuroglia**) are specialised cells that surround neurons, hold them in place (*glia* means glue) and supply them with nutrients and oxygen. There are at least five times as many glial cells as neurons and the different types have different functions, e.g. astrocytes, microglia, ependymal cells and oligodendrocytes (→ Fig. 2.14).

Astrocytes (astroglia) are star-shaped cells found throughout the central nervous system and involved in the regulation of nerve cell activity and processing information. They are also involved in the blood–brain barrier (→ 9.2.2).

Microglia are phagocytes and scavengers. They are usually small and stationary but when brain tissue becomes inflamed, they enlarge, move around and engulf and destroy pathogens and debris from the cells.

Ependymal cells are shaped like columnar epithelial cells (→ Fig. 2.10e), that line the ventricles and canals through which cerebrospinal fluid (CSF) flows. Extensions of their plasma membrane resemble tentacles which make contact with astrocytes. The function of ependymal cells is to allow exchange of materials between the CSF and nervous tissue.

Oligodendroglia form the white matter in the central nervous system. A subgroup called Schwann cells form the white matter (myelin) in the peripheral nervous system, each making a segment of the myelin sheath (→ Fig. 2.13).

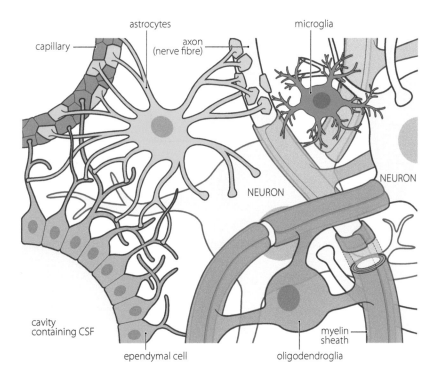

Fig. 2.14 Glia are specialised cells that support and nourish neurons.

2.5.6 Muscle tissue

The muscles in the body carry out all the body's movements because they have the ability to contract (shorten). Muscles are composed of **myocytes** (muscle cells) that form three specialised types of muscle tissue:

- **smooth muscle** is composed of myocytes and found in the walls of hollow organs such as blood vessels and stomach
- **skeletal muscle** is attached to bones and is composed of long muscle fibres (→ 4.16)
- **cardiac muscle** occurs in the walls of the heart and is composed of branching muscle fibres (→ Fig. 2.15) (→ Box 2.17).

Box 2.17 Movements of the skeletal muscles are known as voluntary movements, because they are a response to conscious impulses from the brain.

This is different from smooth and cardiac muscles, which can contract without stimulation by the nervous system and are therefore known as involuntary muscles.

Taking it Further
Contraction of muscle generates force that is needed for movement to take place – a process that requires energy.

In online Chapter 20 you can find out more about respiratory biochemistry and how cells generate energy in the form of adenosine triphosphate (ATP).

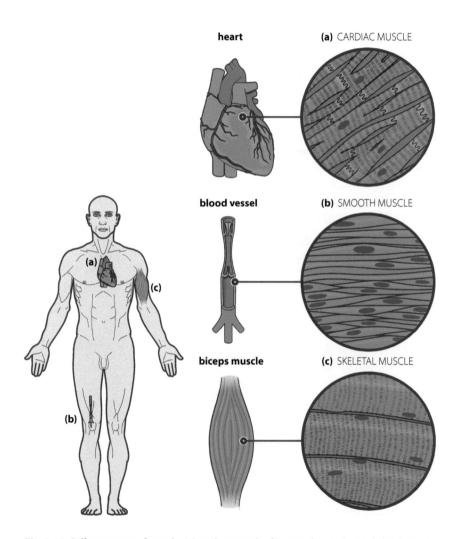

Fig. 2.15 Different types of muscle: (**a**) cardiac muscle, (**b**) smooth muscle, (**c**) skeletal muscle.

Smooth muscle

The myocytes in smooth muscle are elongated, each with a nucleus, and interlaced to form sheets of tissue (→ Fig. 2.15). This type of muscle forms layers in the walls of hollow organs such as the oesophagus, stomach and intestines, bladder, uterus, ducts of glands and the walls of blood vessels. Smooth muscle is under the control of the autonomic nervous system (→ 9.8) and the movements are involuntary, i.e. not controlled by the brain. Smooth muscle is **myogenic**; that is, it can initiate rhythmic muscle contractions without any stimulus from the nervous system; e.g. this type of contraction ensures movement of food through the digestive tract.

Skeletal muscle

Skeletal (**striated**) muscle tissue is composed of long, thin **muscle fibres** containing many nuclei and striated with alternate light and dark bands (→ Fig. 2.16). The muscle fibres contain parallel **microfibrils** enclosed in a sarcolemma (→ Fig. 2.16) and they form the most abundant tissue in the body, forming about 700 named muscles.

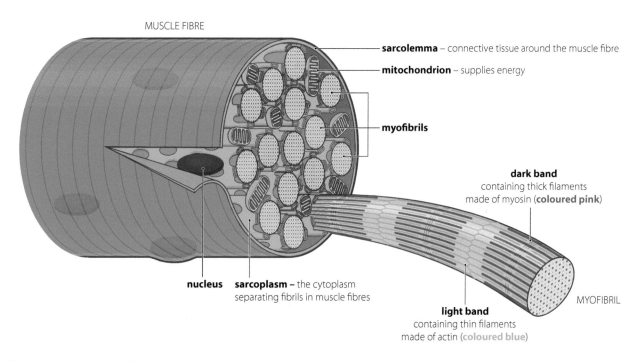

MUSCLE FIBRE

sarcolemma – connective tissue around the muscle fibre

mitochondrion – supplies energy

myofibrils

dark band containing thick filaments made of myosin (**coloured pink**)

light band containing thin filaments made of actin (**coloured blue**)

MYOFIBRIL

nucleus

sarcoplasm – the cytoplasm separating fibrils in muscle fibres

Fig. 2.16 Skeletal muscle fibre with details of one of the myofibrils.

Skeletal muscle is sometimes referred to as **voluntary** muscle as it is under conscious control by the nervous system; it cannot spontaneously contract and only does so when stimulated by impulses from the central nervous system. During contraction, the light and dark bands are pulled closer together, making the muscle shorter and fatter, thus generating the force which pulls on the bone to which the muscle is attached. When the muscle relaxes, the light and dark bands move apart and return to their original positions.

Cardiac muscle

Cardiac muscle (**myocardium**) is found only in the heart wall and is composed of **cardiomyocytes** (cardiac muscle cells), each with its own nucleus, and alternate light and dark bands similar to skeletal muscle, but less pronounced. They are joined together by **intercalated discs** to form a network of branching fibres that enables the heart to function as a single unit (→ Fig. 2.17). Cardiac muscle is **myogenic** – the cardiomyocytes generate electrical impulses spontaneously and rhythmically without tiring, which produces the heartbeat.

nucleus

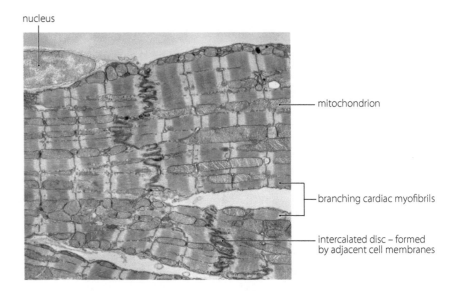

mitochondrion

branching cardiac myofibrils

intercalated disc – formed by adjacent cell membranes

Fig. 2.17 Electron micrograph showing branching cardiac muscle cell containing many mitochondria; magnification × 3000.

Key points

1. Histology reveals the internal structure of cells when examined under the microscope.
2. More than 250 different cell types make up the human body, each having a complex structure comprising nucleus, cytoplasm, intracellular organelles and a plasma membrane.
3. The plasma membrane is a semipermeable structure that regulates movement of substances into and out of the cell.
4. Stem cells are non-specialised cells that can divide and give rise to more specialised cells and tissue.
5. Four major tissue groups make up the organs and systems of the human body – epithelium, connective tissue, muscle and nervous tissue.

Test yourself! Go to *www.lanternpublishing.com/AandP* and try the questions to check your understanding.

CHAPTER 3
THE SKIN

The skin is the sensory organ that covers the body's surface and forms a barrier between the internal and external environment. It also provides information about its owner's life history with its scars and blemishes, wrinkles and colouring, hair and nails, corns, warts, tattoos, and can also show the state of the person's health.

3.1 Skin

The skin is the largest organ in the body, varying in thickness from 0.5 mm on the lips to 4 mm on the soles of the feet, and accounting for about 15% of body weight (→ Fig. 3.1; Box 3.1).

Box 3.1 The condition of the skin – its texture, appearance, colour and **integrity** (whether it is intact or broken) – often reflects underlying disease processes. Health care professionals need to observe a patient's skin because it is the one body system that can be readily inspected without access to special equipment or surgical procedures.

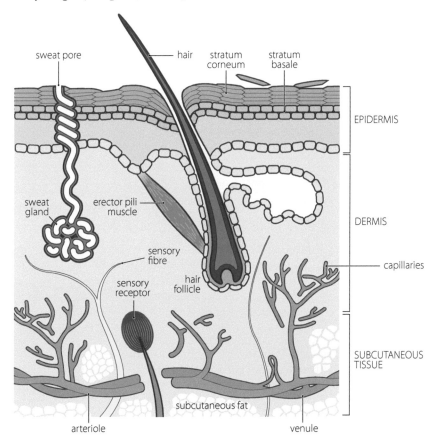

Fig. 3.1 Structure of the skin.

3.1.1 Functions of the skin

Despite being thin, the skin has a complex structure and carries out a number of functions important to the survival of the body (→ Box 3.1). It:
- covers the body and protects it from damage and disease
- plays a key role in regulating body temperature

- regulates the amount of fluid lost through the skin via sweat
- produces vitamin D and melanin
- plays a part in blood pressure regulation
- is sensitive to touch, temperature and pain, making the body aware of external environmental conditions
- is able to repair itself after damage.

3.2 Epidermis

The epidermis continuously renews itself by an orderly process in which cells are removed and replaced. The innermost cells of the **stratum basale** (basal layer) continuously produce new cells by mitosis (→ 13.4.2) which migrate towards the skin surface. As they move outwards they lose moisture, become filled with **keratin** and die. This keratinised layer forms part of the tough, waterproof surface of the skin (→ Box 3.2). It protects the delicate tissues underneath before flaking off or being rubbed away. On average it takes about 60 days for new cells to migrate to the surface and to be shed. In this way, the epidermis continuously renews itself every few weeks (→ Fig. 3.2).

Box 3.2 Keratin is the tough, fibrous protein in the outermost part of the epidermis, giving it strength and durability. The layer of keratin prevents heat loss by evaporation from the tissues in the skin and is a barrier to bacterial entry. The formation of corns and calluses is the skin's way of protecting itself from rubbing and pressure, e.g. the thickening on the fingertips of musicians who play stringed instruments, and on the hands of people who use tools repetitively. Keratin is also the key structural component of hair and nails.

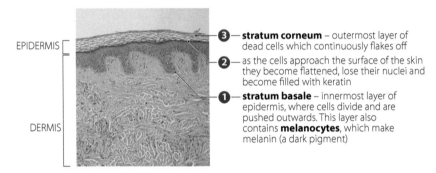

EPIDERMIS

DERMIS

3 — **stratum corneum** – outermost layer of dead cells which continuously flakes off

2 — as the cells approach the surface of the skin they become flattened, lose their nuclei and become filled with keratin

1 — **stratum basale** – innermost layer of epidermis, where cells divide and are pushed outwards. This layer also contains **melanocytes**, which make melanin (a dark pigment)

Fig. 3.2 Keratinisation in the skin: stages 1–3.

3.2.1 Skin colour

Skin colour ranges from almost black to white with a pinkish tinge and is due largely to the activity of **melanocytes** – cells that produce **melanin**. This is a dark pigment that occurs in two forms in the stratum basale:

- **eumelanin** has two sub-types – black and brown – found in the skin of both light- and dark-complexioned people, but in different amounts
- **pheomelanin** – a reddish-yellow colour that occurs in the lips, nipples, glans of the penis and the vagina (→ Box 3.3).

In pale-skinned individuals skin colour is also affected by the amount of blood flowing close to the skin's surface.

Box 3.3 It is essential that healthcare professionals are familiar with variations in presentation of skin conditions in people with skin of colour. For example, areas that appear red or brown on light skin appear black or purple on dark skin, so assessment must be carried out in good light.

Cyanosis

Cyanosis is bluish discolouration of the skin and mucous membranes, seen in fair-skinned people, that results from an inadequate amount of oxygen (**hypoxia**) in the blood. It is associated with heart failure and lung diseases, but can occur in skin of the lips in cold conditions.

Erythema

Erythema is redness of the skin caused by increased blood flow in the capillaries in the lower layers of the dermis. It occurs with any skin injury, infection, or inflammation. Dark pigment can block cues of persistent redness, but may be hot, swollen and firm (induration).

Tanning

The melanocytes in the stratum basale have photosensitive receptors that absorb ultraviolet (UV) radiation from the sun and, in response, produce melanin within a few hours of exposure. Melanin protects the skin from the sun's radiation by absorbing the UV rays and is the body's natural attempt to prevent skin damage through the process called tanning.

Exposure to UV radiation

Exposure to UV radiation can induce mutations in skin cells that interfere with the skin's normal repair mechanisms; this can lead to premature ageing, wrinkling (→ 3.3.6), discolouration such as 'liver spots' and increased risk of skin cancer. The main risk factor for any type of skin cancer is exposure to the sun or light reflected from snow. For this reason, people are encouraged to limit their exposure to sunlight (→ Box 3.4).

3.2.2 Skin biota

The skin biota (flora), also known as **commensal bacteria** (→ 15.5), are the microbes that live on the epidermis of the skin – mainly different strains of bacteria, but microscopic fungi are also present (→ Box 3.5). Most are harmless to their host and some are beneficial because their presence can prevent pathogenic (disease-causing) microbes from infecting the skin. However, when a person's immune system is suppressed or when the skin is wounded, bacteria may enter the bloodstream and cause disease, e.g. methicillin-resistant *Staphylococcus aureus* (MRSA) – a dangerous infection with multiple resistance to antibiotics (→ Box 3.6).

3.3 Dermis

The **dermis** lies underneath the epidermis, is about four times thicker and is composed of connective tissue containing blood vessels, hair roots, sweat glands, sebaceous glands and nerves.

3.3.1 Connective tissue

The connective tissue in the dermis contains **collagen fibres** which prevent the skin from being over-stretched and **elastin fibres** which pull the skin back into shape after it has been stretched. If the skin is subject to prolonged stretching, e.g. the skin of the abdomen during pregnancy or through obesity, the fibres may sometimes become damaged and cannot recoil, leaving scars called stretch marks (→ 2.5.2).

3.3.2 Blood supply

The blood supply in the dermis generally takes the form of small capillary loops in the outer region of the dermis which are linked to a deeper layer of larger blood vessels. Blood supply is under the control of the hypothalamus and cardiovascular centres in the brain. Signals are sent to the arterioles in the dermis to either:
- dilate and allow more blood to flow into the capillary loops, or
- constrict and reduce the blood flow (→ Box 3.7).

3.3.3 Sweat glands

Sweat (perspiration) is the watery fluid made by the sweat glands in the dermis. There are up to 4 million sweat glands distributed around the body

Box 3.4 The sun's rays can penetrate clouds, light clothing, windows, car windscreens; they can also be reflected by water (e.g. sea and lakes), snow, ice and the pavement. People who burn easily, e.g. those with fair skin, are more likely than others to have had severe, blistering sunburn as children, but burning as an adult can also cause damage that leads to skin cancer. The individual's total lifetime exposure to UV rays is the important risk factor. This is why artificial sources of UV light from tanning booths or sunlamps are no safer than sunbathing.

Box 3.5 The number of bacteria on the surface of skin and mucous membranes is greater than the number of cells in the human body.

Box 3.6 Hand hygiene is essential to control infection by skin biota and prevent the transmission of antibiotic-resistant infections such as methicillin-resistant *Staphylococcus aureus* (MRSA) and *Clostridium difficile* (*C. diff*) by ingestion, inhalation or through injured skin (→ 15.5.6).

Box 3.7 When blood supply to the skin capillaries increases, heat loss to the environment is increased, which helps people to cool down.

When blood supply to skin capillary loops is reduced, heat loss is minimised.

and the rate of sweat secretion is determined by thermosensitive neurons in the hypothalamus of the brain, which match sweat production to core temperature (→ Box 3.8).

Eccrine sweat glands (**merocrine glands**) are found in nearly all parts of the dermis, with the highest density on the soles of the feet, forehead, palms and cheeks. They secrete a clear, odourless fluid consisting mainly of water and salt (NaCl) that cools the body as it evaporates. Besides their function in thermoregulation, these glands are also active in **emotion-induced sweating** caused by strong feelings such as anxiety, fear, stress, pain and embarrassment.

Apocrine sweat glands are located in subcutaneous fat layers of the dermis. They develop in association with the hair follicles in the axilla (armpits) and uro-genital region and undergo enlargement and secretory development at puberty. The sweat they produce is mixed with sebum and supports bacterial growth, and it is the action of the skin bacteria that produces the strong characteristic odours associated with this type of sweat (→ Box 3.9).

3.3.4 Hairs

Hairs grow in hair follicles (pits) found in nearly every part of the dermis (→ Fig. 3.1). They show considerable variation in different parts of the body and between genders, the colour depending on the types of melanin present. On some parts of the body, e.g. soles of the feet and palms of the hands, the hairs are very small and fine, giving the appearance of baldness (→ Box 3.10).

Sebaceous glands

Sebaceous glands are attached to the hair shaft and produce a greasy liquid called sebum which spreads over the surface of the skin and keeps it supple. Too much sebum makes the skin greasy and too little makes it dry and rough (→ Box 3.11).

Hair growth

Growth of a hair takes place at the hair root, being faster in the summer (→ Box 3.12). The layer of cells around the hair papilla constantly produces new cells which become added to the base of the hair, making it grow. Each hair follicle has its own growth cycle, which varies in length in different parts of the body. After about ten hair growth cycles have been completed, at approximately 40 years of age, the ability to synthesise pigment becomes exhausted, causing hair to go grey.

Alopecia (baldness)

Alopecia is the medical term for hair loss. There are many types of hair loss with different symptoms and causes, e.g.:
- **male-pattern baldness** affects about 50% of men by 50 years of age as hair recedes from the temple and crown
- **female-pattern baldness** is less pronounced than baldness in men and affects the anterior scalp
- **telogen effluvium** is widespread **thinning of the hair**, rather than specific bald patches. There are many causes, e.g. stress, illness, hormone changes, medication and crash dieting. In most cases, the hair stops falling out and grows again within six months
- **anagen effluvium** is widespread **hair loss** that can affect the scalp, face and body; one of the most common causes is chemotherapy treatment for cancer (→ Box 3.13)

Box 3.8 Physical training and a high level of fitness can encourage sweat glands to become more efficient at temperature regulation by sweating.

Box 3.9 In animals, apocrine secretions function as **pheromones** – chemical signals that elicit specific responses from members of the opposite sex, but which may play only a minor role in human sexuality.

Box 3.10 Lanugo is the first hair to be produced by the foetal hair follicles at about 5 months of gestation. It is very fine, soft, usually unpigmented, and normally shed before birth. If present at birth, it disappears of its own accord within a few days or weeks.

Box 3.11 Acne vulgaris is a common inflammatory disease of the sebaceous glands, most frequently occurring during adolescence. It is characterised by blackheads with **papules** (small, raised spots) and **pustules** (pus-containing blisters). These appear on the face, the upper part of the chest, and the back. Various effective treatments are available.

Box 3.12 The rate of hair growth can also change during pregnancy when higher levels of the hormone oestrogen prolong the growth phase, resulting in less shedding of hair and thicker tresses. The hair may become shinier or change its texture, e.g. become straighter.

Box 3.13 Chemotherapy may cause hair to fall out all over the body. Besides attacking the cancer cells, the powerful drugs also attack other rapidly growing cells including those in the hair roots. The extent of hair loss is related to the type and dosage of the drug, and regrowth can be expected in three to six months after the treatment ends.

- **alopecia areata** causes **patches of baldness** about the size of a large coin that usually appear on the scalp but can occur anywhere, mainly affecting teenagers and young adults.

Hirsutism

Hirsutism is the growth of coarse pigmented hair on the face, chest, upper back or abdomen of women and results from the excessive production of androgen (the male hormone) (➔ Box 3.14).

Box 3.14 Excessive hair growth can affect a woman's quality of life when it causes embarrassment and other psychological effects. Hirsutism is also associated with polycystic ovarian syndrome (➔ 12.9.2) and insulin resistance (➔ 16.1.3).

3.3.5 Nails

Nails are outgrowth of the epidermis and are made of hard, tough keratin. They protect the tips of the fingers and toes and enable the hands to grasp small objects more easily. Like hairs, nails grow at their root where special epidermal cells divide, grow and become filled with keratin. Growth is faster in summer than winter, with fingernails growing about 1 mm per week, three times as fast as toenails.

Nail abnormalities

The condition of the nails is an indication of a person's state of health. Their colour, shape or brittleness can be clues to disease, e.g.:
- **ridging.** Any severe illness may slow the rate of growth and cause a ridge to form across the nail. This is pushed forward as health is restored and nail growth returns to normal
- **spooning.** Severe anaemia causes nails to become concave
- **colour.** Yellow may indicate a fungal infection (ringworm ➔ 3.5.2), brown nails can be caused by thyroid disease, pregnancy, malnutrition or the frequent use of nail varnish
- **root damage.** Severe damage to the root may cause the nail to come away within a week or two. It takes several months for the new nail to grow, and it may be permanently misshapen.

Box 3.15 Medications, in particular steroid drugs, weaken the collagen fibres, causing thinning of the skin in the long term and an increased tendency to bruising.

3.3.6 Ageing of the skin

Generally, skin structure and texture are determined genetically and natural changes take place. As skin ages:
- it becomes less effective at regeneration and therefore thinner (➔ Box 3.15)
- the blood vessels become more visible and bleed easily
- liver spots – brownish patches of melanin – also gradually develop on skin exposed to the sun, especially the hands.

Box 3.16 Over time, the sun's ultraviolet (UV) rays damage the elastin fibres in the skin and they lose their ability to go back into place after stretching, so the skin begins to sag.

Wrinkles

Wrinkles are folds, ridges and creases in the skin that develop as the collagen fibres lose their strength and the skin becomes less elastic. Wrinkles become most prominent in areas that have been exposed to sunlight (➔ Box 3.16), particularly in people who have fair skin, and the process is accelerated by smoking (➔ Box 3.17).

Box 3.17 The appearance of wrinkles can have a profound effect on the self-esteem of some individuals, and has given rise to a multimillion-pound industry producing anti-wrinkle creams.

3.4 Thermoregulation

The skin plays an important part in maintaining homeostasis of body temperature by keeping it more or less constant (➔ Box 3.18). In healthy adults, it stays within the range of 36.0–37.4°C. It is usually a little lower

Box 3.18 The heat that keeps the body warm is produced mainly by core organs such as the liver, heart and brain, and also by active muscles. It is lost mainly through the skin. There are slight variations in temperature when measured on the forehead or in the mouth, armpit, ear or rectum.

in the morning and a little higher in the late afternoon, and also varies in women during the menstrual cycle.

The set point of the core body temperature is controlled by the **thermoregulatory centre** in the hypothalamus in the brain (→ 9.3.4). It acts as the body's thermostat by switching on its temperature regulators that control sweating and shivering using two sets of thermoreceptors:

- receptors in the hypothalamus itself that monitor the temperature of the blood as it passes through the brain (**core temperature**)
- receptors in the skin, especially those on the trunk, that monitor the external temperature.

The thermoregulatory centre compares the information from both sets of receptors and adjusts body temperature as necessary by sending impulses (messages) to several different effectors, mainly the blood vessels and sweat glands in the skin (→ Fig. 3.3) (→ Box 3.19).

Box 3.19 Drinking a hot beverage like coffee or tea on a hot summer's day has a cooling effect because the thermoreceptors in the mouth, throat and stomach inform the brain that body temperature is rising more than it actually is. The body then reacts to this by instantly cooling down.

Taking it Further
Core body temperature is one of several vital signs.

The skills needed to record a person's body temperature accurately, and to understand how and why it can change, are an essential aspect of healthcare practice. You can find out more about this and other physiological observations in online Chapter 17.

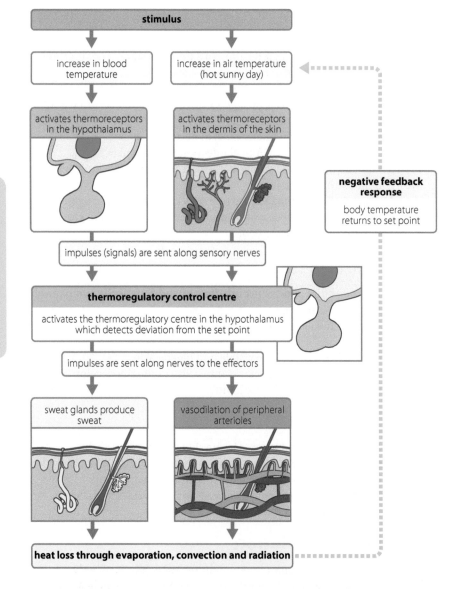

Fig. 3.3 The body's response to heat.

3.4.1 Hyperthermia

Hyperthermia occurs when the temperature rises above that required for normal metabolism and causes the body's systems to malfunction. It differs from fever in that the body's temperature set point remains unchanged (→ 14.3.5).

Heat exhaustion is caused by a loss of body fluids and salts after exposure to heat for a prolonged time. This lowers blood volume and therefore blood pressure, producing symptoms of headache, nausea, vomiting, muscle cramps and fatigue. If steps are not taken to reduce body temperature, heat exhaustion can worsen and become heat stroke (→ Box 3.20).

Box 3.20 Heat exhaustion affects elderly people more than younger ones as they do not adjust as well to sudden changes in temperature.

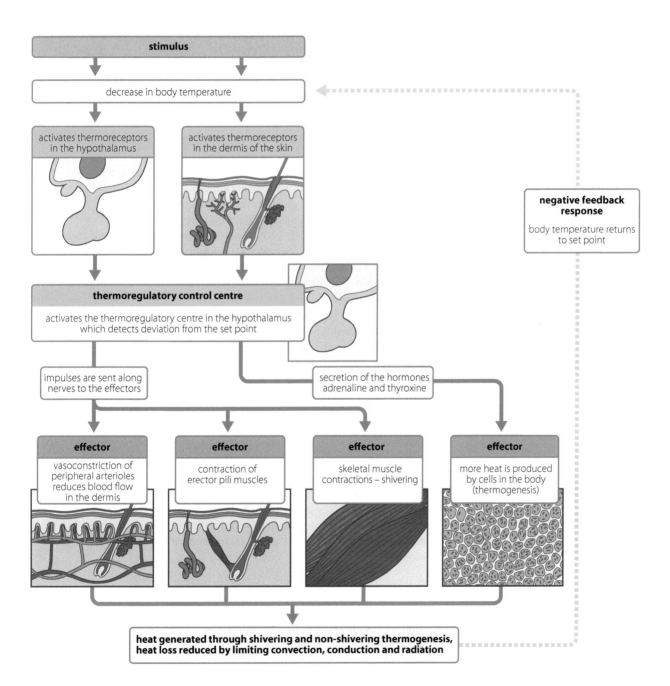

Fig. 3.4 The body's response to cold.

Heat stroke occurs when the body's temperature rises above 40°C and the body is no longer able to cool itself. The extreme heat begins to affect the functioning of proteins in the body's cells, especially in the brain, causing mental confusion or unconsciousness (→ Box 3.21).

3.4.2 Hypothermia

Hypothermia occurs when body temperature drops below 35°C, which is the temperature required to maintain normal metabolism (→ Fig. 3.4). Those most at risk from hypothermia are the severely ill or elderly if they are living in poorly heated homes and unable to move around easily. Babies are also prone to developing hypothermia because their ability to regulate their body temperature is not fully developed.

3.5 Wounds

A wound (**traumatic injury**) is a breakdown in the continuity of the skin's integrity caused by cuts, grazes, ulcers, burns or punctures (→ Box 3.22).

3.5.1 Wound healing

Damage to the dermis starts the process of **haemostasis** (→ 5.5.1) (stoppage of blood flow), beginning with the sudden vasoconstriction of damaged blood vessels. Platelets adhere to the site of injury and activate the formation of a blood clot over the wound, and the healing process starts (→ Box 3.23). Four phases of would healing have been identified, which may overlap (→ Fig. 3.5).

1. **Inflammation.** Signalling factors (→ 14.3.2) are released by damaged tissue, which attracts white cells to the wound where they phagocytose and remove debris and bacteria.
2. **Proliferation.** This phase begins from the edges of the wound where **granulation tissue** forms a thin, delicate layer of new skin that gradually fills the damaged area beneath the scab (→ Box 3.24).
3. **Epithelialisation.** This stage occurs when fine, delicate new epithelium forms to take the place of the scab and cover the surface of the wound.
4. **Remodelling** of the granulation tissue takes place as it becomes stronger, a process that may take up to a year. Scarring may occur, leaving more fibrous tissue than before the wound occurred.

Rate of healing

The rate at which wounds heal can be affected by:

Nutrition. People who are malnourished, very thin or obese can have a slower rate of healing because:

- a poor quality diet, a poor appetite or undernourishment does not supply enough amino acids for rapid healing
- adipose (fat) tissue in large amounts underneath the skin has a reduced blood supply.

Age. Wounds take longer to heal in elderly people due to:
- a general slowing of the body's metabolism
- changes in the structure of the skin, making it more fragile
- reduced padding over bony prominences
- reduction in the intensity of the immune response.

Box 3.21 Groups that are more at risk of heat stroke and dehydration include:
- children under two years of age
- elderly people
- people with kidney, heart or circulation problems
- people with diabetes using insulin.

Box 3.22 Skin integrity means that the skin is healthy, undamaged and able to perform its basic functions.

Box 3.23 For **minor cuts and grazes**, cleaning them thoroughly and covering with a plaster or dressing is usually all that is needed. **Serious bleeding** needs different management (→ 5.6).

Box 3.24 Granulation tissue (→ Fig. 3.5) is new connective tissue and tiny blood vessels that form on the surfaces of a wound during the healing process. A scab is formed from clotted and dried blood over the surface of the wound.

Taking it Further
Nutrition (from the Latin *nutrix* = nurse) is the science of food composition, and the processes by which the human body digests and assimilates food and uses it for growth, homeostasis and repair. You can find out more in online Chapter 19.

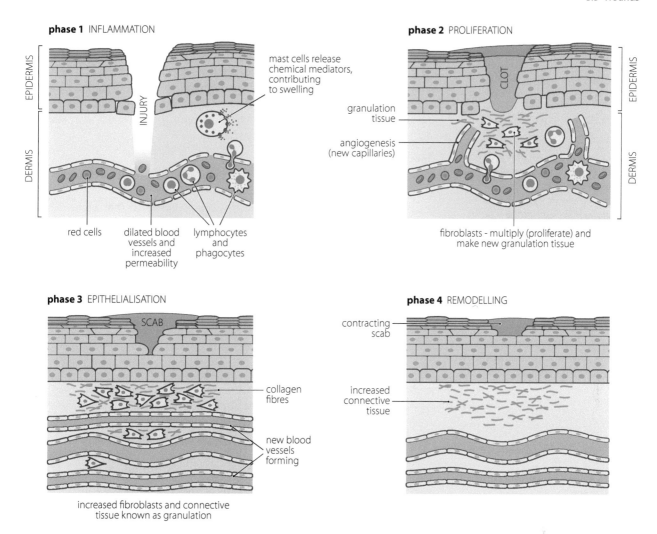

phase 1 INFLAMMATION

EPIDERMIS

DERMIS

INJURY

mast cells release chemical mediators, contributing to swelling

red cells

dilated blood vessels and increased permeability

lymphocytes and phagocytes

phase 2 PROLIFERATION

EPIDERMIS

DERMIS

CLOT

granulation tissue

angiogenesis (new capillaries)

fibroblasts - multiply (proliferate) and make new granulation tissue

phase 3 EPITHELIALISATION

SCAB

collagen fibres

new blood vessels forming

increased fibroblasts and connective tissue known as granulation

phase 4 REMODELLING

contracting scab

increased connective tissue

Fig. 3.5 Phases of wound healing.

Medical conditions. Some disorders can affect the body's ability to heal, e.g.:

- anaemia reduces the body's ability to carry oxygen
- diabetes increases the risk of wound infection
- malignant disease can cause malnourishment
- cardiovascular disease reduces the blood supply to the skin.

3.5.2 Some examples of skin disorders

Rash

Rash is an outbreak of red spots or patches on the skin. It can be due to an infectious disease, an allergy or other causes (→ Box 3.25). A rash is a change of the skin which affects its colour, appearance and itchiness; it can make it warm or cold, bumpy, chapped, dry, cracked, blistered or swollen, and it may be painful. The rash may be localised in one particular area or affect all the skin (→ Box 3.26). In people with darkly pigmented skin, rashes may appear darker brown, purple or grey.

Box 3.25 Diagnosis of a rash must take into account such things as natural skin tone, the appearance of the rash, other symptoms, occupation, what the person may have been exposed to, and any occurrence in family members.

Box 3.26 Nappy rash often develops in babies. It is caused by the baby's skin coming into contact with urine and faeces when nappy changing is delayed or hygiene has been neglected. A mild rash can be treated with simple skin care. If the rash persists, erythema (rash), candida (thrush) or bacterial infection may be investigated. A severe rash needs medication.

Eczema

Eczema (**dermatitis**) is a condition of dry skin that becomes scaly, red and itchy, and constant scratching can cause the skin to split, bleed and be open to infection. On black skin, eczema can cause purple, grey or darker brown patches. People of all ages can be affected by eczema but it is often seen in children. Some may grow out of it, but those who 'grow out of it' may see it recur in later life.

There are different types of eczema, e.g.:
- **atopic eczema** is the most common form of eczema that can affect people of all ages but is most often seen in children (→ Box 3.27)
- **contact eczema** (**contact dermatitis**) refers to eczema that occurs after contact with irritants or allergens in the environment (→ Box 3.28)
- **seborrhoeic eczema** appears in areas of the skin containing large numbers of sebaceous glands, often starting in the scalp, and it may spread to the neck, sides of the nose and behind the ears. Other areas that can be affected are the armpits, under the breasts, in the groin and between the buttocks and genitals. Affected skin becomes inflamed and sheds small white flakes; in severe cases it forms thick crusts.

Psoriasis

Psoriasis is a relatively common autoimmune condition (→ 14.9.3) which leads to rapid growth of skin cells, commonly producing scaly patches on the top-most layer of skin. It tends to run in families and is probably triggered by a particular stimulus, e.g. exposure to streptococcal throat infections, alcohol and some medicines.

Intertrigo

Intertrigo is inflammation (rash) in folds of the skin. It usually appears red and raw-looking, and may itch, ooze and be sore. It can develop from the chafing of warm, moist skin in the areas of the inner thighs and genitalia, the armpits, under the breasts, behind the ears, and in the web spaces between the toes and fingers. The condition occurs more often among overweight individuals, those with diabetes, or who are restricted to bed rest or who use nappies. It can also occur in those who use medical devices, e.g. artificial limbs that trap moisture against the skin.

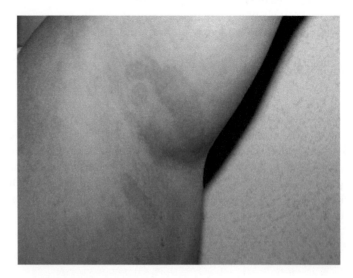

Fig. 3.6 Axillary (armpit) intertrigo due to erythrasma.

Box 3.27 Atopic eczema is the hereditary tendency to experience immediate allergic reactions, e.g. asthma or rhinitis, due to the presence of an inherited antibody to particular allergens.

Box 3.28 Contact eczema can be a form of occupational disease but lots of people have contact dermatitis that is not caused by work. For example, many health professionals develop, over time, skin reactions to the latex (rubber) in gloves, so alternatives are now available made of other materials.

Several skin diseases can also cause an intertrigo to develop, e.g. **erythrasma** – a bacterial skin infection that occurs in areas where skin surfaces are in contact, e.g. armpits, groin and toes (→ Fig. 3.6).

Ringworm

Ringworm is a common fungal infection that feeds on keratin in the outer layer of skin, hair, and nails, causing a ring-shaped red rash. It thrives on warm, moist skin, with the various species of fungus infecting different parts of the body, e.g.:
- **Tinea pedis** (athlete's foot) – fungal infection of the skin of the feet
- **Tinea capitis** – fungal infection of the scalp and hair
- **Tinea unguium** – fungal infection of the fingernails and toenails.

Pressure ulcers

An **ulcer** is a break in a surface, either inside or outside the body, that fails to heal. There are many types of ulcer, the most common being:
- **pressure ulcers** – inflamed patches of skin on the buttocks, heels or elbows of people confined to bed, e.g. following surgery. The constant pressure of the weight of the body stops blood from reaching those areas. Unless the pressure is relieved, ulcers rapidly develop (→ Box 3.29)
- **venous** (**hypostatic**) **ulcers** of the leg are caused by increased pressure in the veins (→ Box 3.30).

Corns and calluses

Corns and calluses are areas of hard, thickened skin that develop when the skin is exposed to excessive pressure or friction. **Corns** are small circles of thick skin that usually develop on the tops and sides of toes. **Calluses** are hard, rough areas of skin that most often develop around the heel area or on the skin under the ball of the foot. They can also develop on the palms of the hands and knuckles.

Warts

Warts are small lumps of keratin that develop in the epidermis due to infection with the human papillomavirus (HPV). They vary in appearance and may develop singly or in clusters in any part of the body, and are slightly contagious. **Verrucas** are warts that usually develop on the soles of the feet. **Genital warts** are small, fleshy growths that develop around the genital or anal area and can be spread during sexual intercourse (→ Box 3.31).

Melanocytic naevi

Melanocytic naevi are **moles** – collections of melanocytes (pigment cells) that are rare in infancy, increase in childhood and adolescence, and decline in old age. These skin lesions (→ Box 3.32) can be under the skin or raised above and are non-malignant. But any change in the shape, texture or colour of an existing mole, bleeding, or the appearance of a new mole, may be an early sign of melanoma, a type of skin cancer (→ 15.10.5), which needs early investigation.

Box 3.29 Pressure ulcers are almost entirely prevented by good nursing. Treatment options may include:
- changing the patient's position frequently, or using special mattresses to relieve the pressure, to allow blood to flow to the areas at risk
- keeping the skin clean and dry
- dressings to protect the skin
- surgery if needed.

Box 3.30 Venous ulcers can be healed by the application of strong sustained compression with a bandage or a stocking, and treating the underlying cause of the ulcer.

Box 3.31 A wart or other growth on the skin needs investigation if it:
- bleeds
- changes in appearance
- spreads
- causes significant pain, distress or embarrassment.

Box 3.32 A skin lesion is a part of the skin that has an abnormal growth or appearance compared to the skin around it.

(a) HEAD LICE

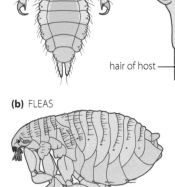

'nit' (egg)

hair of host

(b) FLEAS

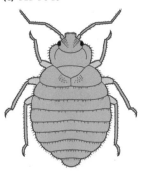

(c) BED BUGS

(d) SCABIES ('THE ITCH')

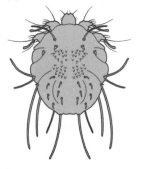

Fig. 3.7 Skin parasites (not drawn to scale): (**a**) louse and nit; (**b**) flea; (**c**) bed bug; (**d**) itch mite.

Insect bites are puncture wounds made by midges, mosquitoes, fleas and bedbugs when they make a hole in the skin and inject anticoagulant in order to feed on the host's blood, which causes the skin around the bite to become red, swollen and itchy. In certain tropical countries mosquito saliva can contain *Plasmodium* parasites that cause **malaria**.

Insect stings are made by bees and wasps when they feel threatened, and their venom causes pain and swelling. The severity of bites and stings varies depending on the type of insect involved and the sensitivity of the person. In rare cases, some people can have a serious allergic reaction (anaphylaxis) to a bite or sting that requires immediate medical treatment (→ 17.4).

3.6 Skin parasites

Skin parasites feed on the blood or skin of their host (→ Fig. 3.7). They may live on the skin, burrow into it, or live outside the body, only feeding every once in a while. An **infestation** occurs when large numbers of parasites are present, causing irritation, itching, scratching and restlessness. Skin parasites are found worldwide and include head lice, fleas, bed bugs and itch mites.

Head lice

Head lice (singular: louse) live amongst the hairs of the head. Eggs (nits) are laid attached to hairs. They can be removed by wet combing, using hair conditioner and a fine-toothed comb. Pubic lice live among the pubic hair and are more crab-shaped.

Fleas

Fleas live in clothing next to the skin and feed by piercing the skin to suck blood, leaving small red marks. They are controlled by personal cleanliness, including clean clothes. The eggs do not survive long in clean buildings or bedding.

Bed bugs

Bed bugs live in bedding and crevices in the bedroom, and give off an unpleasant smell. They come out at night to suck blood from sleeping humans. Bed bugs can be killed by an insecticide spray.

Scabies ('the itch')

Scabies is caused by mites which burrow into the epidermis, feeding on the keratin and laying their eggs there. Infected areas look scaly with pimples, septic spots and boils, usually on the palms, between the fingers and on the wrists. The mites can be killed by applying a special lotion to all parts of the skin, and washing bedlinen and underclothes.

Key points

1. The skin is the largest organ system in the human body and plays a key role in thermoregulation (homeostasis of body temperature) and sensation.
2. The outer layer of skin, the epidermis, is continually renewed by mitosis (cell division).
3. The dermis contains connective tissue, blood vessels, hair follicles, glandular tissues and nerves.
4. Wounds are caused by a break in the skin's integrity and they heal through a highly ordered process involving inflammation, proliferation, epithelialisation and remodelling of the damaged tissues.
5. The rate of healing of skin depends on many factors including age, nutritional status and general levels of wellbeing.

Test yourself! Go to *www.lanternpublishing.com/AandP* and try the questions to check your understanding.

CHAPTER 4
THE MUSCULOSKELETAL SYSTEM

The musculoskeletal system gives shape and support to the body and enables it to move. The skeleton provides support, and movement is achieved by the combined action of muscles, tendons and ligaments attached to the bones. Many components of blood are made in bone marrow, and calcium and other minerals are stored in bone tissue.

4.1 The skeleton

The adult skeleton consists of 206 bones (→ Box 4.1). The bones fit together to form a framework for the body (→ Fig. 4.1) and are held in place by muscles and ligaments.

Box 4.1 There are approximately 270 bones at birth but during development some of the bones fuse together, e.g. the cranium (the upper part of the skull).

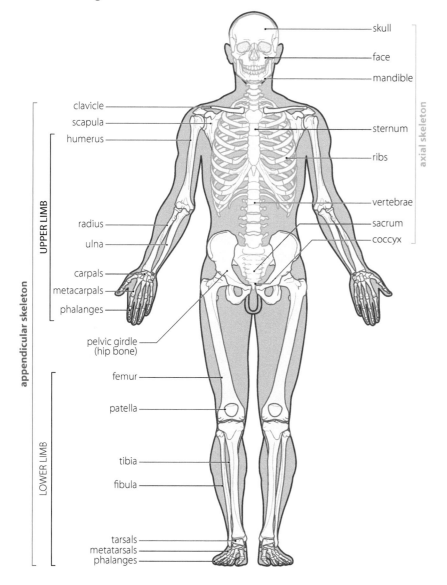

Fig. 4.1 Anterior view of the adult skeleton.

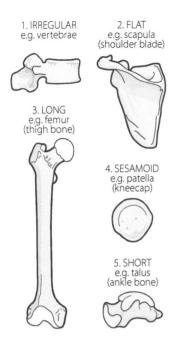

1. IRREGULAR
e.g. vertebrae

2. FLAT
e.g. scapula
(shoulder blade)

3. LONG
e.g. femur
(thigh bone)

4. SESAMOID
e.g. patella
(kneecap)

5. SHORT
e.g. talus
(ankle bone)

Fig. 4.2 Classification of bones by shape.

4.1.1 Functions of the skeleton

Although hard and rigid, bones are living structures built and maintained by living cells. If damaged they bleed and are painful, and if broken they can mend. Continuous activity takes place inside the bones as they carry out their functions. They:

- **support** the body, using bones of various shapes (→ Fig. 4.2)
- **provide attachment for muscles** that enable movement of the body
- **protect the internal organs**: the skull protects the brain, the spine protects the spinal cord, the ribcage protects the heart and lungs, and the pelvis protects intestines, urinary bladder and female reproductive organs
- **produce blood cells**: all the red cells, white cells and platelets in the blood are made in the red bone marrow
- **store calcium and other minerals** so that there is always a supply readily available for release when needed by the cells.

4.1.2 Growth of bones

Bones consist of two types of tissue – bone tissue (→ 2.5.3) and hyaline cartilage (→ 2.5.2). At birth, they consist mainly of cartilage, which is firm but flexible. As the child grows, cartilage is replaced with bone tissue in all parts of the skeleton except the articular surfaces (→ Fig. 4.3). Blood supply to bones is abundant because, like all living cells, bone and cartilage cells need a continuous supply of nutrients and oxygen, and must excrete their waste.

Growth in length of a bone occurs in the **epiphyseal plates** – plates of hyaline cartilage at each end of the long bones in children and adolescents. In adults who have stopped growing, these **ossify** (become replaced by bone) at the **epiphyseal line** (→ Box 4.2).

Box 4.2 Genetic and environmental factors (diet, hormones, compression) can affect bone growth, e.g. cleft palate, spina bifida, acromegaly, gigantism.

Taking it Further
Most of the nutrients required for growth of bone and other tissues are consumed in the diet.

You can find out more about the science of nutrition in online Chapter 19.

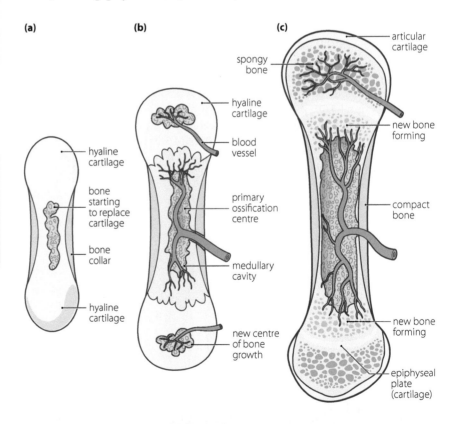

(a)

(b)

(c)

articular cartilage

spongy bone

hyaline cartilage

blood vessel

hyaline cartilage

bone starting to replace cartilage

bone collar

primary ossification centre

medullary cavity

hyaline cartilage

new centre of bone growth

new bone forming

compact bone

new bone forming

epiphyseal plate (cartilage)

Fig. 4.3 Stages in the formation of a long bone (**a**) embryo, (**b**) foetus, (**c**) child.

Growth in width is due to the addition of cells on the inside of the periosteum (→ Fig. 4.4), and is more active in children.

4.1.3 Structure of bones

A bone is a complex structure, shaped for its particular position in the skeleton and the stress it has to bear. The outside of a bone is solid with only a few small canals; the inside contains spaces filled with soft bone marrow which makes blood cells and some fat cells (→ Fig. 4.4).

Articular cartilage covers the places where the bone forms a synovial joint with another bone.

Compact bone forms an outer layer to the bone and is thickest in those places that receive the greatest stress. Its dense texture gives it strength but makes it heavy.

Spongy bone gets its name because of the numerous small spaces within it and not because it is soft and sponge-like. It is neither as strong nor as heavy as compact bone because the spaces are filled with red marrow or fat, which gives it a pinkish colour (→ Box 4.3).

Box 4.3 Most bones consist of both compact bone and spongy bone, thus optimising the balance between strength, rigidity and weight (mass).

Osteoporosis is the loss of bony tissue that makes bones brittle and liable to fracture. It is common in the elderly and in women after the menopause. There is also a high risk amongst people who have had anorexia and also in heavy drinkers. A diet with adequate calcium helps to prevent or delay the disorder.

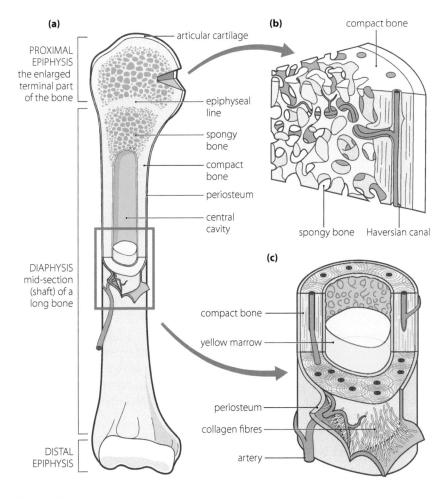

(a)

PROXIMAL EPIPHYSIS the enlarged terminal part of the bone

articular cartilage

epiphyseal line

spongy bone

compact bone

periosteum

central cavity

DIAPHYSIS mid-section (shaft) of a long bone

DISTAL EPIPHYSIS

(b)

compact bone

spongy bone   Haversian canal

(c)

compact bone

yellow marrow

periosteum

collagen fibres

artery

Fig. 4.4 Structure of a long bone.

A **medullary cavity** is present in long bones as this region is not required to take any load or other stress, which makes the bone lighter without any loss of strength. The space contains bone marrow.

Periosteum – the thin, tough connective tissue that covers the outside of the bone not covered by cartilage. It is firmly attached to the bone tissue underneath and contains blood vessels and nerves with branches which penetrate throughout bone tissue in the Haversian canals.

4.1.4 Ossification

Ossification is the formation of bone tissue. The process takes place continuously as the bones are remodelled to meet the demands of:
- growth and development
- repair of damaged tissue
- physical pressures placed on bones (→ Box 4.4)
- homeostasis of blood calcium (→ 4.1.5).

Bone remodelling

The bone remodelling cycle adjusts the structure of bone to meet the demands placed on it and the parathyroid **hormone** regulates the process (→ 11.5).

The two key phases in bone remodelling are:
❶ **osteoclasts** secrete enzymes and acid to dissolve the bone matrix, releasing calcium
❷ **osteoblasts** secrete new **osteoid tissue** (bone tissue) by producing a gel in which a matrix of collagen fibres are laid down. Minute crystals of calcium and phosphate are deposited in the matrix to harden the bone (→ Fig. 4.5).

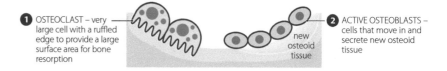

❶ OSTEOCLAST – very large cell with a ruffled edge to provide a large surface area for bone resorption

new osteoid tissue

❷ ACTIVE OSTEOBLASTS – cells that move in and secrete new osteoid tissue

Fig. 4.5 Ossification and remodelling of bone.

4.1.5 Homeostasis of blood calcium

Blood calcium needs to be kept at a constant level for the healthy functioning of cells, and this is achieved by continuous interchange between the large store of calcium in bones and the calcium in blood. When there is a shortage, calcium moves from bone to blood; when there is an excess, it moves in the opposite direction (→ Box 4.5) under the influence of the endocrine system (→ 11.10.1).

4.1.6 Myeloid tissue

Myeloid tissue, also known as **bone marrow**, can be red or yellow. The red colour is due to the presence of blood and the yellow colour is due to

Box 4.4 Bones need the stress of movement and gravity to keep healthy, e.g. bones in limbs which are paralysed or in patients who are on extended bed rest lose calcium, weaken, and are subject to fracture. When astronauts are weightless, calcium is rapidly lost from bones and is removed from the body through the kidneys.

Box 4.5 Bone marrow transplants are carried out in people who are no longer able to produce normal blood cells. Healthy stem cells from the bone marrow of a donor are transferred to the bone marrow of the recipient to take over blood cell production. A bone marrow transplant is used to treat, e.g.:
- severe **aplastic anaemia** – failure of the bone marrow to produce new red cells;
- **leukaemia** – cancer of the white blood cells;
- **non-Hodgkin's lymphoma** – cancer of the lymphatic system;
- genetic blood disorders such as **sickle cell anaemia** and **thalassaemia**.

the presence of fat. At birth, the central cavity in long bones and the spaces in spongy (cancellous) bone are all filled with red marrow. This gradually becomes replaced by fat in the central cavities of long bones so that in adults, red marrow and blood cell production occurs mainly in the flat bones. In cases of severe blood loss, the body can convert yellow marrow back to red marrow to increase blood cell production.

Red marrow contains specialist stem cells which produce three important types of blood components haematopoiesis (→ 2.4.1):
- red cells, which lose their nuclei as they mature
- white cells which help fight infection
- platelets which help stop bleeding.

The rate of red cell production in the bone marrow can be increased by the hormone **erythropoietin** (EPO) which is produced in the kidneys and released into the bloodstream in response to **hypoxia** (shortage of oxygen), as can happen at high altitudes.

4.2 Axial skeleton

The axial skeleton forms the main axis of the body and consists of the skull, vertebral column and ribcage. It also includes the hyoid bone in the neck and the tiny ossicles of the middle ear (→ Fig. 10.12).

4.2.1 Skull

The skull consists of 22 bones interlocked to form a very firm structure with the only movable part being the **mandible** (lower jaw) (→ Fig. 4.6). The largest part of the skull – the **cranium** – surrounds and protects the brain. The shape of the cranium follows the shape of the brain and, as a child's brain grows, the cranium enlarges (→ Box 4.6). The brain connects with the spinal cord through a large hole in the floor of the cranium, and ear openings in the side of the skull lead to the middle and inner parts of the ears, which are inside the floor of the cranium.

Box 4.6 The names of the bones of the cranium correspond to the lobes of the brain (→ Fig. 9.6).

The mandible is horseshoe-shaped and articulates (forms a movable joint) with the temporal bones on the sides of the skull.

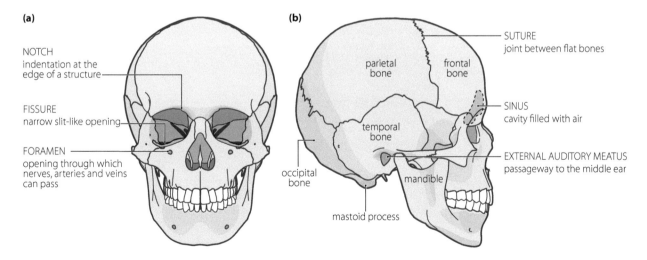

Fig. 4.6 (**a**) Anterior view of the skull; (**b**) Lateral view of the skull.

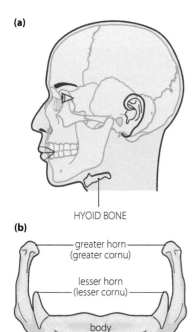

HYOID BONE

greater horn
(greater cornu)

lesser horn
(lesser cornu)

body

Fig. 4.7 The hyoid bone: (**a**) lateral view; (**b**) anterior view.

Facial bones

The views of the skull (→ Fig. 4.6) show the bones of the face arranged so that they surround the cavities of the eyes, ears, nose and mouth. The sinuses are four connected air cavities in the cranial bones near the nose. They help to humidify inhaled air and give resonance to the voice. They also lessen the weight of the skull.

Hyoid bone

The hyoid bone (→ Fig. 4.7) is a small U-shaped bone in the neck which is held in position by muscles and ligaments attached to the mastoid process (→ Fig. 4.6). The hyoid bone supports the tongue and raises the larynx, which enables them to work together to produce a large variety of distinct sounds that makes speech possible.

Fontanelles and sutures

Fontanelles are the 'soft spots' in a baby's skull – the areas between the bones that are covered by a tough but flexible membrane (→ Fig. 4.8a). They allow the skull to change shape slightly (mould) as the baby is pushed through the birth canal (→ Box 4.7). The fontanelles disappear as the skull bones enlarge and join together, the posterior fontanelle by the age of 2 months, and the anterior fontanelle by about 18 months.

Sutures in the cranium refer to the fibrous joints that hold the bones firmly together to form a strong, protective case for the brain (→ Fig. 4.8b). During infancy and childhood, the sutures are flexible, allowing the skull to change shape as it grows and develops. The relative positions of the bones continue to change slowly during adult life until, in old age, the sutures may ossify (turn to bone) completely (→ Box 4.8).

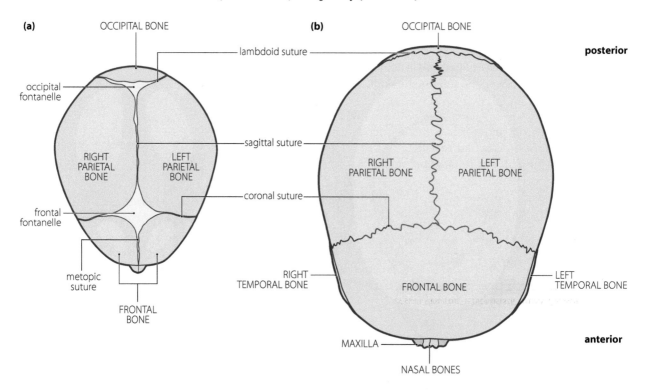

Fig. 4.8 Superior view of the skull of (**a**) an infant; (**b**) an adult.

4.2.2 Vertebral column

The vertebral column (**spine**; **backbone**) is a column of 33 small bones called **vertebrae** (each is a vertebra). The top 24 are separate bones, the next five are fused to form the **sacrum** and the lowest four are fused to form the **coccyx**, which is the remnants of a tail (→ Fig. 4.9). Viewed from the side, the spine has an S-shaped curve and behaves rather like a spring by absorbing vibrations and jolting, with the cartilage discs between the vertebrae acting as shock absorbers.

Box 4.7 Newborn head moulding is an abnormal head shape that results from pressure on the baby's head during childbirth. The normal shape returns within a few days.

Box 4.8 In surgery, a suture refers to a stitch or row of stitches holding together the edges of a wound or surgical incision.

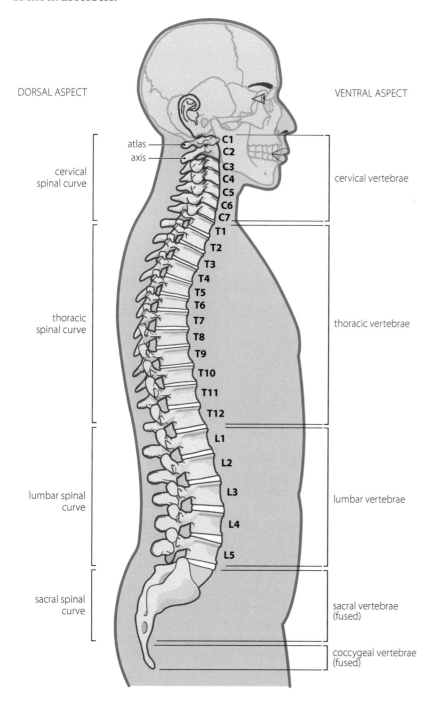

DORSAL ASPECT   VENTRAL ASPECT

atlas — C1
axis — C2
C3
C4
C5
C6
C7

cervical spinal curve / cervical vertebrae

T1–T12 / thoracic spinal curve / thoracic vertebrae

L1–L5 / lumbar spinal curve / lumbar vertebrae

sacral spinal curve / sacral vertebrae (fused)

coccygeal vertebrae (fused)

Fig. 4.9 Regions and curves of the vertebral column. C1–C7 are the cervical vertebrae of the neck; T1–T12 are the thoracic vertebrae, each connected to one pair of ribs; L1–L5 are the largest, strongest vertebrae; the sacrum is a large triangular bone that connects with the pelvis.

Functions of the spine:

- supports the upper part of the body
- encloses and protects the spinal cord
- provides points of attachment for the ribs and the muscles of the back
- the joint between the skull and the top vertebra (**atlas**) allows the head to move backwards and forwards
- the joint between the first and second vertebrae (**atlas** and **axis**) allows the head to turn from side to side
- cartilage discs between the vertebrae allow a small amount of movement, and their combined movements allow the trunk to bend and turn (→ Box 4.9).

Curvature of the spine

- **Kyphosis** is excessive outward curvature of the thoracic spinal curve, causing hunching of the back (→ Fig. 4.10a). This can make it difficult to stand up straight, cause worries about appearance, and may cause pain.
- **Lordosis** is excessive inward curve of the spine, usually in the lower back, particularly in the lumbar region just above the buttocks, leading to an exaggerated posture (→ Fig. 4.10b).

> **Box 4.9** Back pain associated with the spine is a common cause of absence from work, due perhaps to:
> - **whiplash** – neck injury caused by sudden movement forwards, backwards or sideways that follows sudden impact;
> - **ankylosing spondylitis** – pain and stiffness where the spine meets the pelvis;
> - **lumbago** – pain in the lower back;
> - **sciatica** – irritation or compression of the sciatic nerve causing pain, numbness and tingling that travels down one leg:
> - **prolapsed disc** (→ 4.2.5).

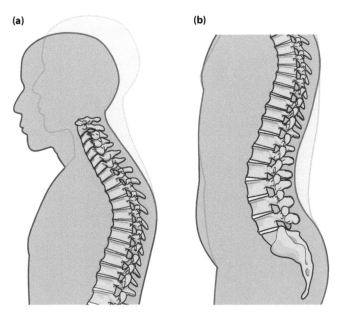

(a) **(b)**

Fig. 4.10 Excessive curvature of the spine (**a**) kyphosis, (**b**) lordosis.

4.2.3 Vertebrae

A vertebra is an irregularly shaped bone with a hole in the centre for the spinal cord to pass through. The sturdy part of bone is called the '**body**' with bony **spinous processes** extending from it (→ Box 4.10). Each vertebra has two pairs of **facets** – flat surfaces that form joints with the neighbouring vertebrae, one pair facing upwards and one downwards (→ Fig. 4.11).

> **Box 4.10** On the outside of the back, the spinous processes can be felt as bumps along the spine.

The **spinal canal** is the passage that runs through the spine containing the spinal cord and cerebrospinal fluid (→ Fig. 4.11). Nerve fibres branch off from the spinal cord to form pairs of **spinal nerves** that pass through

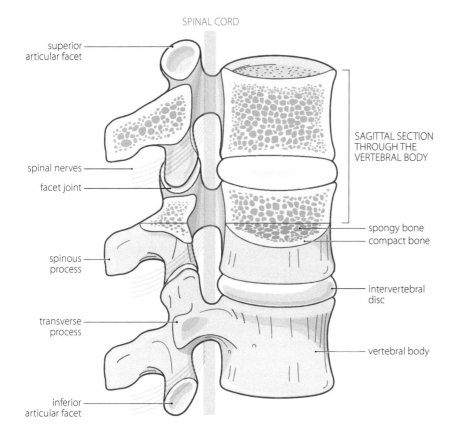

SPINAL CORD

superior
articular facet

SAGITTAL SECTION
THROUGH THE
VERTEBRAL BODY

spinal nerves

facet joint

spongy bone

compact bone

spinous
process

intervertebral
disc

transverse
process

vertebral body

inferior
articular facet

Fig. 4.11 Lateral view of 3 lumbar vertebrae with the upper part in sagittal section showing compact bone enclosing spongy bone and the annulus and nucleus of an intervertebral disc.

openings between adjacent vertebrae in the thoracic, lumbar and sacral regions (→ Fig. 9.15). This is why damage to the spinal cord can cause pain or paralysis in certain areas and not others, depending on which spinal nerves are affected.

4.2.4 Intervertebral discs

The individual bones of the spine are joined together by **intervertebral discs** which make up about a quarter of the length of the backbone, making the spine flexible but strong. Each disc has a strong outer ring of fibrocartilage called the **annulus**, and a soft, jelly-like centre called the **nucleus pulposus** which has a high water content, helping the discs to act as shock absorbers.

As people get older, small changes in the structure of discs and surrounding tissues can lead to subtle changes in the flexibility of the spine so that it loses elasticity and becomes stiffer (→ Box 4.11). Osteoporosis may accompany these changes, leading to spinal compression (→ 4.5.1).

Box 4.11 Degeneration of intervertebral discs is a major cause of loss of mobility in people over 60, causing pain in some people. However, others with greater degenerative changes may not experience any pain.

4.2.5 Prolapsed intervertebral disc

A prolapsed intervertebral disc (herniated disc; slipped disc) occurs when pressure on the disc causes a portion of the the nucleus to push through a crack in the annulus and press on the roots of an adjoining nerve. The pressure is often the result of sudden bending or twisting of the spine and can cause severe pain (→ Fig. 4.12).

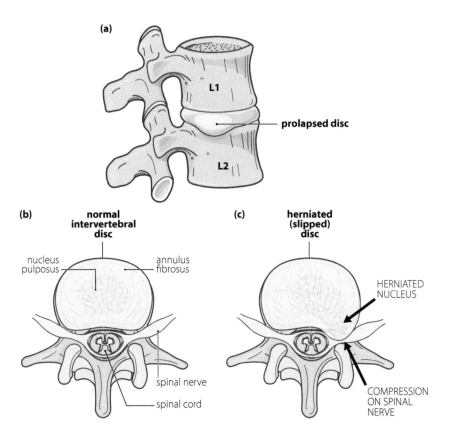

Fig. 4.12 Intervertebral disc: (**a**) lateral view of a prolapsed disc, (**b**) normal disc in cross-section. (**c**) cross-section of a prolapsed disc pressing on a spinal nerve.

4.2.6 Thoracic cage

The thoracic cage (ribcage) is formed by the sternum, ribs and the thoracic vertebrae. It encloses the thoracic cavity containing the heart and lungs (→ Fig. 4.13). Twelve pairs of ribs are joined to the twelve thoracic vertebrae; the upper seven pairs are also joined directly to the sternum by costal cartilage and are called 'true ribs'; rib pairs 8–10 do not join the sternum directly but are connected to rib 7 by cartilage, and are known as 'false ribs'; the two lower pairs of ribs are sometimes called 'floating ribs' because they have no connection with the sternum although they are firmly held in place by the muscles of the back.

Costal cartilage refers to the cartilages that connect the ends of the ribs to the sternum, and the spaces between the ribs – **intercostal spaces** – contain the **intercostal muscles.** Numerous muscles of the neck, thorax, upper abdomen and back are attached to the thoracic cage and, together with the costal cartilages, give the cage the elasticity that enables it to move during the respiratory cycle.

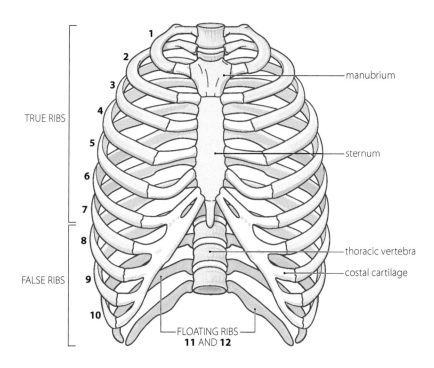

Fig. 4.13 The thoracic cage.

4.3 Appendicular skeleton

The appendicular skeleton consists of bones which are arranged to form the the pectoral and pelvic girdles and the limbs attached to them.

4.3.1 Pectoral girdle

The pectoral girdle is composed of four bones (→ Fig. 4.14):
- two **clavicles** which are attached to the sternum. Their function is to support the scapula; one end of a clavicle is attached to the sternum, the other end forms joints with the scapula

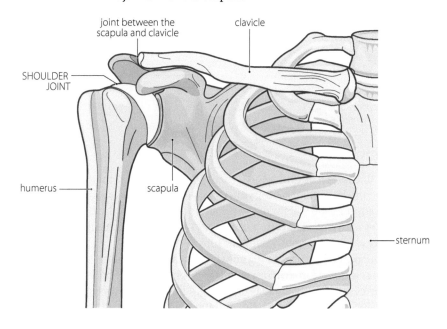

Fig. 4.14 Right pectoral girdle.

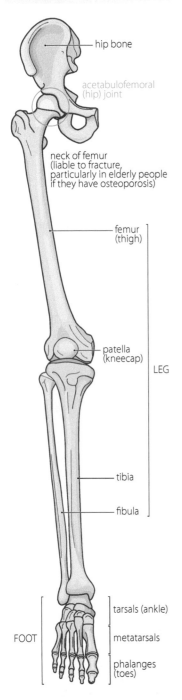

Fig. 4.16 Anterior view of the right leg attached to the right pelvis by a ball and socket joint.

- two **scapulae** (sing. scapula) commonly called **shoulder blades**, provide a large surface area for attachment of the muscles of the arm, back and chest that hold the shoulder joint in place. The scapula moves by sliding over the rib cage, taking the arm with it
- the **shoulder joint** is formed where the end of the humerus (long bone of the upper arm) fits into a bony socket of the scapula (shoulder blade). This arrangement allows for a wide range of movement of the arm, although the area is also prone to injury.

4.3.2 Pelvic girdle

The pelvic girdle consists of three bones – the **right pelvis**, **left pelvis** and **sacrum** (the lower part of the spine). They form a ring of bone strong enough to support the weight of the upper part of the body and take the strain of the attached muscles of the legs, spine and abdominal wall. The right and left pelvis meet at the **pubic symphysis** where they are held together by tough, fibrous connective tissue. In males the pubic symphysis is rigid, but in females, it allows slight movement to occur during childbirth (→ Fig. 4.15).

The shape of the pelvic girdle depends on gender. It is wider and flatter in females and adapted to the needs of childbirth (→ Box 4.12). Males are more muscular than females and have a larger and stronger pelvis to which their powerful leg muscles are attached.

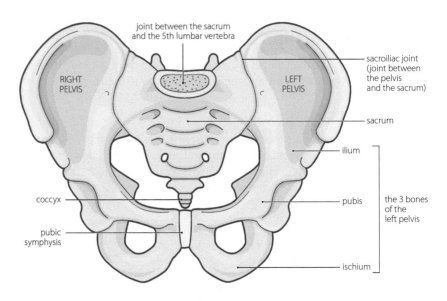

Fig. 4.15 Pelvic girdle.

4.3.3 Limbs

The upper limbs – **arms and hands** – function to grasp and manipulate objects and the lower limbs – **legs and feet** – enable locomotion. The lower limbs also support the weight of the upper body and helps the body adapt to gravity. They are pentadactyl (five-fingered) limbs with a common pattern. Moving outwards from the shoulder or hip:

- the upper part of the arm or leg consists of a single bone
- the next segment (forearm or lower leg) has two parallel bones
- next comes a cluster of small bones – eight in the wrist, seven in the ankle
- five parallel bones form the palm and foot
- the limb ends with five jointed digits (fingers and toes) (→ Figs. 4.16 and 4.17).

4.4 Joints

A joint is the place where two bones meet and are linked together by ligaments (→ Fig. 4.18). A **ligament** is a band of tough fibrous tissue which limits the amount of movement that can take place between the two bones (→ Box 4.13). Joints are classified according to the amount and type of movement between the bones.

Fixed joints (immovable joints) The bones interlock where they touch each other and are firmly held together by fibrous tissue, with no movement between them, e.g. bones of the skull (→ Fig. 4.8b).

Cartilaginous joints The bones are firmly held together by tough cartilage which is flexible enough to allow a slight amount of movement when squeezed or stretched, e.g. the joints between the vertebrae, between the sternum and ribs, and the pubic symphysis.

Synovial joints are freely movable joints (→ Figs. 4.18 and 4.19). Movement between two bones is possible because:
- **smooth and hyaline cartilage** covers the ends of the bones where they touch each other
- a smooth, moist **synovial membrane** lines the inside of the joint: secretes **synovial fluid** which lubricates the joint
- a tough **capsule** encloses and seals the joint
- **muscles** attached to the bones by tendons enable movement to take place at the joint (→ Box 4.14).

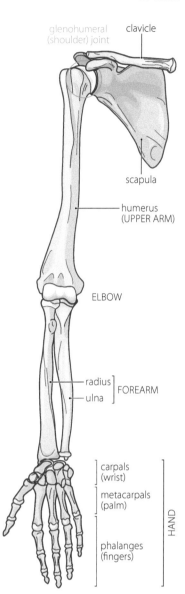

Fig. 4.17 Anterior view of the right arm attached to the right pectoral girdle by a ball and socket joint.

Box 4.13 Hypermobility (double-jointedness) means that the ligaments can allow a larger range of movements because the ligaments can stretch more than usual.

A **sprain** is an over-stretched ligament, which is painful but gradually heals.

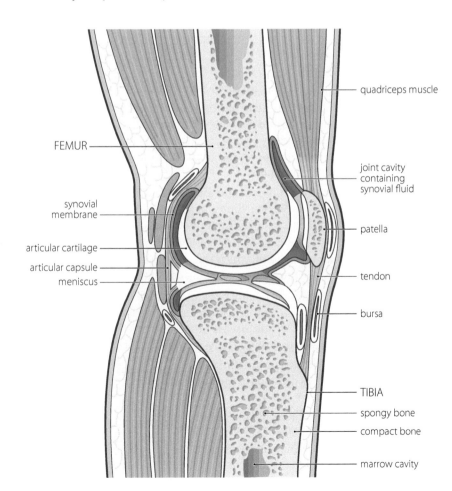

Fig. 4.18 Section through the knee joint.

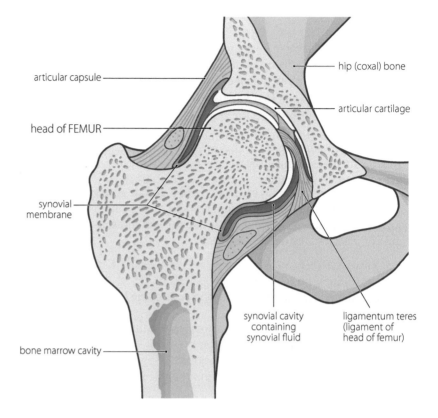

Fig. 4.19 Section through the hip joint.

Types of synovial joint

The two main types of synovial joint are:

- **ball and socket joints**. The end of one bone is rounded and fits into a hollow in the other bone and movement in nearly all directions is possible, e.g. shoulder and hip joints
- **hinge joints**. These act like door hinges and allow movement in one plane only, e.g. finger joints, knee joint.

4.5 Joint disorders

4.5.1 Arthritis

Arthritis is inflammation of a joint, which causes pain and limits movement. There are many types, the most common being osteoarthritis and rheumatoid arthritis.

Osteoarthritis

Osteoarthritis is a degenerative disease of the joints caused by wear and tear of the joint cartilage. In this type of arthritis:

- the smooth cartilage at the ends of the bones becomes worn away and gradually disappears (→ Box 4.15)
- the condition is restricted to the joints
- it tends to occur in the weight-bearing joints of the hips, knees and spine, and to increase with age.

Rheumatoid arthritis

Rheumatoid arthritis (**RA**) is an autoimmune disease that usually starts in the wrists, hands or feet, making the affected joints look swollen, red and warm to the touch due to increased blood flow. It can spread to other joints and make the sufferer feel generally ill with fever and exhaustion, and it can cause weight loss (→ 14.9.3).

Some people with an acute episode of rheumatoid arthritis recover completely; with others, the condition is intermittent with weeks or months when the joints improve, followed by pain and stiffness again. Others may have permanent changes to the joints, usually seen in the hands (→ Box 4.16).

4.5.2 Other joint disorders

Gout

Gout is a type of arthritis in which small crystals of uric acid form inside and around one or more joints. The condition develops when either the body produces too much uric acid or the kidneys fail to filter enough out. The uric acid then builds up in the blood and is precipitated in the joints as tiny, sharp crystals, causing sudden attacks of severe pain, swelling and redness. The symptoms develop rapidly over a few hours and typically last three to ten days. After this time the pain should pass and the joint should return to normal (→ Box 4.17).

Bunion

A bunion is a swollen joint on the big toe. It is caused by **bursitis** – inflammation of one or more **bursae** (small sacs) of synovial fluid within the joint due to pressure and rubbing by shoes.

4.6 Skeletal muscles

Skeletal muscles form the flesh of the body (→ 2.5.6). There are about 600 of them and they vary considerably in size and shape, ranging from those in the middle ear that contain only a few muscle fibres to the many **fascicules** (bundles of muscle fibres) that form the large gluteal muscles of the buttocks (→ Fig. 4.20).

4.6.1 Functions of skeletal muscles

- **Movement**. Skeletal muscles generate force when they contract, which pulls on bones and results in movements either of the whole body (locomotion) or of its parts.
- **Posture**. Standing, sitting and other postures are maintained by the continuous partial contraction of skeletal muscles known as **muscle tone**.
- **Heat production**. Like all cells in the body, muscle cells produce heat. As skeletal muscle is more abundant and active than other types, much of the body's heat is produced by this tissue.

4.6.2 Tendons

Tendons are tough cords that attach muscles to bones. They are whitish in colour and sometimes known as gristle (→ Box 4.18). Usually there is a tendon at each end of a muscle, although in some cases muscles are attached directly to a bone (→ Fig. 4.21).

Box 4.16 Rheumatoid arthritis usually affects younger people, mainly women, often before the age of 40. Some affected joints can be replaced with artificial ones, especially the finger joints.

Box 4.17 Gout is caused by a combination of diet and genetic factors, mainly affecting men over 30. It occurs more commonly in those who eat a lot of meat, drink a lot of alcohol, or are overweight.

Box 4.18 Tendons and ligaments are both made of strong, fibrous, flexible connective tissue. They differ in that:
- **tendons** attach muscles to bones;
- **ligaments** attach bones to bones at a joint.

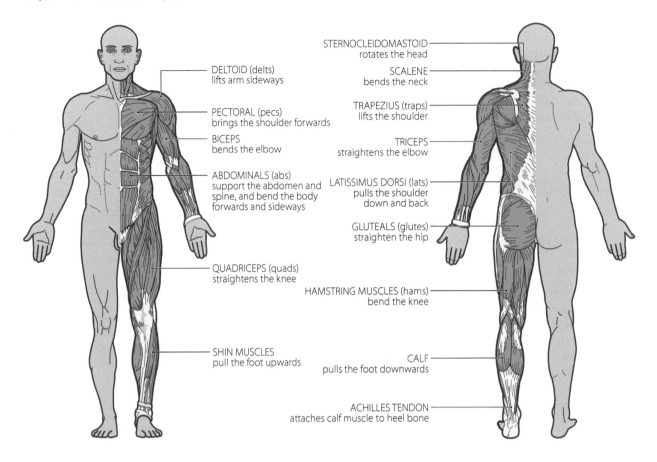

Fig. 4.20 Anatomy of skeletal muscles.

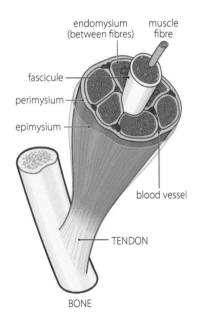

Fig. 4.21 Section through a skeletal muscle showing tendon attachment to bones at a joint.

4.6.3 Microstructure of muscle fibres

Skeletal muscle is formed from bundles of muscle fibres (→ Fig. 4.21) bound together by fascia (singular: fascicule) (→ Box 4.19). Each muscle fibre contains a number of parallel, contractile threads called **myofibrils** enclosed in a thin, transparent membrane called the **sarcolemma** which is similar but not identical to plasma membrane (→ Fig. 4.22).

Sarcomeres

The sarcomere is the basic unit of a myofibril and each myofibril contains many thousands of them placed end to end. Sarcomeres contain:

- thick myofilaments composed of **myosin** – a protein with the properties of elasticity and contractility
- thin myofilaments are predominantly **actin** – a protein that plays an important role in the process of contraction.

Muscle contraction

During muscle contraction, the myosin and actin filaments slide over each other and cause the sarcomeres to shorten (see Fig. 4.23). Movement in the sarcomeres is controlled by nerves that branch many times so that each muscle fibre has its own nerve ending called the **motor end plate** or **neuromuscular junction**. When impulses from the brain pass along the motor nerve to tell the muscle to contract, all the sarcomeres receive the impulses from the spinal cord at the same time, and they contract together to shorten the muscle, perhaps by as much as half its length. When the impulses cease, the sarcomeres relax and the muscle returns to its original shape and length. Although each sarcomere is very tiny, their combined action is able to generate enough force to move limbs and maintain posture.

4.6.4 Sliding filament theory

The sliding filament theory explains the mechanism by which muscles are thought to contract. The theory is based on the **contraction cycle** – a series of events within skeletal muscle. The contraction cycle is closely linked to the excitation of motor units (→ Box 4.20) and takes place in several stages.

Stages in the contraction cycle, 1–8

❶ An impulse arrives at the membrane of the motor end plate and depolarises it. **Depolarisation** is loss of the difference in electric charge between the inside and outside of the plasma membrane, so permeability to calcium ions increases (→ Fig. 4.22).

Box 4.19 Fascia are sheets or bands of fibrous connective tissue. **Plantar fasciitis** (jogger's heel) is a cause of heel pain due to inflammation of the plantar fascia that runs across the bottom of the foot and connects the calcaneus (heel bone) to the toes.

Box 4.20 A **motor unit** is a motor neuron and its terminal end plates. Motor units are all the muscle fibrils and their sarcomeres that are innervated by a single motor nerve.

Motor unit recruitment refers to the activation of additional motor units to accomplish an increase in contractile strength in a muscle. In general, the smallest motor units are recruited first.

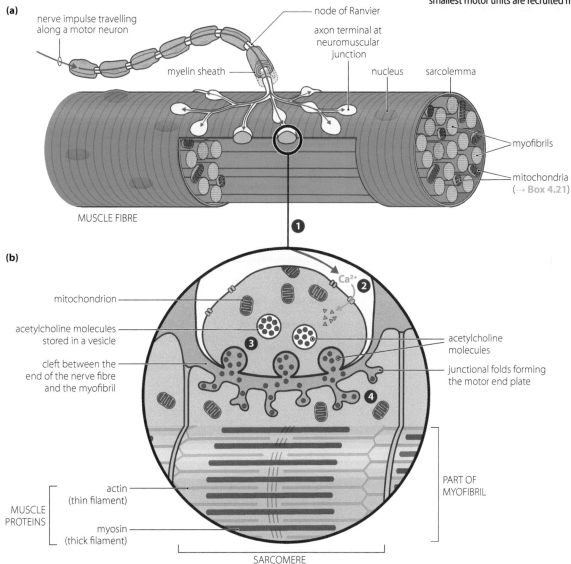

Fig. 4.22 (**a**) Section of a muscle fibre; (**b**) neuro-muscular junction and sarcomere.

❷ **Calcium ions** are also released from intracellular storage sites and trigger the contraction cycle.

❸ **Acetylcholine is released** into the cleft.

❹ **Acetylcholine binds to specific receptors** on the sarcolemma (muscle fibre membrane), initiating a wave of excitation that travels along the fibre (→ Fig. 4.22a).

❺ **Myosin filaments** (the thick ones) remain constant in length during the contraction cycle; they are able to break down the high energy bond of adenosine triphosphate (ATP) to release energy that is used to generate force (→ Fig. 4.23).

❻ The energy pulls the **actin filaments** (the thin ones) towards each other so that they slide over the myosin filaments in a process called the **power stroke**.

❼ Because the actin filaments are tethered to the **Z-disc**, when they slide past the myosin filaments, the **sarcomere shortens** and the muscle contracts.

❽ When the impulse stops, calcium ions are transported back into the intracellular storage sites and the contraction ends. The muscle fibres slide back to their original length and the muscle relaxes.

Box 4.21 Muscle fibres contain many mitochondria to supply the energy needed for contraction (shortening), when the actin filaments slide over the myosin filaments in the sarcomeres.

Taking it Further

All skeletal muscles are able to produce ATP that is needed for the contraction cycle.

Some muscle fibres can generate ATP very rapidly by glycolysis; others have many mitochondria and have the capacity to produce ATP through aerobic respiration. Both fibre types are found in all skeletal muscles, although their relative proportions can vary.

You can find out more about these biochemical processes in online Chapter 20.

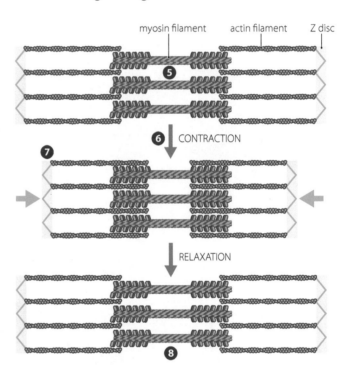

Fig. 4.23 Excitation triggers the contraction cycle in skeletal muscle fibres.

4.7 Movement

The function of skeletal muscles is to move bones (→ Box 4.22). Each skeletal muscle has one end – **origin** – attached to a bone that does not move; the other end – **insertion** – is attached to the bone that moves when the muscle contracts. For example, the biceps muscle has its origin in the scapula (shoulder blade) and its insertion in the radius of the forearm so that, when the biceps muscle contracts, the forearm moves.

Because skeletal muscles can only pull bones but not push them, they always work in **antagonistic pairs** – one muscle pulls the bone that can

Box 4.22 The study of body movement is a very broad discipline called **kinesiology** which includes orthopaedics, biomechanics, electrophysiology, strength and conditioning, rehabilitation, occupational therapy and sport psychology.

cause movement at a joint, another muscle pulls the bone back to its original position, e.g.:
- the **biceps muscle** bends the arm and the **triceps** muscle straightens it
- the **shin muscle** bends the ankle and the **calf muscle** straightens it.

Flexor muscles are those that cause the joint to bend; **extensor muscles** straighten the joint.

4.7.1 Levers

Muscle contraction enables bones to act as levers, a **lever** being a rigid rod that is able to pivot about a fixed point (**fulcrum**) when a force is applied to it. In the body:
- the **lever** is a bone
- the **fulcrum** (**F**) is a joint – the point at which the lever pivots
- the **effort** (**E**) is the force exerted by contracting muscles
- the **load** (**L**) is the resistance to the pull of the muscles, e.g. weight of an object or the pull of gravity (→ Fig. 4.24).

Levers are classified as first, second, and third class according to the positions of the fulcrum, effort and load or resistance.

(a) FIRST CLASS LEVER

the fulcrum is between the effort (neck muscles) and the load (weight of the head)

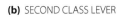
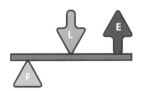
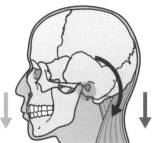

> **Taking it Further**
> Some drugs and medications act at neuromuscular junctions. You can find out more about their effects in online Chapter 18.

(b) SECOND CLASS LEVER

the ankle is the fulcrum, the load is the body weight and the effort is the contracted calf muscles

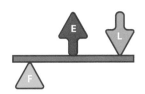
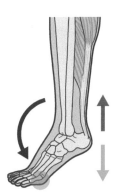

(c) THIRD CLASS LEVER

the elbow is the fulcrum as the effort (contracted biceps) lifts the load (forearm)

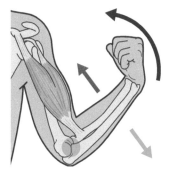

Fig. 4.24 The range of levers used in the human body.

4.7.2 Muscle tone

Muscle tone is the state of slight tension in which muscles are maintained that keeps them ready for action. Movement of the skeleton takes place at the joints and action can only occur when the muscle on one side of the joint contracts and pulls harder than the muscle on the other side. Gradual relaxation keeps the movement smooth and under control.

Because of muscle tone, healthy muscles are never fully relaxed and the body is able to maintain its posture when standing or sitting upright. Muscle tone decreases during sleep and, if a person falls asleep while sitting up, the head may flop forward.

4.7.3 Muscle growth and development

No new myocytes (→ 2.5.6) are formed in the foetus after the sixteenth week of development, and growth of muscle tissue occurs as the myocytes increase in length and diameter. At one year of age, the diameter of myocytes is roughly 30% of adult size, and at 5 years, it is 50%.

Muscle repair and regeneration after injury follow a pattern very similar to the prenatal development. If muscle tissue is damaged and myocytes die, repair at the site of an injury is by growth of the surrounding undamaged myocytes, leaving a scar.

The effects of exercise

Exercise involves muscle contractions that can be of shorter or longer duration, lower or higher intensity depending on the type of activity. Muscles respond to physical activity in ways that lead to physiological changes, including increased muscle mass (hypertrophy), that strengthen and alter the muscle and make repeat exercise easier. When not used, they waste away (**atrophy**); people confined to bed can lose around 1% of muscle strength for each day in bed.

Muscles that are stretched too far by overuse, strain or pressure will swell and be painful, especially in the wrist, legs and shoulder areas (→ Box 4.23).

Muscle atrophy

Muscle atrophy is a decrease in the mass of the muscle tissue, which leads to muscle weakness. It is a natural process, accelerated by a sedentary lifestyle, that generally starts after the age of 30. The biggest changes occur during the 40s and 50s, with about 1% of lean muscle mass being lost per year after the age of 40. Muscle atrophy also affects astronauts, who spend much time in a weightless state. **Neurogenic atrophy** is muscle atrophy that results from damage to the motor nerve that stimulates the muscle.

4.7.4 Adaptations to physical activity and exercise

When physical tasks are undertaken, other systems in the body are involved besides muscles.

Metabolic changes

As the activity proceeds and/or becomes more intense, core body temperature begins to rise. The involuntary response of the sympathetic system is to dilate the arterioles in the dermis (→ Fig. 3.1) for heat loss by radiation and to increase the activity of the sweat glands. When the period of activity is over, the parasympathetic nervous system restores the resting state.

Box 4.23 Simple treatment advice for helping muscle damage to heal is called RICE, which stands for:
- **R**est – to allow the injured muscles to recover
- **I**ce packs – to reduce swelling
- **C**ompression by a bandage – helps to keep the swelling small
- **E**levation of a damaged limb to waist level helps to reduce swelling.

Circulatory system

Blood flow to skeletal muscles and the skin increases dramatically when a person moves from a sedentary state to exercise, the magnitude of the changes depending on the intensity of the activity and its duration. Blood flow to skeletal muscles is increased and blood flow to less active organs is decreased. This is an involuntary response of the sympathetic division of the nervous system (→ 9.8.2) and results in:

- increased heart rate, stroke volume and blood pressure increases the volume of blood in circulation
- vasodilation of arterioles in skeletal muscles increases the muscles' blood supply
- vasodilation of coronary blood vessels increases the heart's blood supply, enabling the heart muscle to beat harder and faster
- vasoconstriction of blood vessels in the gastrointestinal tract reduces their blood supply, allowing more blood to be diverted to where it is needed.

4.8 Physiotherapy

Physiotherapy is treatment that aims to improve a person's flexibility, mobility and quality of life (→ Box 4.24). It involves a range of techniques to ease pain and promote healing, e.g. massage, joint manipulation, remedial exercises, ultrasound, hydrotherapy, acupuncture and transcutaneous electrical nerve stimulation (**TENS**) (→ Box 4.25).

Physiotherapists treat physical problems linked to many of the body's systems, e.g.:

- **musculoskeletal therapy** identifies and treats the underlying causes of about 200 different conditions affecting the skeleton, skeletal muscles and joints, e.g. to help recovery from broken legs and head injuries
- **cardiovascular therapy** improves blood circulation though the heart and blood vessels and helps fluid drain more efficiently through the lymphatic system, e.g. rehabilitation following myocardial infarction (heart attack), angioplasty, heart bypass surgery and heart transplantation (→ Box 4.26)
- **respiratory therapy** involves the treatment and management of acute and chronic breathing disorders, e.g. to help patients to expand and clear their lungs after operations and encourage people with chronic obstructive pulmonary disorder (COPD) to feel confident about exercise.

4.8.1 Exercise

Remedial exercises are designed to strengthen and lengthen muscles and improve the range of movement at the joints. Therapists will advise people about which exercises to do for their condition and how to do them safely. Exercises of the right type can:

- strengthen muscles and joints and increase the range of movement after ligament tears, fractured bones or joint replacement surgery
- enable patients to walk normally after having a leg in a plaster cast following a fracture (broken bone) in the leg or foot
- help people who have had a heart attack, heart failure, heart valve surgery or coronary artery bypass grafting
- help stroke victims recover the use of affected muscles
- enable asthmatics to breathe more efficiently
- help recovery from back pain and sciatica and prevent recurrence.

Box 4.24 Physiotherapists form the third largest health profession after doctors and nurses, working in the NHS, in private practice, for charities, and in the workplace. As well as treating specific disorders, physiotherapists may also suggest ways to improve general wellbeing, e.g. regular exercise and maintaining a healthy weight.

Box 4.25 TENS is a method of pain relief using a mild electrical current. Leads from a small, battery-operated, hand-held device are connected to electrodes attached to the skin. TENS may be able to help reduce pain and muscle spasms caused by a wide range of conditions including knee, neck and back pain, arthritis, period pain and sports injuries. It is also sometimes used as a method of pain relief during labour.

Box 4.26 Physiotherapy-led cardiac rehabilitation (CR) programmes are clinically effective in improving health and quality of life, reducing length of stay in hospital, the number of hospital readmissions, and mortality.

Hydrotherapy (aquatic therapy)

Box 4.27 Hydrotherapy is often used with children and adults who have physical and learning disabilities.

Hydrotherapy (→ Box 4.27) is physiotherapy exercises carried out in warm water. The water supports the body so that weak muscles and stiff joints can move more easily and activities that are not possible on dry land can be performed. Exercises against the resistance of water can improve muscle strength, balance and co-ordination, e.g.:

- restore function to a fractured limb after immobilisation in a cast for several weeks
- strengthen weak muscles following a stroke
- loosen stiff muscles of children with cerebral palsy.

4.8.2 Manual therapy

Manual therapy uses 'hands-on' treatment techniques to mobilise joints and soft tissues to:

- relieve pain
- improve blood circulation and lymphatic drainage
- improve the movement of different parts of the body.

Therapeutic massage

Massage involves manipulating the soft tissues of the body to aid relaxation and circulation for the improvement of many disorders. There are different types of massage that can be applied with the hands or a massaging device such as ultrasound, e.g.:

- **clinical massage** focuses on medical issues and pain relief
- **massage therapy** is used for relaxation and stress relief.

Joint manipulation

Joint manipulation is the skilled use of the hands to improve or restore movement to stiff and painful joints. It is often applied on the back and neck, and also to other joints such as shoulders, elbows and knees. It helps to relieve tension in the muscles, which allows the joints to move freely again and is useful for people of all ages who have stiff joints.

4.9 Posture

Posture is the way the body is held when standing, sitting, walking, bending or lifting (→ Fig. 4.25).

Good posture allows the body to move easily and without putting undue strain on the muscles.

Poor posture puts the muscles out of balance and gives rise to a wide range of common ailments such as back pain or stiff neck. It:

- throws more work on to muscles to counteract the pull of gravity, leading to fatigue
- puts abnormal strain on bones and may in time produce deformities
- interferes with various functions such as respiration, heart action and digestion.

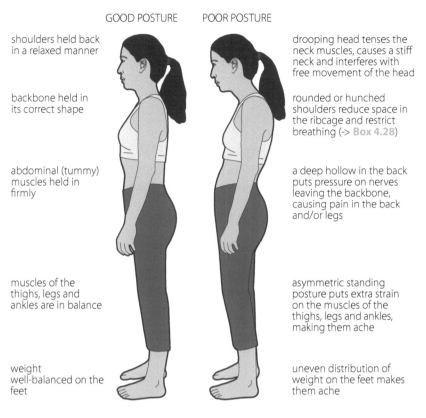

GOOD POSTURE   POOR POSTURE

shoulders held back in a relaxed manner

backbone held in its correct shape

abdominal (tummy) muscles held in firmly

muscles of the thighs, legs and ankles are in balance

weight well-balanced on the feet

drooping head tenses the neck muscles, causes a stiff neck and interferes with free movement of the head

rounded or hunched shoulders reduce space in the ribcage and restrict breathing (-> **Box 4.28**)

a deep hollow in the back puts pressure on nerves leaving the backbone, causing pain in the back and/or legs

asymmetric standing posture puts extra strain on the muscles of the thighs, legs and ankles, making them ache

uneven distribution of weight on the feet makes them ache

Box 4.28 Postural kyphosis can be caused by slouching all day in an office chair which tightens chest muscles and pulls the spine and shoulders forwards; this condition is reversible with appropriate exercise.

Fig. 4.25 Comparison of good and poor posture.

4.10 Myopathies

Myopathies are diseases of skeletal muscle which are not related to problems with the nervous system. A wide range of factors including inheritance, infections, inflammation, drugs and toxicity, contribute to the cause(s). Common features of myopathy are muscle weakness, fatigue and impaired activity to carry out activities of daily living, e.g. difficulty getting up from a sitting position, climbing the stairs or walking.

4.10.1 Muscular dystrophy

Muscular dystrophy is a rare inherited disorder in which muscles are weak and waste away. A common form is **Duchenne muscular dystrophy**, which only occurs in boys. The disease cannot be cured, but physiotherapy and support equipment such as calliper splints can help in living with the condition.

4.10.2 Tendonitis

Tendonitis is inflammation of a tendon. It is commonly caused by repeated overuse or injury to a particular tendon, especially those of the shoulder, elbow, wrist, finger, thigh, knee and Achilles tendon. Symptoms include pain when the affected tendons are being used.

4.10.3 Polymyositis

Polymyositis is a systemic connective tissue disorder characterised by inflammatory and degenerative changes in the muscles, leading to weakness and some degree of muscle atrophy. It affects all age groups but is more common in women and tends to affect people aged 30 to 60 years.

4.10.4 Rhabdomyolysis

Rhabdomyolysis is the breakdown of damaged skeletal muscle resulting in the release of myocyte contents into the circulation. Some of this is toxic to the kidney and frequently results in further tissue damage.

4.11 Neuromuscular disorders

Neuromuscular disorders include a large group of conditions which affect the nerves that control the muscles.

4.11.1 Dyspraxia

Dyspraxia is clumsiness due to the poor coordination of muscle movements by the brain. The condition does not affect a child's intelligence but it does reduce the ability to learn skills that involve coordination of muscles, e.g. riding a bicycle.

4.11.2 Repetitive strain injury

Repetitive strain injury (RSI) is an umbrella term referring to injuries involving muscles, tendons, ligaments and nerves caused by repetitive movements or overuse, usually of the tendons or ligaments of the hands, wrists or shoulders, e.g. by computer use. Symptoms include:

- inflammation of the tendons and joints of the hands and arms
- tenderness or pain in the muscles and joints
- tingling ('pins and needles') or numbness in the hand or arm
- loss of strength or sensation in the hand.

4.11.3 Myalgic encephalomyelitis

Myalgic encephalomyelitis (ME) is also known as **chronic fatigue syndrome**. The main symptom is persistent tiredness and exhaustion that does not go away with sleep or rest. Other symptoms can include muscle and joint pains, headaches and poor concentration. It tends to last for months or years, but most people eventually recover.

4.11.4 Fibromyalgia

Fibromyalgia is a debilitating chronic illness characterised by widespread muscle pain with stiffness, tenderness at specific points in the body, and fatigue. The condition is probably genetic, affecting more women than men, mostly between the ages of 20 and 50.

Key points

1. The skeleton provides a rigid, bony framework that supports the human body, protects internal organs and enables locomotion (movement).
2. Bones are complex structures that provide strength, produce blood cells and store minerals including sodium and calcium.
3. Bones continually undergo the process of remodelling to enable their physical structure to match the demands placed upon them.
4. Joints are the places where two bones make contact and are linked by means of ligaments.
5. Skeletal muscles, which are attached to bones by tendons, contract (shorten) and generate the force that enables bones to move.

Test yourself! Go to *www.lanternpublishing.com/AandP* and try the questions to check your understanding.

CHAPTER 5
THE CARDIOVASCULAR SYSTEM

The function of the cardiovascular system is to pump blood continuously around the body in the blood vessels. As the blood passes through the tissues, it helps to maintain homeostasis of the internal environment by delivering essential substances to the body's cells and removing waste and harmful substances. The pressure of blood must be maintained at an optimal level to ensure an adequate flow to every cell in the body.

5.1 Blood

Blood is a viscous (thick) red liquid that circulates around the body within a closed system of blood vessels but, if it comes into contact with air or with damaged tissues within the body, it becomes sticky and coagulates (→ Box 5.1). The amount of blood in the body depends on the person's size, e.g. an average adult weighing 70 kg will have 5–6 litres, whereas a child weighing 12 kg will have about 1 litre (→ Box 5.2).

5.1.1 Composition of blood

Blood is composed of four elements – plasma, red cells, white cells and platelets (→ Fig. 5.1). Plasma is the liquid part of blood with the other elements suspended in it. The red cells, white cells and platelets are all produced by the process of haematopoiesis that takes place in red bone marrow (→ 2.4.1).

5.1.2 Functions of blood

The function of blood is to transport substances and heat from one part of the body to another (→ Box 5.3). As blood travels round the body it:

- collects oxygen from the respiratory system and carries it to cells all over the body; arterial blood is oxygenated and bright red in colour while venous blood is deoxygenated and dark purplish-red
- collects nutrients from the digestive system and carries them to the liver and then to the cells in all parts of the body
- collects waste substances such as carbon dioxide and urea from the cells and delivers them to the lungs and kidneys
- collects hormones from the endocrine glands and delivers them to the target cells
- carries white cells and antibodies in the bloodstream, which help to protect the body against infection
- carries platelets that play an essential part in the clotting of blood
- helps to maintain body temperature by absorbing the heat generated by the liver and muscles and transferring it to colder parts of the body; when the body is over-hot, heat is lost from blood to the external environment as it circulates close to the skin surface.

Box 5.1 Blood is red because it contains the red pigment haemoglobin, hence the origin of terms such as **haematology** – the study of blood.

Box 5.2 The volume of blood increases during pregnancy so that a pregnant woman will have about 1.5 litres more blood than when not pregnant. Most of this increase is plasma, with a smaller increase in red cell volume – a process called **haemodilution**.

Box 5.3 As blood is the major transport system of the human body, it plays a vital role in homeostasis because it is involved in the physiological processes of every organ and tissue.

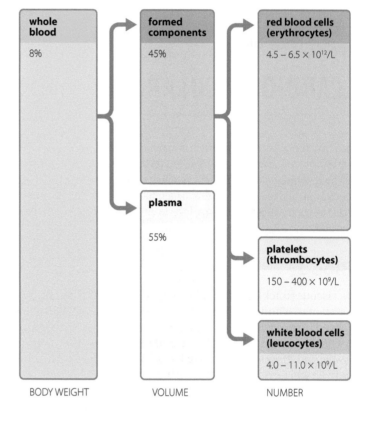

Fig. 5.1 Blood composition.

5.2 Plasma

Plasma is a straw-coloured fluid consisting of 90% water and 10% **solutes** – substances in solution. It helps to regulate the body's osmotic pressure (→ 20.5.1), plays a role in the immune system and in blood clotting (→ Box 5.4). Plasma also transports the many different solutes needed by the body, which can be grouped into:

- plasma proteins
- food substances – mainly glucose, amino acids and lipids
- respiratory gases – mainly dissolved carbon dioxide, as the amount of dissolved oxygen is very small
- compounds formed by metabolism, e.g. urea, uric acid, creatinine and lactic acid
- regulatory substances, e.g. hormones and enzymes
- inorganic salts, e.g. sodium, potassium, calcium and magnesium.

5.2.1 Plasma proteins

Box 5.4 When a sample of plasma is required for analysis, an anticoagulant such as heparin is added to the blood to prevent it from clotting. The plasma – which contains all the clotting factors – can then be separated from the cells (→ 17.5.1).

Plasma proteins account for the majority of the solutes in plasma and most are made in the liver (→ Box 5.5). There are many different types of plasma proteins, each with its own particular function, e.g.:

- **albumin** helps to maintain osmotic pressure of the blood and normal circulation
- **immunoglobulins** (antibodies) are involved in immunity (→ 14.6.1)
- **transferrin** binds to iron and acts as a carrier for iron in the bloodstream.

Box 5.5 When a blood clot forms it uses the clotting factors in the blood. The cells and platelets become trapped in the clot, leaving a straw-coloured fluid, which is **serum**. Serum is plasma with fibrinogens and other clotting factors removed.

5.3 Erythrocytes

Erythrocytes are commonly called **red cells** (→ Fig. 5.2).

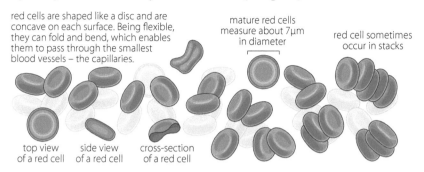

Fig. 5.2 Red cells.

The structure of red cells is related to their function of carrying oxygen to the tissues:

- the large surface area allows for the rapid diffusion of oxygen
- the cells are packed with haemoglobin – a pigment that absorbs oxygen in the lungs and then releases it to the rest of the body, changing colour from bright red to dark purplish-red as it does so (→ Fig. 5.3).

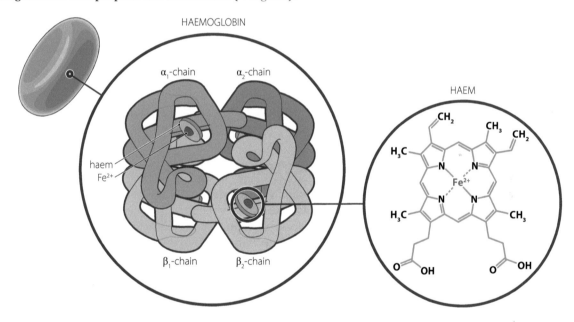

Fig. 5.3 Haemoglobin molecule – consists of four protein sub-units and a haem component containing iron. It can carry up to four oxygen molecules.

5.3.1 Red cell maturation

Red cells are produced from stem cells (→ 2.4) at a rate of about 2 million per second in a healthy adult. As they develop, the nucleus is expelled so that when mature, red cells have no nucleus or organelles (→ Fig. 5.4).

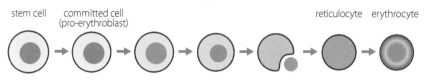

Fig. 5.4 Maturation of a red cell.

5.3.2 Life cycle of red cells

Box 5.6 The term 'mononuclear phagocytic system' means that the system uses cells with one nucleus that carry out phagocytosis (→ Fig. 5.6).

It takes about 7 days for red cells to mature. They then circulate continuously around the body for about 100–120 days before being broken down by the **mononuclear phagocytic system**, also called the **reticulo-endothelial system**. The iron which is released is recycled to make more red cells (→ Fig. 5.5) (→ Box 5.6).

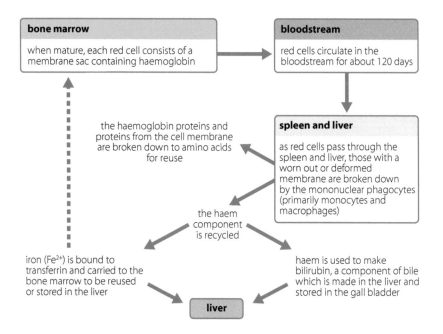

Fig. 5.5 Mononuclear macrophage system (reticulo-endothelial system).

5.4 Leucocytes

Box 5.7 White cells make up about 1% of the total blood volume in a healthy adult. Their number in the blood is often an indicator of disease.

Box 5.8 Diapedesis is the movement of white cells through the intact walls of capillaries (tiny blood vessels).

Leucocytes, commonly called **white cells**, are larger than red cells, but there are fewer of them, and they retain their nucleus (→ Box 5.7). Like red cells, white cells develop from stem cells in the bone marrow but then migrate to all parts of the body, accumulating in large numbers in the lymphatic system (→ 5.17). They are more or less spherical when carried in the blood stream but change shape as they crawl along the inside walls of blood vessels, squeeze through the capillary walls, and move around between the cells of the tissues (→ Box 5.8). The five types of white cell shown in Table 5.1 are part of the immune system (→ Ch 14), where they help to protect the body against disease by:

- **phagocytosis** – the process of removing pathogens, mainly bacteria and viruses, by engulfment and using digestive enzymes to destroy them (→ Fig. 5.6)
- **producing antibodies** – protein molecules which confer immunity by identifying and neutralising pathogens
- **killing cells** that have been attacked by viruses or are potentially cancerous.

Table 5.1 White cells stained with various dyes that enable the different parts of the cell to be seen

Type	Shape	Life span	Function
Granulocytes (cytoplasm has granules)			
(a) Neutrophils	multi-lobed nucleus / granular cytoplasm	6 hours–few days	• Phagocytosis of bacteria (→ Fig. 5.6) • Take part in the inflammatory response, which is the first stage in the healing process (→ 14.3.3)
(b) Eosinophils	bi-lobed nucleus / granular cytoplasm	8–12 days	• Phagocytosis • Found in unusually high numbers at sites of ectoparasite infection and in allergy
(c) Basophils (called a **mast cell** when it settles in connective tissue)	large nucleus / granular cytoplasm	few hours–few days	• Granules contain the vasodilator histamine, which promotes blood flow to the tissues; also causes itchiness and inflammation
Agranulocytes (cytoplasm lacks granules)			
(d) Monocytes (called **macrophages** when they leave the blood-stream)	kidney-shaped nucleus / clear cytoplasm	hours to days	• Phagocytosis • Recognition of foreign or dangerous matter • Initiation of wound healing
(e) Lymphocytes (B and T cells; natural killer cells)	large nucleus / clear cytoplasm	weeks to years	• B cells produce antibodies • T cells coordinate the immune response • Natural killer cells attack some virus-infected and tumour cells

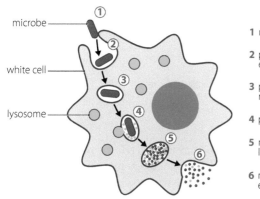

1 microbe adheres to phagocyte

2 phagocyte forms pseudopods that engulf the microbe

3 phagocytic vesicle containing microbe (phagosome)

4 phagosome fuses with a lysosome

5 microbe is killed and digested by lysosomal enzymes

6 residual material is expelled by exocytosis

Fig. 5.6 Stages of phagocytosis.

5.5 Platelets

Platelets (**thrombocytes**) are very small disc-like fragments of cytoplasm much smaller than red cells (→ Fig. 2.9) with a lifespan of up to 10 days. They circulate freely in the blood and play an important role in the formation of blood clots. (→ Box 5.9). When activated, platelets become sticky and aggregate (clump) to form platelet plugs. The same conditions will also trigger formation of fibrin, which forms a gel. This then creates the sticky, tangled mass that is known as a clot, which allows healing and repair to take place underneath.

Box 5.9 Aspirin inhibits platelet action and in low doses is used as medication to prevent the formation of blood clots and reduce the risk of heart attacks and strokes.

Box 5.10 Even while a clot is forming, the coagulation cascade triggers action by another enzyme – **plasmin**, which can destroy fibrin and prevent the clot from becoming too large. The balance between fibrin and plasmin is an important example of homeostasis.

Box 5.11 Prothrombin time (PT) is a blood test that measures how long it takes blood to coagulate (clot) and can be used to check for bleeding problems. Low PT time can be caused by:

- disease or injury of the liver, where clotting factors are made
- shortage of vitamin K, which is needed to make prothrombin and other clotting factors.

The international normalised ratio (INR) is another laboratory measurement of how long it takes blood to form a clot. Along with PT test, INR may be used to check the effect on patients of anticoagulant medicine such as warfarin (→ 18.9.1). While taking warfarin, the patient's blood will be regularly tested to make sure that the dose is correct.

Box 5.12 Bilirubin is the waste product formed from the breakdown of the haem component during the disintegration of old red cells.

As the body heals, bruises change in colour as a part of the healing process, so the age of a bruise can be estimated by healthcare professionals because bilirubin, which is a greenish-yellow colour, remains in the skin.

People with medium skin tones tend to have more red and yellowish colouration of bruises, while people with darker skin tones often display darker bruises. Most bruises disappear without treatment within about two weeks, fading to a light brown.

5.5.1 Haemostasis

Haemostasis (blood clotting) is the process that causes bleeding to stop when blood vessels are injured (→ Box 5.10). It involves a coordinated response between platelets and numerous blood clotting factors, plasma proteins and enzymes – which results in blood clot formation (→ Fig. 5.7).

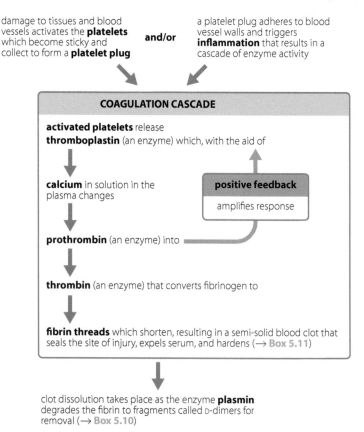

Fig. 5.7 Haemostasis is the body's response to blood vessel damage.

5.5.2 Clots in the skin

When skin is damaged, bleeding helps to carry bacteria away from the site of the wound, and the formation of a blood clot stops blood leaking from the body and prevents dirt from entering the wound. As the clot dries out it hardens and forms a scab over the wound. The scab falls off when the skin underneath has healed (→ 3.6.5).

Haematoma (bruise)

A haematoma is bleeding under the skin that occurs when the tiny capillaries are damaged and blood leaks into the soft tissue. At first it looks red or pink, then becomes a blue-black colour as it loses oxygen, although natural skin tone will affect the colour. As the blood is gradually broken down and removed, the bruise changes to a greenish colour due to bilirubin before disappearing (→ Box 5.12).

5.5.3 Clots inside blood vessels

Thrombosis

Thrombosis is the formation of a blood clot called a **thrombus** inside a blood vessel. It can happen when the lining of the blood vessel becomes roughened or inflamed (→ atherosclerosis 5.16.1) and when the blood flow becomes very slow or stops. The thrombus blocks circulation in the area partly or completely, a normal process in the body because, by sealing off the area, healing can take place. However, this normal clotting process can lead to complications when:

- the clot forms an **obstruction in an artery** and the tissue served by the artery gets little or no oxygen and dies. When this happens in an artery in the heart it causes **coronary thrombosis** (a heart attack), and in an artery to the brain it causes **cerebral thrombosis** (a stroke).
- the clot forms an **obstruction in a vein** so that the blood cannot get back to the heart, the tissues behind the blockage become swollen. When this happens in the legs it causes **deep vein thrombosis** (**DVT**) (→ Box 5.13).

Thrombosis is more likely in older people and becomes more common with age (→ Box 5.14). Other factors that make the development of thrombosis more likely include:

- family history (→ Box 5.15)
- diabetes
- obesity
- sedentary lifestyle
- raised blood cholesterol
- surgery and immobilisation.

Embolism

An embolus is a thrombus that breaks away from where it was formed and travels in the bloodstream until it becomes trapped in a small artery and is prevented from moving any further. It causes:

- **pulmonary embolism** in the lungs
- **heart attack** in the coronary arteries
- **stroke** in the brain
- **gangrene** in the legs.

5.6 Haemorrhage

Haemorrhage is loss of blood (→ Box 5.16). Each type of blood vessel – artery, vein and capillary – has its own bleeding characteristics.

- **Arterial bleeding** is characterised by spurts (pulses) of bright red blood that correspond with the heart beat. Bleeding from arteries can be difficult to control because the blood flows so quickly. Severe haemorrhage can cause hypovolaemic shock due to the loss of circulating blood (→ 16.5.1).
- **Venous bleeding** is usually a slow, steady flow and is dark red in colour.
- **Capillary bleeding** comes from small cuts and grazes. The blood oozes out, but soon stops because the surrounding blood vessels undergo **vasospasm** – sudden constriction – that cuts off most of the blood supply and allows a blood clot to form over the wound.

Box 5.13 Treatment for thrombosis uses an anticoagulant, e.g. warfarin, to prevent any clot from getting larger, and new clots from forming. The body's own healing mechanisms then get to work to break up the clot.

Box 5.14 Virchow's triad describes three elements, at least two of which are thought to be essential for thrombosis to occur:

- **blood stasis** – stoppage or slowdown in the flow of blood
- **endothelial injury** – trauma of the inner lining of blood vessels
- **hypercoagulability** – increased tendency towards blood clotting.

Box 5.15 Some people are born with an inherited tendency for blood to form clots too easily – a state called **hypercoagulation** – which means that thickened blood can be deposited in blood vessels.

Risk factors for clotting also include:

- prolonged bed rest after a fall or surgery
- sitting for a long time on a plane
- smoking
- cancer
- pregnancy.

Box 5.16 The body can cope with the loss of small volumes of blood because homeostatic mechanisms are able to compensate for the loss, as occurs when blood is donated to a blood bank. A relatively small proportion of blood – about 13% – of total blood volume is taken from the donor, who can easily replace all the cells and fluids lost in the donated blood.

Box 5.17 The cause of anterior nosebleeds can include a minor injury to the nose, picking the nose, blowing the nose very hard, excessive use of nasal decongestants, high altitude, or use of illegal drugs that are snorted such as cocaine.

Box 5.18 Nosebleeds require immediate medical attention when:
- the bleeding doesn't stop after 10 minutes of home treatment
- they happen after a severe head injury or a blow to the face
- the person is taking anticoagulants or has a bleeding disorder.

Box 5.19 Viral haemorrhagic fevers are rare and sometimes deadly diseases found across the world, e.g. Ebola, dengue, Lassa and Marburg fevers. All are complex multisystem disorders that affect the lining of blood vessels, causing bleeding which can lead to hypovolaemic shock (→ 16.5.1).

Box 5.20 The cranium is a rigid structure and bleeding within it, e.g. by a haemorrhagic stroke, increases **intracranial pressure (ICP)**. This can lead to cognitive changes including irritability, aggression, loss of consciousness or coma. The effect of rising ICP can be assessed by means of the Glasgow Coma Scale (GCS) (→ 17.1.10). As the ICP rises, the GCS score falls.

Box 5.21 During pregnancy, the maternal blood volume increases in line with the increasing foetal weight. There is also an increase in coagulation factors to enable the blood to clot quickly and minimise the loss of blood from the placental site during and after the delivery. The hyper-coagulation state can also contribute to the tendency of pregnant women and newly delivered mothers to form blood clots because of an increase in coagulation factors. When the rapid loss of a very large volume of blood occurs – **post-partum haemorrhage** – there is a real risk of mortality. PPH is a major cause of maternal mortality across the world.

5.6.1 Nosebleeds

Nosebleeds (**epistaxis**) are fairly common, particularly in children. Blood flows from one nostril or both, and a nosebleed can start just inside the nose (anterior area) or at the back of the posterior nose.

Anterior nosebleeds come from the wall – **septum** – that separates the two nasal passages in the front part of the nose that contain many delicate blood vessels which can be easily damaged (→ Box 5.17).

Posterior nosebleeds can be more serious and are more common in adults than children. The bleeding is heavier and comes from arteries that supply blood to the space inside the nose between the roof of the mouth and the brain (→ Box 5.18). The risk of posterior nosebleeds can be increased by:

- a broken nose
- nasal surgery
- hypertension (high blood pressure)
- exposure to irritant chemicals
- a tumour in the nasal cavity
- leukaemia
- medicines such as anticoagulants, which inhibit the blood clotting process, e.g. warfarin, heparin and aspirin.

5.6.2 Internal haemorrhage

The severity of an internal haemorrhage depends on the bleeding rate and its location: e.g. brain, lungs, abdomen and uterus. Bleeding that takes place within a body cavity may be substantial, as happens when the spleen is ruptured after an accident or fight. Severe internal bleeding is a medical emergency as it can result in circulatory shock (→ 16.5), cardiac arrest or death if proper treatment is not received quickly (→ Box 5.19).

Cerebral haemorrhage

Cerebral haemorrhage (**haemorrhagic stroke**) occurs when a blood vessel bursts within the brain. A major risk factor is high blood pressure, which makes the arteries in the brain more prone to rupture. This kind of stroke is also often caused by rupture of an aneurysm (→ 5.16.4). The long-term effects of a brain haemorrhage depend on the part of the brain where bleeding occurs. (→ Box 5.20)

Post-partum haemorrhage

Contraction of the uterus after delivery is intended to stop bleeding from the site of attachment of the placenta. However, women giving birth beyond twenty weeks of gestation are at risk of post-partum haemorrhage (PPH), which is the loss of more than 50 cm³ of blood, and which could lead to circulatory shock (→ 16.5). The most common cause of PPH is failure of the uterus to contract fully after delivery of the baby (→ Box 5.21).

5.6.3 Coagulation disorders

Coagulation disorders (inherited or acquired) disrupt the body's ability to control blood clotting. They are usually caused by deficiencies of one or more clotting factors.

- **Vitamin K deficiency** results in insufficient production of prothrombin. It can lead to bruising and serious bleeding problems if not supplemented.

- **Haemophilia** is an inherited condition that leads to the blood's inability to clot (→ 13.7.4). Bleeding from a wound continues for longer than normal because there are insufficient clotting factors in the blood to enable coagulation to take place.
- **Thrombocytopenia** refers to a reduced number of platelets, which increases the potential for haemorrhage associated with minor injuries.
- **Disseminated intravascular coagulopathy** (**DIC**) is a rare, life-threatening condition in which blood clots form throughout the body's small blood vessels. These reduce, or block, blood flow through the tissues and can damage the body's organs. At the same time they exhaust the supply of clotting factors, which leads to uncontrolled bleeding.

5.7 Blood groups

Blood group is inherited and does not change throughout life (→ Box 5.22). A person's blood group:
- belongs to one of the four groups in the ABO system, A, B, AB or O (→ Fig. 5.8)
- will be either Rh-positive or Rh-negative
- will contain other subgroups. There are at least 33 subgroups with more than 200 different subtypes, some of which are extremely rare.

Box 5.22 The genes that determine the A and B blood group antigens are located on chromosome 9. These genes, as well as haemoglobin variants and red cell enzymes, can vary amongst races and nations. Many studies have investigated relationships between blood groups and diseases including cancer, diabetes, rheumatoid arthritis and psoriasis, with the aim of trying to shed light on the disease processes.

erythrocytes	antigen A	antigen B	antigen A and antigen B	neither antigen A nor antigen B
plasma	**anti-B** antibodies	**anti-A** antibodies	**neither** anti-A nor anti-B antibodies	both **anti-A and anti-B** antibodies
blood types	**type A** erythrocytes with type A surface antigens and plasma with anti-B antibodies	**type B** erythrocytes with type B surface antigens and plasma with anti-A antibodies	**type AB** erythrocytes with both type A and type B surface antigens and plasma with neither anti-A nor anti-B antibodies	**type O** erythrocytes with neither type A nor type B surface antigens and plasma with both anti-A and anti-B antibodies

Fig. 5.8 Main blood cells and blood groups.

5.7.1 ABO system

The ABO system is used internationally and the four groups in the system depend on the presence or absence of:
- two **blood group antigens** called **A** and **B** which are found on the surface of erythrocytes (red cells) (→ Box 5.23)
- two **antibodies** called anti-A and anti-B found in plasma (→ Table 5.2).

People inherit blood group antigens from their parents. Those who inherit A antigens are blood group A; if they inherit B antigens, they are group B; if they inherit both antigens they are Group AB and if they inherit neither antigen they are group O. The distribution of these four different blood groups varies around the world according to ancestral origin and ethnicity.

Antigens and antibodies are discussed further in *Chapter 14: Immunity*.

Box 5.23 Antigens are proteins that cause the immune system to produce **antibodies** – immunoglobulins (→ 14.6.1). Because of the great variety of blood group antigens to be found in blood, it is possible to identify a person from a blood sample. In paternity cases, a blood sample can show whether a man is the father of a child.

5.7.2 The RhD system

Rhesus factor system is a different system of grouping blood from the ABO system. Whether someone is RhD positive or RhD negative is determined by the presence of the rhesus D (RhD) antigen – a molecule found on the surface of red blood cells. People who have the RhD antigen are RhD positive, and those without it are RhD negative. In the UK, around 85% of the population are RhD positive.

The mother's Rhesus group is important in pregnancy when the mother is RhD negative and the father is RhD positive. If the child is RhD negative like the mother there is no problem, but if the baby is RhD positive like its father, and maternal and foetal blood come into contact during pregnancy or delivery, the mother will become sensitised to the RhD positive antigen and the immune system will recognise it if it meets it again. Should the mother have another RhD positive baby, she would immediately produce antibodies against the RhD antigens, with the risk of causing **Rhesus disease** in the unborn baby (→ Fig. 5.9) (→ Box 5.24). Rhesus disease is uncommon because it can be prevented by injections of anti-D.

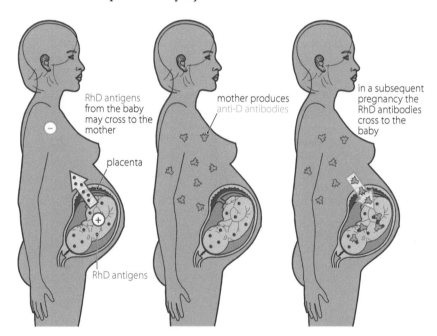

RhD antigens from the baby may cross to the mother

placenta

RhD antigens

mother produces anti-D antibodies

in a subsequent pregnancy the RhD antibodies cross to the baby

Fig. 5.9 Rhesus factor: mother and baby implications.

5.8 Blood transfusion

Blood transfusion is the transfer of blood or one of its components from a healthy person (the donor) into the bloodstream of a patient (the recipient).

- An **autologous blood transfusion** is the collection and re-infusion of the patient's own blood or blood components.
- An **allogenic blood transfusion** involves infusing the blood of a compatible donor into the recipient (→ Box 5.25).

Cross-matching before a transfusion takes place refers to the safety procedures that are carried out prior to a blood transfusion. These procedures ensure that the transfused blood is compatible with the recipient's own blood for ABO type, rhesus type and certain other factors

(→ Table 5.2). When the receipient's blood is incompatible with the donor's blood, **agglutination** (clumping) of red cells will occur rapidly. This reaction leads to haemolysis – disintegration of red blood cells and the release of haemoglobin, a condition that can lead quickly to death.

Table 5.2 The results of cross-matching donor and recipient blood

			Normal blood		Agglutinated blood	
Recipient's blood			**Donor's blood group**			
	Antigens on red cells	Plasma antibodies	Donor group **O**	Donor group **A**	Donor group **B**	Donor group **AB**
Group **O**	none	anti-A anti-B	(normal)	(agglutinated)	(agglutinated)	(agglutinated)
Group **A**	antigen A	anti-B	(normal)	(normal)	(agglutinated)	(agglutinated)
Group **B**	antigen B	anti-A	(normal)	(agglutinated)	(normal)	(agglutinated)
Group **AB**	antigen A antigen B	none	(normal)	(normal)	(normal)	(normal)

In an emergency

- Blood group O RhD negative can be given to everyone; people with this blood group are **universal donors**.
- People with blood group AB RhD positive are **universal recipients** because they can receive blood of any group.

5.8.1 Fractionated blood

Blood used for transfusion can be whole blood or it can be fractionated (separated) into its component parts and then stored and preserved for later use in a 'blood bank'. Transfusing a fractionated part of blood instead of whole blood:

- allows the treatment to be specific – patients receive only the blood component they need, which reduces the risks of side-effects
- means that the different components from a single unit of blood can be used to treat several people.

5.8.2 Blood bank

A 'blood bank' typically refers to the place where blood and blood components are prepared by techniques that preserve sterility. They are then stored in specially-designed fridges and freezers (→ Fig. 5.10).

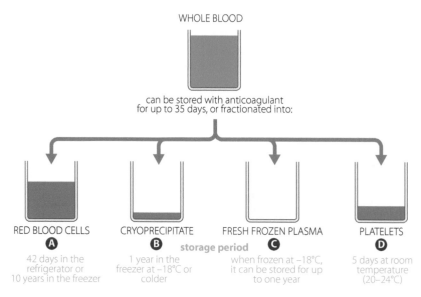

Fig. 5.10 Items stored in a blood bank.

Ⓐ RBCs are used to increase the number of circulating red blood cells after trauma or surgery, or to treat severe anaemia.

Ⓑ Cryoprecipitate is a frozen blood product prepared from plasma (→ Box 5.26).

Ⓒ Used to correct a deficiency in coagulation factors or to treat shock due to plasma loss, e.g. from massive bleeding or burns.

Ⓓ Used to treat or prevent platelet disorders, e.g. thrombocytopenia (low platelet count), which can result from leukaemia or from medical treatment, including chemotherapy.

Box 5.26 Cryoprecipitate is prepared from plasma and contains fibrinogen and clotting factors useful for bleeding abnormalities.

5.9 Blood disorders

5.9.1 Anaemia

Anaemia is a shortage of haemoglobin, the red pigment in blood that carries oxygen. Because the blood cannot then supply the tissues with enough oxygen (**hypoxia**), anaemia often causes tiredness, weakness and breathlessness (→ Box 5.27).

Iron-deficiency anaemia is the most common cause of anaemia. The absence of enough iron in the body to make the required amount of haemoglobin can result from:
- **insufficient intake of iron**:
  – a diet lacking enough meat, eggs and vegetables
  – feeding babies entirely on milk for more than a few months.
- **an increased need for iron** during:
  – rapid growth at puberty
  – pregnancy, due to the baby's need to make haemoglobin.
- **excess loss of blood** caused, for example, by:
  – heavy menstrual bleeding
  – piles and the prolonged loss of small quantities of blood
  – peptic ulcers due to bleeding into the stomach or bowel.
- **occult blood loss** refers to the hidden ('occult') slow and unnoticed drips of blood from a stomach ulcer or a cancer into the gut – a common cause of iron-deficiency anaemia.
- **surgery** (→ Box 5.28).

Vitamin B$_{12}$ deficiency causes:
- **pernicious anaemia.** A deficiency of vitamin B$_{12}$ in the body prevents the bone marrow from making enough red cells. This type of anaemia develops when the stomach fails to make a substance called **intrinsic factor** (→ 7.5.1) which enables vitamin B$_{12}$ to be absorbed from the small intestine.

Box 5.27 Pulse oximetry measures oxygen saturation (%) of blood (→ Fig. 17.2). It is possible for an individual to have 100% saturation while displaying signs of anaemia, because although all of the haemoglobin is saturated, there may simply be an inadequate amount of it.

Box 5.28 Management of iron-deficiency anaemia is based on dietary advice and supplementation.

Pre-operative management of iron-deficiency anaemia is important as it reduces risks associated with surgery.

- **megaloblastic anaemia.** A deficiency of vitamin B$_{12}$ or folate can cause the body to produce abnormally large red cells (**megaloblasts**) that cannot function properly (→ Box 5.29).

Anaemia caused by parasites includes:
- **malaria**, which is spread by mosquitoes infected with *Plasmodium* – a single-celled parasite. When an infected mosquito bites a human (the host), the parasites pass into the host's bloodstream and make their way to the liver. Here, they multiply many times before returning to the bloodstream and invading and destroying red cells, causing anaemia and other symptoms (→ Box 5.30)
- **hookworm and other intestinal parasites** that damage the gut wall and lead to a serious loss of blood.

Haemoglobinopathies – inherited genetic defects that produce abnormal types of haemoglobin, e.g.:
- **thalassaemia** is an inherited anaemia caused by the synthesis of abnormal haemoglobin. It is found mainly in countries bordering the eastern Mediterranean, the Middle East, India and Asia, or in people who have originated from these areas (→ Box 5.31)
- **hyperbilirubinaemia (neonatal non-haemolytic jaundice)** is the most common diagnosis in neonatal medicine and arises because of the yellowish pigmentation of the skin in many newborn infants, especially breastfed babies (→ Box 5.32)
- **sickle cell anaemia.** This inherited disease gets its name because the red cells of affected people change to a sickle shape when there is a shortage of oxygen and become trapped in capillaries, leading to hypoxia. They contain an abnormal type of haemoglobin – **haemoglobin S** – and do not last as long as that found in normal red cells (→ Fig. 5.11).

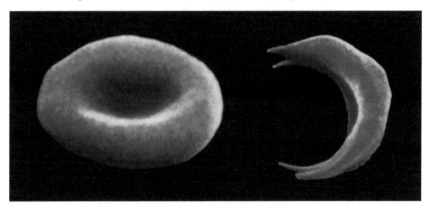

Fig. 5.11 Scanning electron micrograph (SEM) showing normal and sickle red blood cells.

5.9.2 Disorders of white cells

White cell disorders are chiefly due to altered levels of circulating white cells caused by infection or cancer, e.g.:
- **human immunodeficiency virus (HIV)** infects and kills white cells and reduces the body's immunity and its ability to fight infections. This can lead to **acquired immunodeficiency syndrome (AIDS)**, a condition in which progressive destruction of the immune system allows life-threatening infections and cancers to thrive
- **blood cancers.** These affect the function and production of white cells and immunity. The three main types of cancers of the immune system are leukaemia, lymphoma and myeloma (→ 15.10.5).

White cell disorders are also discussed in the chapter on immunity (→ 14.9.4).

Box 5.29 A megaloblast is an abnormally large, nucleated red blood cell found especially in people with pernicious anaemia or certain vitamin deficiencies.

Box 5.30 Malaria is found in more than 100 countries, mainly in tropical regions. The World Health Organization (WHO) states that in 2012 there were 207 million cases of malaria worldwide and 627 000 deaths.

Mosquitoes in the UK do not transmit malaria parasites but people returning to the UK from abroad are sometimes diagnosed with the disease, which can be fatal. Malaria can also be spread through blood transfusions and sharing needles, but these cases are rare.

Box 5.31 Most babies that inherit the thalassaemia gene do not show symptoms until about six months of age. This is because all babies begin life with **foetal haemoglobin** and it takes six months for it to be completely replaced by the inherited adult form.

Box 5.32 Neonatal **hyperbilirubinaemia** is universal and seen in about 80% of all babies. It occurs when there is extra bilirubin in the blood soon after birth because the liver of the newborn is immature. Normally, the levels of bilirubin begin to decline by the end of the first week of life.

In some babies, the bilirubin levels continue to rise to a level that leads to **kernicterus** – bilirubin-related injury to nerve tissue. **Kernicterus** remains a leading cause of preventable death and disability amongst newborns in sub-Saharan Africa and other poorly-resourced countries where treatment is hampered by lack of devices, erratic electrical supplies or financial constraints. The standard treatment is by **phototherapy** – the newborn's skin is exposed to lamps that generate blue light.

5.10 Heart

The heart and blood vessels form the **cardiovascular system** – the transport system of the body that carries nutrients to and from the cells and removes their waste products. The heart is situated in the thoracic cavity between and in front of the lungs with its lower surface adjacent to the diaphragm. It is centrally placed, but tilted so that most of the heart muscle is left of centre, which causes the heartbeat to be heard on the left side (→ Fig. 5.12) (→ Box 5.33).

The heart has four chambers: left and right atria, and left and right ventricles (→ Fig. 5.12). Cardiomyocytes (cardiac muscle cells) make up 30% of all heart cells but account for about 75% of the heart mass. The rest of the heart comprises endothelial (lining) cells, fibroblasts, smooth muscle and immune cells.

5.10.1 Pericardium

The **pericardium** is the sac of connective tissue that surrounds and encloses the heart and the roots of the attached blood vessels (→ Box 5.34). It consists of two parts: the outer part is the tough **fibrous pericardium** while the inner part is the **serous pericardium**, the double layer of serous membrane forming an enclosed sac with the pericardial cavity between them (→ Fig. 5.13). The cavity contains a small quantity of **pericardial fluid** that acts as a lubricant and allows the two layers to easily slide over one another with each heartbeat (→ Box 5.35).

Box 5.33 From the outside the human body appears to be mostly symmetrical but some organs, e.g. heart, stomach and spleen, all lie towards the left side of the body, and the liver towards the right side. **Situs inversus** is an inherited condition in which major organs are transposed (inverted to the opposite side of the body).

Box 5.34 Pericarditis is inflammation of the pericardium, the main symptom being a sharp, stabbing pain. There are several causes including viral infection.

Box 5.35 Cardiac tamponade is a build-up of fluid or blood in the pericardial cavity. This prevents the ventricles from expanding to their full filling capacity, and the body does not receive enough blood for its needs.

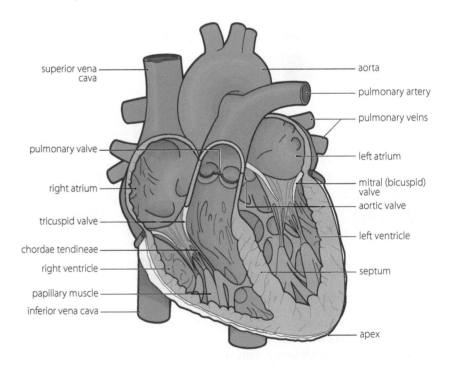

Fig. 5.12 Section through the heart showing the major structures.

5.10.2 Heart wall

The heart is a muscle about the size of the closed fist. Its wall is composed mainly of cardiac muscle – a specially adapted form of muscle with particular properties that enable the heart to act as a pump. Three distinct layers make up the heart wall (→ Fig. 5.13):

- **endocardium** – the lining of the interior surface of the heart chambers, consisting of a layer of endothelium and an underlying layer of connective tissue
- **myocardium** – composed of cardiac muscle tissue that forms the greater part of the heart wall, being thicker in the ventricles than the atria
- **epicardium** – a layer of connective tissue that forms the inner layer of the serous pericardium.

Energy requirements

The heart wall has a high demand for energy because it is beating continuously. Every day, the heart consumes about 15–20 times its own weight in adenosine triphosphate (ATP) – a high-energy molecule produced by the mitochondria in the cells (→ 2.3.1). Because the heart has a high demand for energy, mitochondria make up about 30% of the volume of cardiomyocytes (→ Box 5.36).

Box 5.36 Heart failure is one of the most prevalent, debilitating disorders in the western world and impaired generation of energy by heart muscle is a common feature of the disease. The muscle of an adult heart has only limited capacity to regenerate after injury so it has been suggested that implantation of stem cells (→ 2.4) to the failing heart could cause regeneration and improve cardiac function.

Taking it Further
You can find out more about energy and ATP production in the online biochemistry chapter (→ 20.13).

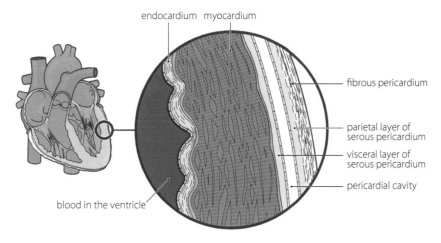

endocardium   myocardium

fibrous pericardium

parietal layer of serous pericardium

visceral layer of serous pericardium

pericardial cavity

blood in the ventricle

Fig. 5.13 Wall of the heart.

5.10.3 Blood flow through the heart

Although the right and left sides of the heart are joined together and beat at the same time, the blood flowing through them belongs to two different separate circulations (→ Box 5.37).

- The **pulmonary circulation** receives deoxygentaed blood from the upper and lower parts of the body and transmits it to the lungs and then back to the heart.
- The **systemic circulation** receives oxygenated blood from the lungs and transmits it to all parts of the body and then back to the heart (→ Fig. 5.14).

Box 5.37 The right side of the heart is completely separate from the left side, and blood flowing through one side does not mix with blood flowing through the other side.

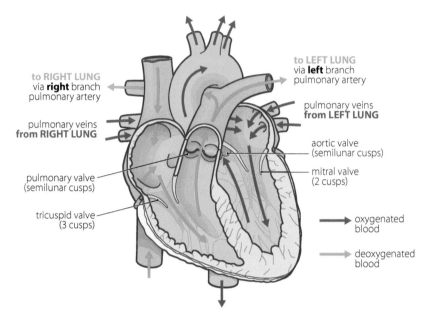

Fig. 5.14 Direction of blood flow through the heart.

5.10.4 **Heart valves**

The valves in the heart are composed of small **cusps** (flaps) of thin, tough, connective tissue which surround an opening (→ Box 5.38).

- The **atrioventricular (AV) valves** – **tricuspid** and **mitral** – separate the upper and lower chambers of the heart.
- The **semilunar valves** – **pulmonary** and **aortic** – are located where the arteries leave the heart.

The function of the valves is to ensure a one-way flow of blood through the heart, opening and closing with each heartbeat. The cusps are pressure-sensitive and open and close in response to pressure differences. When blood is flowing in the correct direction, the pressure forces back the cusps and allows the blood to pass through the opening. When the pressure drops, the blood has a tendency to flow in the opposite direction, and the backward flow catches the cusps and presses them tightly together to block the opening so that no blood leaks back into the chambers (→ Box 5.39).

Box 5.38 The **cardiac skeleton** is a framework of dense collagen fibres that forms four fibrous rings that surround the four valves, and anchors them in the heart. The position of the cardiac skeleton electrically isolates the atria from the ventricles.

Box 5.39 A valve that fails to close properly allows blood to leak backwards, thus reducing the forward flow of blood, e.g. leakage from the mitral valve is called **mitral regurgitation**. Defective valves may need to be repaired or replaced by surgery.

(a)
when the pressure in the atrium is greater than that in the ventricle, the tricuspid valve opens to allow blood to flow into the ventricle

(b)
when the pressure in the ventricle is greater than that in the aorta, blood is ejected through the semilunar valves into the arteries

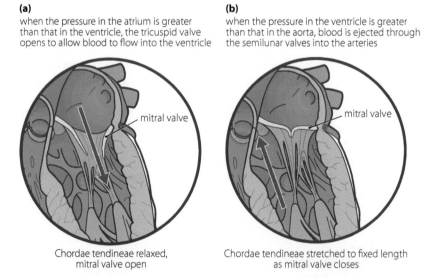

Chordae tendineae relaxed, mitral valve open

Chordae tendineae stretched to fixed length as mitral valve closes

Fig. 5.15 Action of the chordae tendineae as the mitral valve (**a**) opens; (**b**) closes.

Chordae tendineae

The chordae tendineae (heart strings) are thin, strong cords, mostly of collagen fibres, which anchor the tricuspid and mitral valves to the ventricle walls (→ Fig. 5.15). These cords prevent the valves from being turned inside out – like a blown umbrella – during heartbeat.

Heart sounds

As the heart valves shut they make rhythmical sounds described as

LUB---DUP pause LUB---DUP pause LUB---DUP pause

LUB is a soft sound made when the tricuspid and mitral valves close. DUP is a shorter, sharper sound made when the pulmonary and aortic valves close.

Heart murmurs are abnormal sounds made by the blood as it flows through the heart; they indicate that the blood flow is not smooth, as may be the case when a heart valve is damaged.

Taking it Further
Gathering information about the function of the heart is an important example of physiological measurement. To find out more, see online Chapter 17.

5.11 Heartbeat

Heartbeat is generated by the alternate contraction and relaxation of the muscular walls of the heart chambers – the atria and ventricles in turn (→ Box 5.40). **Heart rate** (HR) is the number of beats per minute. When resting, the heartbeat of an adult is about 70 times a minute, slower in an athlete and faster in a child. The rate can increase up to 200 beats a minute when exercise is being taken in order to supply the muscles with extra oxygen and nutrients; the increase will be less in the fit than the unfit.

Box 5.40 With every heartbeat, the atria contract first and help to fill the ventricles with blood. The ventricles then contract and eject blood into the arteries. Thus the familiar, characteristic rhythm of the heart is produced.

5.11.1 Control of electrical activity of the heart

The heartbeat is controlled by a series of impulses produced by a group of pacemaker cells (specialised cardiomyocytes) called the **sinoatrial (SA) node** or **pacemaker**, which is one of the main elements in the cardiac conducting system. Pacemaker cells are excitable cells because they are able to spontaneously generate an electrical impulse known as depolarisation. Impulses follow a clearly defined pathway along conducting fibres and travel to every part of the heart muscle wall, causing it to contract (→ Fig. 5.16).

❶ The **sinoatrial node (SA node)**, located in the upper wall of the right atrium, contains pacemaker cells that generate impulses roughly 70 times a minute in an adult and which spread through the atria (→ Boxes 5.41 and 5.42).

❷ The **atrioventricular node (AV node)** is a bundle of specialised fibres situated in the septum that separates the atria. It receives impulses from the SA node and transmits them onwards via the atrioventricular bundle. The AV node acts like a gate that slows the electrical signals before they enter the ventricles. This delay gives the atria time to contract before the ventricles do.

❸ The **atrioventricular bundle (AV bundle; bundle of His)** is a bundle of conducting fibres that carries the impulses rapidly from the AV node to the septum separating the ventricles.

❹ The AV bundle then divides into **right and left bundles**, one for each ventricle.

❺ These bundles conduct the impulse to the **apex** of the heart.

❻ **Purkinje fibres** transmit impulses from the apex of the heart to every part of the ventricles, which contract in less than one-tenth of a second later.

Box 5.41 Although the SA node normally sets the rate of heartbeat, the rate can be altered by various factors. For example, it is increased by means of activity in the sympathetic nervous system, e.g. exercise and excitement, and by some diseases and medications (→ 18.8.3).

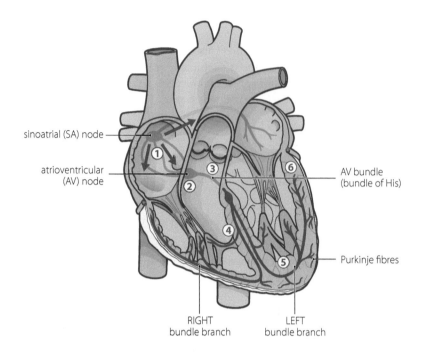

Fig. 5.16 Cardiac conducting system of the heart.

Electrocardiogram

An electrocardiogram (ECG) records the heart's rhythm and electrical activity. Electrodes (sensors) placed on the skin detect and amplify the electrical impulses produced by the heart each time it beats (→ Fig. 5.17). The ECG is recorded on a screen or a paper tracing and shows the characteristic P wave, QRS complex and T wave and can reveal any **arrhythmias** – heartbeats with an irregular or abnormal rhythm (→ Box 5.42).

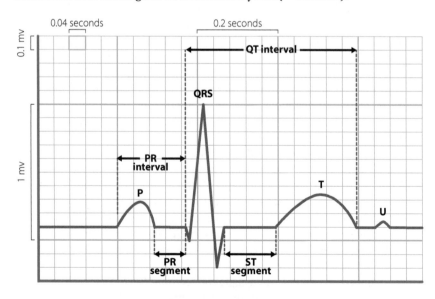

Fig. 5.17 Electrocardiogram (ECG). P wave – depolarisation of atria (→ Fig. 9.11); QRS complex = depolarisation of ventricles; T wave = repolarisation of ventricles.

Box 5.42 Artificial pacemakers are electrical devices that are used to treat and regulate some abnormal heart rhythms (arrhythmias) – such as heart block – that can cause the heart muscle to beat too slowly, miss beats or stop the chambers from beating in time. By doing this, the device can replace or regulate the function of the electrical conduction system of the heart.

An internal pacemaker is one in which the electrodes to the heart, the circuitry and the power supply are all implanted within the body (→ Box 5.63). Sometimes a different kind of device that resembles a pacemaker – called an implantable cardioverter-defibrillator (ICD) – is implanted. These devices are often used in the management of patients at risk from sudden cardiac death.

Taking it Further
Treatment with a **defibrillator** stops the heart by applying electricity across the chest. The SA node may then re-establish the rhythm.

Fewer than 1 in 10 people in the UK survive an out-of-hospital cardiac arrest, so Public Access Defibrillators (PAD) and training in CPR (→ 17.8.3) are sometimes purchased through fundraising activities and business sponsorship. This is especially the case in rural areas of the UK, where ambulance response times may be longer than in urban areas.

5.12 Cardiac cycle

The **cardiac cycle** refers to the sequence of events between one heartbeat and the next. The cycle starts with the generation of cardiac impulses by the sinoatrial node, and has two main phases – diastole and systole (→ Fig. 5.18) (→ Box 5.43).

Diastole is the phase when the ventricles fill up with blood: the atrioventricular valves are open, the semilunar valves are closed, the whole heart is relaxed and blood flows into the heart (→ Box 5.44).

Systole is the phase when the ventricles contract and eject blood at high pressure into the arteries.

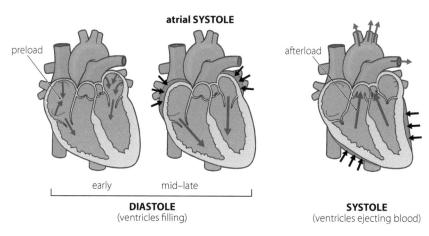

Fig. 5.18 The cardiac cycle.

5.12.1 Cardiac output

Cardiac output (CO) is the volume of blood ejected by the ventricles and is usually expressed in litres per minute. It is always closely matched to the body's demand for blood through the homeostatic control of the following four factors:

- **heart rate** – beats per minute (bpm); a faster heart rate gives more beats per minute, hence increased cardiac output
- **preload** – a bigger (returning) volume of blood creates more stretch and hence more force to eject a greater (stroke) volume from the heart
- **afterload** – determined by the pressure and resistance within the arteries and systemic circulation, hence it reflects the force the heart has to push against
- **contractility** – the mechanical properties of contracting cardiac muscle means that an increase in contractility leads to an increase in cardiac output.

Stroke volume

Stroke volume (SV) is the volume of blood pumped from each ventricle of the heart with each heartbeat. The stroke volume for each ventricle is generally equal, both being approximately 70 ml in a healthy 70 kg man. It is calculated using measurements of ventricular volumes from an echocardiogram (→ 17.3.1) by subtracting the volume of the blood in the ventricle at the end of a beat (end-systolic volume) from the volume of blood just prior to the next beat (called the **end-diastolic volume**).

The cardiac output varies whenever the heart rate or the stroke volume are altered (→ Box 5.45).

Box 5.43 In babies, the cardiac cycle is much shorter than adults, resulting in a much faster heart rate. The heart rate of newborn babies is about 120–160 beats per minute.

Box 5.44 Blood flows because of pressure differences; it therefore flows into a relaxed heart because the pressure inside is low.

Box 5.45 Calculating cardiac output (CO) using the formula:

$$CO = HR \times SV$$

(HR = heart rate; SV = stroke volume)

Examples

a) A person at rest has a normal HR of 72 bpm and SV of 70 cm³/min

$$CO = 72 \times 70 \text{ cm}^3/\text{min}$$
$$= 5040 \text{ cm}^3/\text{min} -$$
about 5 litres/min

b) The person starts to exercise intensely and the HR increases to 120 bpm and SV to 80 cm³/min:

$$CO = 120 \times 80 \text{ cm}^3/\text{min}$$
$$= 9600 \text{ cm}^3/\text{min}$$

The CO has nearly doubled to 9.6 L/min.

c) The person bleeds profusely and HR increases to 140 bpm but the SV is decreased to 40 cm³/min:

$$CO = 140 \times 40 \text{ cm}^3/\text{min}$$
$$= 5600 \text{ cm}^3/\text{min}$$

The normal CO is being maintained (5.6 L/min) but requires additional work by the heart.

Box 5.46 The pulmonary artery is the only artery which carries deoxygenated blood and the pulmonary vein is the only vein which carries oxygenated blood (from lungs to left side of the heart).

Box 5.47 Healthy arteries have elastic walls that expand and recoil as blood pulses through. Loss of elasticity is a normal part of the ageing process, and arteriosclerosis stiffens the artery walls and increases resistance to flow (→ 5.16.1).

5.13 Blood vessels

Blood vessels are tubes through which blood flows as it circulates around the body (→ Fig. 5.19). The **arteries** carry blood away from the heart, the **veins** return blood back to the heart, and **capillaries** link arteries to veins. The three types of blood vessel have different structures (→ Fig. 5.20).

5.13.1 Arteries

Arteries (except the pulmonary artery) carry oxygenated blood away from the heart. As blood pulsates rapidly and at high pressure through the arteries, the elastic tissue in the wall allows the arteries to expand and recoil with each pulse, which normally corresponds to the heartbeat. Bleeding from an artery produces bright red, oxygenated blood which spurts out in time with the pulse (→ Box 5.47). **Arterioles** are tiny arteries which have relatively muscular walls. The smooth muscle tissue in the wall of smaller arteries and arterioles enables them to dilate and constrict and thus control the blood supply to particular organs or tissue.

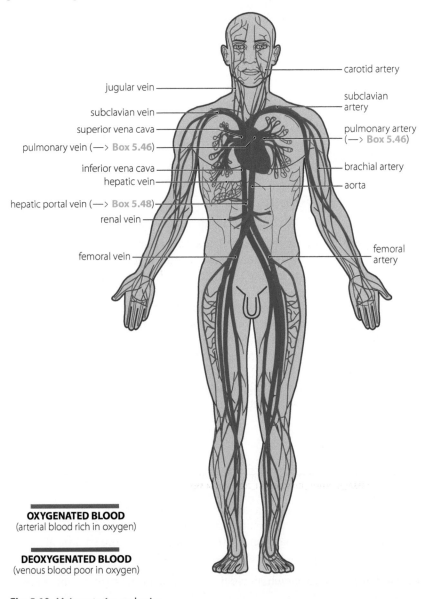

carotid artery

jugular vein

subclavian artery

subclavian vein

superior vena cava

pulmonary artery (—> Box 5.46)

pulmonary vein (—> Box 5.46)

inferior vena cava

brachial artery

hepatic vein

aorta

hepatic portal vein (—> Box 5.48)

renal vein

femoral vein

femoral artery

OXYGENATED BLOOD
(arterial blood rich in oxygen)

DEOXYGENATED BLOOD
(venous blood poor in oxygen)

Fig. 5.19 Major arteries and veins.

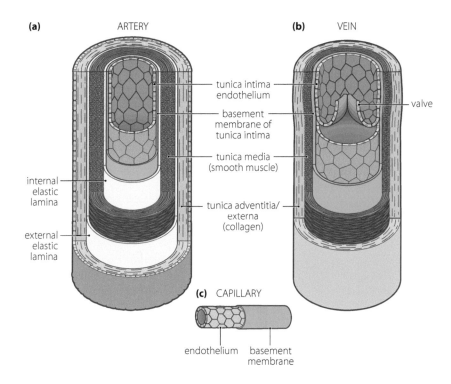

Fig. 5.20 Structure of (**a**) an artery, (**b**) a vein and (**c**) a capillary.

Vasoconstriction is the narrowing of arterioles due to contraction of the muscle tissue they contain. For example, on a cold day, low temperature leads to contraction of the arterioles in the skin; blood is then diverted inwards to conserve body heat.

Vasodilation is the widening of arterioles that results from relaxation of the muscle tissue in their walls. For example, when people are exercising, the dilation of arterioles in muscle tissue ensures that they receive an adequate supply of oxygen and nutrients for the activity, and that carbon dioxide and other wastes are eliminated.

5.13.2 Veins

Veins (except the pulmonary vein) carry oxygen-poor blood towards the heart. Like arteries, veins also have a three-layer wall but the walls are thinner, the lumen is larger, and venous blood is a darker red as much of the oxygen has been removed in the tissues. Because the blood in veins is under low pressure, when they are cut the blood oozes out, but never spurts. The blood moves slowly through veins and many also have valves to prevent the blood from flowing backwards. **Venules** are tiny veins that drain blood from capillaries into larger veins, with many venules uniting to form a vein.

Box 5.48 Blood carried in the hepatic portal vein goes directly from the intestines to the liver, unlike other veins, which carry blood back to the heart.

5.13.3 Capillaries

Capillaries are the network of tiny blood vessels that penetrate throughout all the living tissues and form an interconnecting network between the arterioles and the venules called **capillary beds**. The capillary wall consists of a single layer of endothelium and most of the cells are not far from circulating blood (→ Fig. 5.21). The volume of blood flowing through a capillary bed at any one time depends on smooth muscle activity of the arteriole walls and the **pre-capillary sphincters**, a sphincter being a ring of muscle fibres. When the arterioles and pre-capillary sphincters constrict, blood flow through the capillaries is reduced or stops; when they dilate, blood flow is resumed.

Not all capillaries are open at the same time. The networks open when the tissue is active, but when the tissue is resting many are closed, e.g. the capillary supply to the stomach wall is open when gastric juice is being produced, but most of the network is closed when the stomach is empty.

When the inflammatory response is triggered (→ 14.3.3), blood flow to the tissue is increased by vasodilation and the opening of the capillary beds in the area.

Interstitial fluid

In capillaries, the pressure from the circulating blood filters some of the fluid from plasma though pores in the semi-permeable capillary walls. This fluid is now called **interstitial fluid** (extracellular fluid; tissue fluid) and it surrounds the cells and fills the spaces (interstices) between them (→ Box 5.49). Interstitial fluid is similar to plasma in being a solution of oxygen, sugars, fatty acids, amino acids, salts, vitamins and hormones required by the cells, and it collects carbon dioxide and other waste products from the cells for removal from the tissues. Unlike plasma, interstitial fluid does not normally contain proteins. At the venous end of the capillary, fluid tends to flow back into the blood because the colloid osmotic pressure at this end of the capillary exerts a relatively greater effect. The rest of the fluid drains into the **lymphatic capillaries** and returns to the bloodstream via the thoracic duct and subclavian veins (→ Fig. 5.28).

Box 5.49 Net filtration pressure (NFP) is the sum of all the various forces across the wall of a capillary and is important because it determines the rate at which filtration occurs and hence it drives the rate at which interstitial fluid is formed.

Interstitial fluid is being formed continuously from blood plasma and, in adults, amounts to approximately 25 L/day. If it is not returned to the blood or lymphatic circulation (→ 5.17), it accumulates in the interstitial spaces between cells, causing oedema (→ 5.17.4).

Taking it Further
You can find out more about osmosis in the online biochemistry chapter (→ 20.7).

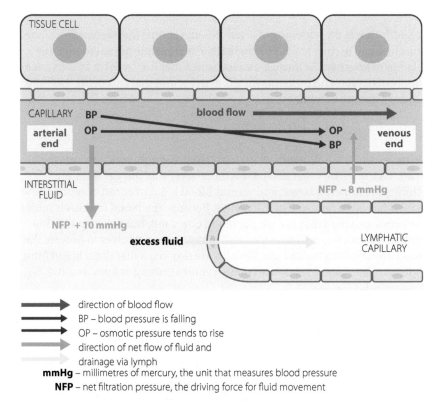

Fig. 5.21 Formation of interstitial fluid in the tissues.

5.14 How blood circulates

The heart is not one pump but two, with the right and left sides of the heart each pumping blood into a different circulation known as the double circulatory system (→ Fig. 5.22). This refers to the two separate circuits through which blood travels, and it must travel through one circuit in order to enter the other circuit, taking about half a minute to complete both circuits.

- The **pulmonary circuit** carries deoxygenated blood from the right side of the heart to the lungs to collect oxygen and release carbon dioxide before returning to the left side of the heart.
- The **systemic circuit** carries oxygenated blood from the left side of the heart to all parts of the body (except the lungs), and delivers deoxygenated blood back to the right side of the heart to be pumped onwards to the lungs.

Taking it Further
Every heartbeat generates a pressure wave (the pulse) that travels through the arteries.

More information about routine physiological observations of cardiovascular function is to be found in online Chapter 17.

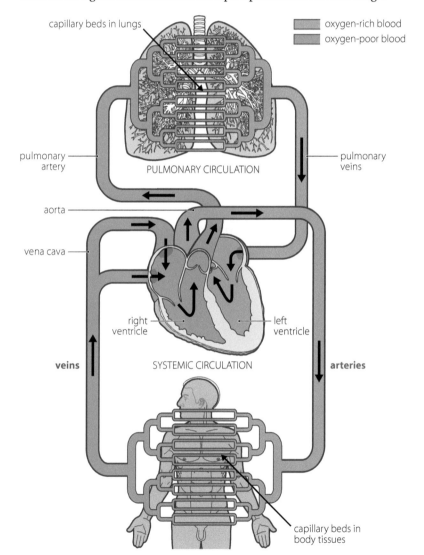

Fig. 5.22 Systemic and pulmonary circulations (not to scale).

5.14.1 Maintaining the circulation

The flow of blood from one area to another is dependent on pressure gradients (→ Box 5.50). **Vascular resistance** refers to the resistance that must be overcome to push blood through the circulatory system and create flow.

Box 5.50 Like any fluid, the flow of blood depends on pressure differences, and blood always flows around the vascular system from an area where the pressure is higher to an area where pressure is lower.

Arterial circulation is the movement of blood through the arteries. It is felt as the pulse and is dependent on the pumping action of the heart. Blood is ejected:

- under **high pressure from the left ventricle** in order to overcome the high vascular resistance (→ Box 5.51) of the systemic circulation
- at **lower pressure from the right ventricle** because there is much less resistance on its journey to the lungs which are close and highly vascular.

Venous circulation is movement of blood back to the heart. At any one time, about 60% of the body's blood volume is contained within systemic veins where the pressure is very low because of the large diameter of the vessels (→ Box 5.51). Venous circulation is assisted by the:

- **respiratory pump** – breathing in expands the thoracic cavity, which in turn lowers the pressure within the cavity and allows for more blood to flow into the heart via the vena cava
- **skeletal-muscle pump** – the compression of veins when skeletal muscles contract forces blood towards the heart against the force of gravity (→ Fig. 5.23). It is especially important in increasing venous return to the heart when the body is upright (→ Box 5.51).

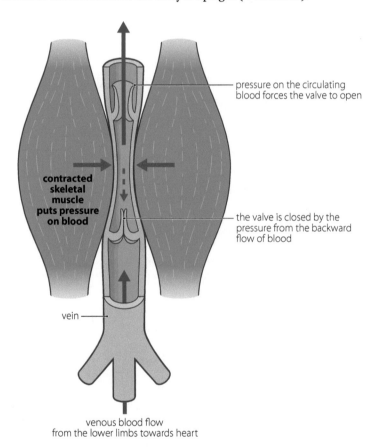

pressure on the circulating blood forces the valve to open

contracted skeletal muscle puts pressure on blood

the valve is closed by the pressure from the backward flow of blood

vein

venous blood flow from the lower limbs towards heart

Fig. 5.23 Skeletal muscle pump.

5.14.2 Special circulations

Hepatic portal system

A **portal circulation** is a special network of blood vessels that connects two organs without blood returning to the heart. In the **hepatic portal system** blood from the intestines travels to the liver via the hepatic portal vein before it returns to the heart (→ Fig. 5.19). This means that, after a meal is absorbed, nutrient-rich blood can be processed in the liver before it reaches the systemic circulation via the hepatic vein.

Hypophysial portal system

This is a system of blood vessels in the brain that connects the hypothalamus with the anterior pituitary via the **pituitary stalk** (→ 11.3). It provides fast communication for the transport and exchange of hormones between these glands, much faster than if the hormones had to travel through the double circulation.

Cerebral circulation

The **circle of Willis** is a system of arteries that encircles the base of the brain and enables circulation between the blood supply of the forebrain and hindbrain (→ Box 9.9). It allows blood to reach all parts of the brain if the supply to either part is interrupted by disease or clot formation.

Placental circulation

The placental circulation operates during pregnancy when the foetal circulation becomes very close to the maternal circulation. The **placenta** is a unique organ which develops during pregnancy. It provides a very large surface area for exchange of substances between the foetus and the mother while ensuring that foetal and maternal blood never actually intermingle.

Maternal blood increases in volume during pregnancy and flows from the uterus into the placenta via the umbilical arteries to deliver oxygen and nutrients to the foetus, before flowing back to the systemic circulation via the endometrial and uterine veins (→ Fig. 12.16).

5.14.3 Pulse

The **pulse** is the rhythmic expansion and contraction of the arteries as a pressure wave pulses through with each heartbeat. It can be felt in places where main arteries come close to the skin and lie over a bone (→ Fig. 5.24a). The cardiac output, and hence the pulse rate, alters according to the body's needs, speeding up during exercise and slowing down during rest. In an adult, the average pulse rate is 60–75 beats per minute when resting. Exercise causes the pulse rate to increase and, during strenuous exercise, the adult rate can increase up to a maximum 200 beats per minute. The pulse rate is also increased by, for example, excitement, fear, fever and circulatory shock (→ 17.4) (→ Boxes 5.52 and 5.53).

Taking the pulse

Taking the pulse provides information about the rate and rhythm of the heartbeat, and the size of the pulse – full, weak or thready.

A **'full' (strong)** pulse is associated with:
- an optimal cardiac output that meets the body's demands
- dilated arteries that commonly occur as a result of heat, exercise, emotion, alcohol or pregnancy.

Box 5.52 Tachycardia is a rapid heart rate (pulse) when a person is resting, usually defined in an adult as greater than 100 beats per minute. It may be due to fever or illness; it may be irregular and accompanied by **palpitations** (awareness of the heartbeat). When due to exercise or excitement, it is not necessarily a cause for concern.

Box 5.53 Bradycardia – a slow heart rate – is normally found in highly trained athletes who develop bigger hearts that deliver larger volumes of blood in each beat. A slow heart rate (pulse) can also be the result of changes in the heart because of ageing, but might also be caused by problems within the electrical conducting system of the heart.

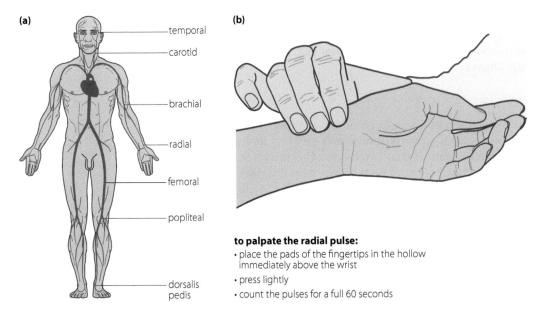

Fig. 5.24 (**a**) Pulse points; (**b**) radial pulse. Note that when the radial pulse cannot be felt, the carotid pulse is used.

A **'thready' pulse** is scarcely perceptible, often very rapid and difficult to feel on palpation. It is caused by low cardiac output that is inadequate for the body's demands and is associated with:

- a heart problem
- circulatory shock due to acute blood loss
- constricted arteries as a result of cold weather or great anxiety.

5.15 Blood pressure

Blood pressure is usually measured as the pressure in a main artery – normally the brachial artery of the upper arm. The pressure rises and falls in time with the heartbeat, being highest just after the ventricular muscle contracts – **systolic pressure** – and lowest at the end of the resting phase – **diastolic pressure** (→ Box 5.54). Blood pressure is measured in millimetres of mercury (mmHg) or kilopascals (kPa). Two numbers are recorded: the top number is the systolic pressure and the bottom number is the diastolic pressure. This is usually recorded as, for example, 120/80 mmHg. Blood pressure can be affected by many factors, and can also alter from minute to minute according to activity and emotional state. For example, strenuous activity, anger or nervousness raise the blood pressure, while rest and contentment lower it (→ Fig. 5.25).

Box 5.54 The formula for calculating the mean arterial blood pressure (MAP) is:

MAP = diastolic BP +
1/3 (systolic BP – diastolic BP).

The reason it is not the average of the two readings is that more time is spent in diastole than in systole during each cardiac cycle.

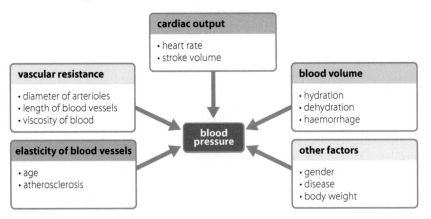

Fig. 5.25 Factors affecting blood pressure.

5.15.1 Hypertension

Hypertension (HTN), often referred to as high blood pressure, is a condition in which the arterial blood pressure is consistently above the normal range for a particular age group. It is a major risk factor for heart attacks, strokes, chronic kidney disease and eye problems, but can be kept under control by medication. HTN has a tendency to run in families and can also result from medical conditions affecting the kidneys, heart, arteries or endocrine glands, but in most people the cause is unknown (→ Box 5.55).

5.15.2 Hypotension

Hypotension (HoTN) is abnormally low blood pressure and it occurs when the arterial blood pressure is insufficient to pump the blood to the head when standing or sitting. A **faint** is sudden unconsciousness caused by low blood pressure in the arteries of the brain. As soon as the head becomes level with the heart – as happens when a person falls down – blood pressure is restored and the person recovers (→ Box 5.56).

5.15.3 Homeostasis of blood pressure

Blood pressure is monitored by the **baroreceptors** – groups of nerve endings that detect stretching in blood vessel walls. The most important arterial baroreceptors are located in the carotid sinuses (at the bifurcation of external and internal carotid arteries) and in the aortic arch. They can identify both the rate of change in pressure on the walls with each arterial pulse, and also changes in the mean arterial blood pressure.

Baroreflex

The baroreflex is an essential part of the body's homeostatic mechanisms that helps to maintain blood pressure at nearly constant levels – the set point. It is initiated by **baroreceptors** (stretch receptors) that detect changes in pressure on blood vessel walls. The cardiac control centre in the brain responds very quickly to maintain a stable blood pressure, and baroreceptors are most effective for remedying short-term changes (→ Fig. 5.26). Their response diminishes with time and when blood pressure is maintained at an elevated level for a long time, the baroreceptors tend to be reset to operate at the higher level, which results in hypertension.

Long-term regulation of blood pressure

Renin–angiotensin–aldosterone system (RAAS) is a hormone system that regulates blood pressure and fluid balance in the longer term. It acts by influencing the diameter of blood vessels and controlling the volume of blood circulating at any one time and by influencing the function of the kidneys (→ Fig. 8.13).

5.16 Cardiovascular disease

Cardiovascular disease (**CVD**); is a group of diseases that involve the heart and blood vessels.

5.16.1 Atherosclerosis

Atherosclerosis is a build-up of fatty plaque on the inner walls of arteries (→ Fig. 5.27). As plaque builds up over time, the arteries become less elastic

Box 5.55 Before hypertension is diagnosed, blood pressure is usually measured on at least three different occasions at the same time each day. The reason for this is that some people become very anxious and need to get used to the procedure of having their blood pressure taken.

Box 5.56 Orthostatic hypotension (postural hypotension) is a form of low blood pressure that is experienced on standing up, causing dizziness and lightheadedness, which lasts for a few minutes. It is due to gravitational stress that results in venous pooling, falling cardiac output and decreased blood pressure. Normal blood pressure is rapidly restored by the baroreceptor reflex.

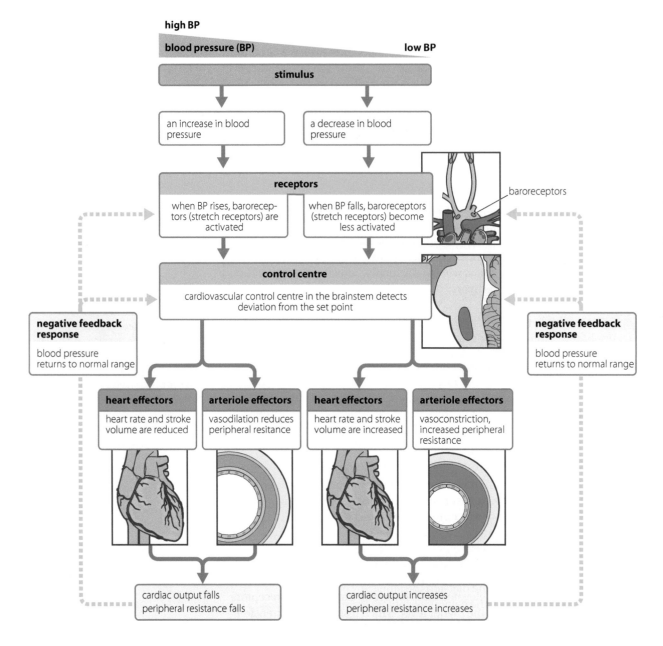

Fig. 5.26 Baroreceptor response (baroreflex) for short-term regulation of blood pressure.

Box 5.57 Coronary angioplasty is a surgical procedure that widens blocked or narrowed coronary arteries. Angioplasty means using a balloon to stretch open a narrowed or blocked artery. Most modern angioplasty procedures also involve inserting a short wire-mesh tube, called a **stent**, into the artery during the procedure. The stent is left in place permanently to allow blood to flow more freely to regions beyond it.

and narrower, with a reduced blood flow to the tissues they supply. If some of the plaque ruptures, a rough surface is left behind on which a blood clot may form and partly or completely block the blood flow through the artery (→ Fig. 5.27). Risk factors for plaques include familial hypercholesterolaemia smoking, high saturated fat intake and sedentary lifestyle. Atherosclerosis in the coronary arteries (the main blood vessels supplying the heart) may sometimes be relieved by angioplasty (→ Box 5.57).

5.16.2 Coronary heart disease

Coronary heart disease (**CHD; ischaemic heart disease**) occurs when the heart's blood supply is blocked or interrupted by a build-up of plaque in the coronary arteries, leading to angina and myocardial infarction (heart attack)

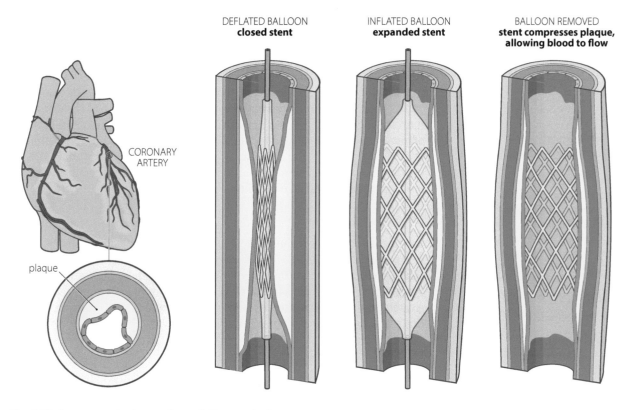

DEFLATED BALLOON
closed stent

INFLATED BALLOON
expanded stent

BALLOON REMOVED
stent compresses plaque, allowing blood to flow

CORONARY ARTERY

plaque

Fig. 5.27 Coronary angioplasty and stent balloon angioplasty.

(→ Box 5.58). Both conditions produce the same kind of pain in the centre of the chest, often spreading to the neck and arms. The difference between angina and a heart attack is that angina is recurring and responds to rest and treatment. Treatment can include coronary angioplasty and the insertion of a stent.

Angina

Angina results when the coronary arteries have become partly blocked ('furred up') and are unable to supply enough oxygenated blood to the heart muscle. Chest pain is experienced as intense dull pressure or squeezing when increased demands are made on the heart by exercise or cold weather; it then disappears with relaxation and warmth (→ Boxes 5.59 and 5.60).

Myocardial infarction

Myocardial infarction (**heart attack**) is the death of a segment of the heart muscle when its blood supply is restricted. This is usually caused by a blood clot in one of the coronary arteries, which reduces or cuts off the blood supply to a part of the heart muscle. A combination of symptoms indicate myocardial infarction – chest pain that can radiate to the jaw, neck, arms and back, shortness of breath, feeling weak, sweaty or lightheaded, and an overwhelming feeling of fear. Tests to confirm the diagnosis can include coronary angiography – a type of X-ray used to examine blood vessels (→ Fig. 17.12).

Box 5.58 CHD is the leading cause of death both in the UK and worldwide. In the UK, an estimated 2.3 million people are living with CHD, mainly angina. In premenopausal women, the incidence of CHD is lower because oestrogen is 'cardio-protective'.

Box 5.59 The main treatment to relieve angina is glyceryl trinitrate (GTN) spray. When sprayed under the tongue it relaxes and dilates blood vessels in the heart and the rest of the body, which lowers the workload of the heart. People with angina may be given anticoagulants to prevent clotting, e.g. aspirin.

Box 5.60 Not everyone with angina experiences severe chest pain; it can be mistaken for indigestion. It is the combination of symptoms that is important in determining whether a person is having a heart attack, and not the severity of chest pain.

5.16.3 Other cardiovascular disorders

Heart failure

Heart failure means that the heart cannot pump as effectively as it should (not that it has failed to work altogether). The condition can develop quickly (acute heart failure) or gradually (chronic heart failure) and can be due to a number of causes, some of which can be corrected (→ Box 5.61). The severity of heart failure can be estimated through the **ejection fraction** – the volume of blood ejected from the heart with each beat. This is normally about 70% of the blood contained within the ventricles but in cases of heart failure, the ejection fraction can fall to less than 40%.

Cardiac arrest

Cardiac arrest occurs when the heart ceases to pump effectively. It commonly happens when the heartbeats are uncoordinated (**ventricular fibrillation**) or when the heart stops beating completely. The result is abrupt loss of consciousness, absence of pulse, and cessation of breathing. Unless treated promptly by **cardiopulmonary resuscitation (CPR)**, irreversible brain damage and death can follow (→ 17.8.3).

Heart valve disease

A diseased or damaged valve can affect the flow of blood and hence cardiac output in two ways:
- **valve stenosis** caused by a valve that does not open fully or has become stiff and obstructs the flow of blood
- **valve incompetence** (**leaky valve**) e.g. **mitral valve prolapse**, caused by a valve that does not close properly and allows blood to leak backwards (regurgitation).

In both these conditions, the workload of the heart has increased and the blood behind the affected valve will be under extra pressure, called 'back pressure'. This can result in a build-up of fluid (oedema) either in the lungs, ankles or legs, depending on which valve is affected (→ Box 5.62).

Arrhythmia

An arrhythmia occurs when the heart loses its ability to synchronise contractions and pump blood effectively. The condition can arise spontaneously or as a result of homeostatic disturbances, e.g. hyperkalaemia (raised plasma potassium levels). Common examples of arrhythmia are:
- **atrial fibrillation (AF)** – the most common type, when the atria beat irregularly and faster than normal
- **supraventricular tachycardia** – episodes of abnormally fast heart rate when resting
- **heart block** – the heart beats more slowly than normal (**bradycardia**) which can cause collapse
- **ventricular fibrillation** – uncoordinated heartbeats, leading rapidly to disruption of blood flow, loss of consciousness and sudden death if not treated immediately (→ Box 5.63).

Congenital heart disease

Congenital heart disease is a general term for a range of birth defects that affect the normal workings of the heart. It affects up to 9 in every 1000 babies born in the UK and, in many cases, can be diagnosed during an ultrasound scan before a baby is born. Congenital heart defects may not cause problems for the

Box 5.61 Acute heart failure – sudden decrease in heart function – could be due to sudden blockage of coronary arteries but might be caused by drug toxicity, anaesthetic or infections. **Chronic heart failure** develops over time and puts a strain on other systems in the body, which then increases the strain on the heart.

Box 5.62 Many people with heart valve disease need little or no treatment. When surgery is recommended it could be for:
- **valve repair** – often used for mitral valves which leak but are not seriously damaged
- **valve replacement** – the diseased valve is removed and replaced with a new one.

Box 5.63 An **artificial pacemaker** is a small battery-powered device implanted under the collar bone with one or more leads to the heart. It sends signals to the SA node to regulate the beating of the heart.

foetus in the uterus because, while the placenta is functioning, the mother's circulation is providing oxygen and nutrients and removing wastes. However, difficulties may arise in the change-over from foetal to neonatal circulation after the birth, when the lungs become active (→ Box 5.64).

Aneurysm

An **aneurysm** is a bulge caused by weakness in a blood vessel wall, usually where it branches. Aneurysms can develop in any blood vessel in the body, but the two most common places for them to form are in the abdominal aorta and the brain (→ Box 5.65).

Haematoma

A **haematoma** is a localised swelling that is filled with blood caused by a break in the wall of a blood vessel.

5.16.4 Blocked blood vessels

Thrombosis

A **thrombus** is a blood clot that forms inside a blood vessel. It can happen when the lining of the blood vessels becomes damaged or when the blood flow becomes very slow or stops. The clot blocks circulation in that area partly or completely when it is in:

- **an artery**. The tissues served by the artery get no oxygen and may die. When this happens in the heart it causes **myocardial infarction** (a heart attack), and in the brain it causes **cerebral thrombosis** (a stroke).
- **a vein**. The blood cannot return to the heart and the tissue becomes swollen behind the blockage. When this happens in the legs it may cause **deep vein thrombosis** (DVT).

Embolism

An **embolus** is a blood clot which breaks away from where it was formed and travels in the bloodstream until it becomes trapped in an artery small enough to prevent it moving any further. It can cause **pulmonary embolism** in the lungs, **heart attack** in the coronary arteries, **gangrene** in the legs and a **stroke** in the brain.

5.16.5 Stroke

A stroke occurs when the normal blood supply to a part of the brain is disrupted. When deprived of oxygen for more than a few minutes, brain cells die and the functions controlled by that part of the brain cease, which may result in paralysis down the opposite side of the body, loss of cognitive function and problems with speech (→ Box 5.66). The two main types are ischaemic stroke and haemorrhagic stroke (→ Box 5.67).

Ischaemic stroke

This is the most common type of stroke and occurs when a blood clot blocks the flow of blood in an artery to the brain, depriving that area of oxygen. If a small area is affected, only minor symptoms may occur. Ischaemia in a large area can cause severe symptoms and even death. The stroke typically forms in an area where the arteries have been narrowed and blocked by plaques (patches of fatty material), or by embolism – a clot which has become trapped.

Box 5.64 Factors that are known to increase the risk of congenital heart disease are:
- Down syndrome
- inherited genes
- rubella during pregnancy
- poorly controlled diabetes in the mother.

Box 5.65 In most cases, a brain aneurysm causes no symptoms and goes unnoticed. If it ruptures, it releases blood into the brain tissue, causing a stroke. An aneurysm may be treated by surgery when the potential benefits outweigh the known risks of the procedure.

Box 5.66 Stroke symptoms and the action to be taken can be remembered using the mnemonic **FAST**
Facial weakness – can the person smile? Has their mouth or eye drooped?
Arm weakness – can the person raise both arms?
Speech problems – can the person speak clearly and understand what you say?
Time to call an ambulance **FAST**

Box 5.67 CT scans for stroke patients are recommended to find out which type of stroke has occurred, because ischaemic and haemorrhagic strokes need to be treated quite differently (→ 17.2.3).

Transient ischaemic attack (TIA) is often referred to as a 'mini stroke' and is caused by a temporary disruption in the blood supply to part of the brain. The lack of oxygen to the affected area can cause sudden symptoms similar to those of a stroke, such as speech and visual disturbance, and numbness or weakness in the face, arms and legs. The effects often only last for a few minutes or hours and are fully resolved within 24 hours. However, small areas of **infarct** remain – localised areas of tissue that are dying or dead. Over time, TIAs can have a cumulative effect, contributing to vascular dementia, and they are often precursors to a major stroke (→ Box 5.68).

Haemorrhagic stroke

Haemorrhagic stroke (**cerebral haemorrhage; intracranial haemorrhage**) usually occurs when a blood vessel in the brain bursts and bleeds into the brain (**intracerebral haemorrhage**). Many bleeds occur in the sub-arachnoid space (→ Fig. 9.3), but in about 5% of cases the bleeding occurs on the surface of the brain (**subdural haematoma**). The main risk factor for haemorrhagic stroke is hypertension, which can alter the structure of arteries in the brain, making them prone to rupture (→ Box 5.69).

5.16.6 Disease of the veins

Varicose veins

Varicose veins are swollen veins usually seen on the legs. They occur when the valves in the veins fail to close properly, allowing some blood to flow backwards and collect, causing the veins to swell and be painful. A tendency to varicose veins often runs in families.

Deep vein thrombosis

Deep vein thrombosis (DVT) is a blood clot in one of the deep veins in the body, usually in the calf or thigh. It is more likely to occur when a person has been in the same position for a long time, e.g. on a long flight, when the blood in a vein moves so slowly that it clots. The person may experience some discomfort, but a risk occurs if the clot becomes loose, travels in the bloodstream through the heart and into the arterial circulation and results in pulmonary embolism or an ischaemic stroke (→ Box 5.70).

5.16.7 Gangrene

Gangrene is death and decomposition of areas of soft tissue (**necrosis**) caused by loss of blood supply. It results from severe hypoxia due to blockage in major arteries, particularly of the lower body. The colour of the affected area changes to dark brown or blackish due to the breakdown of haemoglobin. Gangrene is commonly secondary to peripheral vascular disease such as atherosclerosis or thrombosis. It is also associated with diabetes and long-term tobacco addiction (→ Box 5.71).

There are different types:

- **dry gangrene (coagulative necrosis)** – the affected tissue dries up and shrivels
- **wet gangrene (liquefaction necrosis)** develops in infected, damaged tissue which becomes swollen, soft, dark and produces a foul odour. It is more common in internal organs, and the risk of sepsis is high (→ 16.5.1).
- **gas gangrene** is often caused by infection of the injured tissue with anaerobic bacteria such as *Clostridium perfringens*, found in soil. The bacteria produce enzymes and toxins that destroy connective tissue, causing bubbles of gas to form in muscle tissue (→ Box 5.72).

Box 5.68 Vascular dementia is the second most common type of dementia after Alzheimer's disease, affecting around 150 000 people in the UK.

Box 5.69 Stroke rehabilitation involves a team of specialists which could include physiotherapists, psychologists, occupational therapists, speech therapists and specialist nurses and doctors. The rehabilitation programme offered to a stroke patient will depend on the individual's symptoms and their severity.

Box 5.70 All combined oral contraceptives increase the risk of venous thrombosis.

Although the incidence of DVT is low, the risk is of real concern because of widespread use of the contraceptive pill by women. The effect size appears to depend on both on the progestogen used and the dose of oestrogen in the contraceptive.

Box 5.71 People who have diabetes should frequently inspect their feet for signs of any redness, cuts or infections, particularly if they have diabetic neuropathy (→16.2.3) and decreased sensation of pain. Diabetes also affects the immune system so the body may be less able to fight infectious agents at the site of wounds.

Box 5.72 Dry gangrene eventually requires amputation. **Wet gangrene** requires antibiotic treatment and sometimes surgical drainage. **Gas gangrene** needs surgery to remove dead, damaged, and infected tissue.

5.17 Lymphatic system

The lymphatic system (→ Fig. 5.28) is a network of vessels that form part of the cardiovascular system. It has three main functions:

- it conveys **lymph** from the tissues to join the bloodstream near the heart
- the **lacteals** (lymph capillaries in the small intestine wall) absorb lipids and transport them to the liver (→ 7.6.3)
- **lymphocytes** destroy pathogens and other unwanted particles in the lymph.

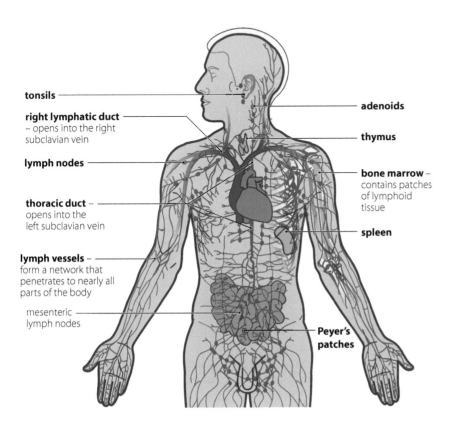

tonsils

adenoids

right lymphatic duct
– opens into the right
subclavian vein

thymus

lymph nodes

bone marrow –
contains patches
of lymphoid
tissue

thoracic duct –
opens into the
left subclavian vein

spleen

lymph vessels –
form a network that
penetrates to nearly all
parts of the body

mesenteric
lymph nodes

Peyer's
patches

Fig. 5.28 The lymphatic system.

Lymphoid tissue

Lymphoid tissue is the tissue that contains lymphocytes. Although lymphocytes are produced in bone marrow, they mature and develop in lymphoid tissue. Here they either stay in discrete groups or move out to other lymphoid tissue in the:

tonsils – two almond-shaped patches of lymphoid tissue, one on each side at the back of the throat; the tonsils are first-line defences against ingested or inhaled pathogens (→ Box 5.73)

adenoids (pharyngeal tonsils) – patches of lymphoid tissue in the nasopharynx; enlargement can obstruct nasal breathing and block the Eustachian tubes, causing glue ear

thymus – situated in the thorax underneath the top of the breastbone; it increases in size during childhood while the immune system is developing and then almost disappears in adulthood

Box 5.73 Tonsillitis is infection and inflammation of the tonsils. It is common in children but not adults because the tonsils have almost disappeared by adulthood.

spleen – situated in the abdomen near the stomach; it removes old red cells (erythrocytes) and platelets from the circulation. It is also very active in helping to develop immunity to disease

lymph nodes – situated along the lymph vessels rather like beads on a string; they are found in clusters in the armpit, neck, groin, etc. and their functions are to filter lymph and to assist the immune system in building an immune response

Peyer's patches – patches of lymphoid tissue in the digestive tract and abdominal wall

groups of cells in other organs.

5.17.1 Lymph

Lymph is the almost colourless fluid that flows through the lymphatic system. It is formed from the fluid that leaves the blood capillaries and becomes called **interstitial fluid** as it moves through interstices (spaces) in the tissues (➔ Fig. 5.29).

Lymph consists mainly of water which moves passively across capillary walls in both directions. The net rate of movement of water across the capillary walls depends mainly on the balance between:
- **hydrostatic pressure** – the pressure of circulating blood that forces water through the capillary walls into the tissues (➔ Fig. 5.21)
- **oncotic pressure** (colloid osmotic pressure) – created by proteins in plasma, which tends to draw water back into the capillaries (➔ Box 5.74).

Other pressures that affect the movement of fluid through the capillary walls are:
- inflammation – which increases permeability of blood vessels
- tissue osmotic pressure – which rises if proteins are allowed to leave blood vessels when blood vessels become more permeable
- changes in water-retaining properties of the tissues themselves; for example, changing levels of oestrogens and progesterone during the menstrual cycle are factors that affect water retention.

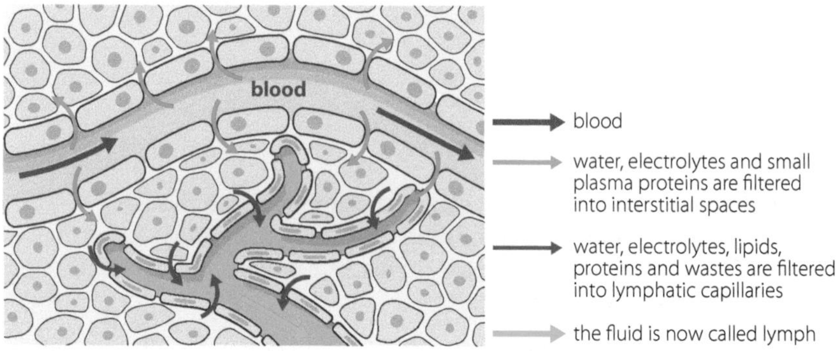

> **Box 5.74** The **Starling equation** is an equation that illustrates the role of hydrostatic and oncotic forces (the so-called Starling forces) in the movement of fluid across capillary membranes (➔ Fig. 5.21).

Fig. 5.29 Formation of lymph.

5.17.2 Movement of lymph

The lymphatic system starts as blind-ended tubes – **lymph capillaries** – situated between the cells of the tissues. They are similar to blood capillaries in having endothelial walls that are one cell thick, but they differ in allowing much larger particles to pass through. About 10% of the interstitial fluid flows into the lymph capillaries instead of back into the bloodstream. As it does so, many bacteria, viruses and other small particles from the interstitial spaces flow with it (→ Fig. 5.29).

The lymph capillaries unite to form lymph vessels and these join up to form a system of increasingly larger vessels which branch and join up freely. As lymph travels through the lymph vessels it has to pass through the lymph nodes where it is filtered and unwanted matter removed.

The main lymph vessel is the **thoracic duct** which lies in front of the vertebral column. This duct collects lymph from all parts of the body except the upper right side because the lymph from this region collects into the **right lymphatic duct**. These two ducts open into the two **subclavian veins** and return lymph to the bloodstream at the base of the neck (→ Fig. 5.28).

5.17.3 Lymph nodes

Lymph nodes (lymph glands) are situated along the course of the lymph vessels (→ Fig. 5.30). They are bean-shaped bodies containing **lymphoid tissue** – tissue in which lymphocytes are made. The tiny passageways in the lymph node are lined with white cells; these are mainly:

- **B-lymphocytes**, which produce antibodies that can identify and neutralise pathogens (germs)
- **T-lymphocytes** (CD4+ and CD8+ cells) which actively respond to a stimulus and coordinate the immune response (→ Box 5.75)
- **macrophages** which phagocytose bacteria and other small particles that flow slowly by, but they do not destroy viruses.

Box 5.75 Lymphocytes are a subset of white cells (→ 14.5.1).

B-lymphocytes have B cell receptors on their surface which allow them to bind to specific antigens against which they will form antibodies (→ 14.5.3).

CD4+ cells are the "helper T-lymphocytes" that assist other white blood cells in the immunological response (→ 14.5.2).

CD8+ cells are the cytotoxic T-lymphocytes which kill viral-infected and tumour cells.

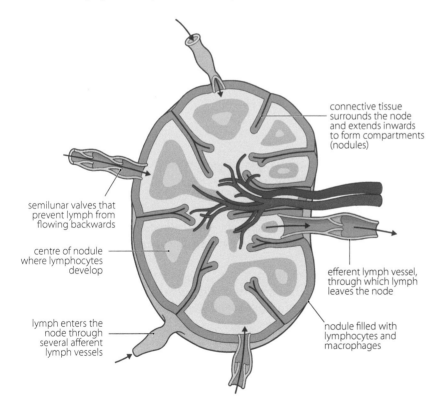

connective tissue surrounds the node and extends inwards to form compartments (nodules)

semilunar valves that prevent lymph from flowing backwards

centre of nodule where lymphocytes develop

efferent lymph vessel, through which lymph leaves the node

lymph enters the node through several afferent lymph vessels

nodule filled with lymphocytes and macrophages

Fig. 5.30 Section through a lymph node.

5.17.4 Oedema

Oedema is the retention of fluid in the body. The build-up of fluid causes swelling and puffiness, which can occur in one or more parts of the body:

- **lymphoedema** is due to a build-up of lymph in the body's tissues caused by obstruction of lymphatic vessels, e.g. by injury, inflammation or a tumour (→ Box 5.76)
- **pitting oedema** is swelling or puffiness of the skin, which temporarily holds the imprint of finger pressure
- **peripheral oedema** affects the feet and ankles (→ Fig. 5.31)
- **cerebral oedema** affects the brain
- **pulmonary oedema** affects the lungs
- **macular oedema** affects the eyes
- **idiopathic oedema** is swelling of the face, hands, trunk and limbs, occurring in premenopausal women and a variety of other conditions.

Box 5.76 Treatment for lymphoedema is exercise and massage to stimulate the flow of lymph into the lymph capillaries and along the lymph vessels, thus reducing its accumulation in the tissues. Wearing elastic support stockings or bandages also stimulates the flow of lymph.

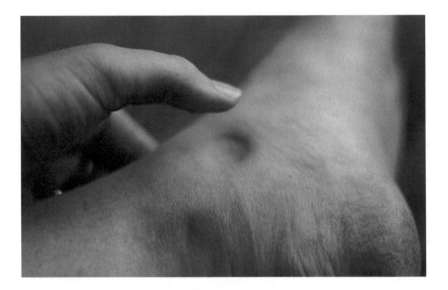

Fig. 5.31 Peripheral oedema with pitting.

Causes of oedema

Oedema is most commonly caused by:

- physical inactivity – no exercise and little walking
- standing or sitting still for a long time
- inflammation
- genes, which may be responsible for macular oedema
- surgery – there is normally some swelling due to inflammation after a surgical procedure
- high altitudes – especially when combined with physical exertion
- heat – in hot weather the body is less efficient at removing fluid from tissues
- fluid retention – pregnant women and women in the premenstrual phase tend to retain much more water than usual
- insect bites.

Oedema may also be a sign of an underlying pathophysiological condition:

- kidney disease
- heart failure

- chronic lung disease
- thyroid disease
- liver disease
- malnutrition
- side-effect of some medications.

5.18 Disorders of the lymphatic system

5.18.1 'Swollen glands'

Lymph nodes (often referred to as 'glands') become inflamed in various infections and diseases that range from throat infections to life-threatening cancers. The infection or disease may be in the lymph node itself or may originate some distance away. For example, when a hand is infected, pathogens from the infection are carried along the lymph vessels and become trapped in the lymph nodes at the elbow or armpit, causing them to swell (→ Box 5.77).

5.18.2 Infectious mononucleosis

Infectious mononucleosis (glandular fever) is an infectious disease caused by a virus mainly occurring in adolescents and young adults. It starts as a sore throat, the lymph nodes, particularly those in the neck, usually swell and abnormal lymphocytes occur in the blood (→ Box 5.78).

5.18.3 Tonsils and adenoids

The tonsils in the throat and the adenoids at the back of the nose contain lymphoid tissue which helps to protect the body from pathogens (germs) which have been inhaled or ingested. They are very active in childhood, normally enlarging at 5–6 years of age and shrinking after the age of 10. If they become chronically infected, they may need to be removed because they are then a source of infection and not a protection against it (→ Box 5.79).

5.18.4 Elephantiasis

Elephantiasis (lymphatic filariasis) is a disease characterised by the thickening of the skin and swelling of the underlying tissues, especially in the legs and male genitals. It is caused by parasitic thread-like roundworms and transmitted by mosquito bites. Elephantiasis results when the parasites lodge in the lymphatic system.

5.18.5 Compartment syndrome

Compartment syndrome arises when the pressure within the interstitial spaces (compartments) increases above the hydrostatic pressure in the capillaries. It develops most often in people who have musculoskeletal injuries. Debris accumulates in the interstitial spaces, which may reduce blood flow to the tissue and prevent lymphatic drainage away from the injury. Failure to relieve the build-up of pressure within the tissue can cause pain and loss of function. It may also lead to necrosis (death) of tissue because cells are deprived of oxygen.

Box 5.77 Swollen and inflamed lymph nodes can be hard to the touch, or tender.

NB Mumps is a viral infection of the parotid glands, not the lymph glands (→ Fig. 7.1).

Box 5.78 Infectious mononucleosis is caused by the **Epstein–Barr virus (EBV)**. Although it can make the patient feel quite ill, full recovery is normal. Most people infected with EBV gain immunity (→ Fig. 14.10).

Box 5.79 Tonsillectomy and adenoidectomy (surgical removal of tonsils and adenoids, respectively) is sometimes performed to break cycles of repeated infections of the throat. However, the operation is not without pain and other longer-term consequences for immunity, so the operation is now performed much less than in the 1960s.

Key points

1. Blood is a complex fluid comprising four components – plasma, erythrocytes, leucocytes and platelets – that circulate around the human body within a closed system of blood vessels.
2. The function of the heart is to generate the force required to pump blood through two essential circuits – the pulmonary circulation and the systemic circulation.
3. The sinoatrial node (pacemaker) generates the impulses which travel through the heart and initiate rhythmic contraction of the muscular chambers in every heartbeat.
4. Valves within the circulatory system prevent backflow and ensure one-way flow of blood through the heart and veins.
5. Cardiac output and blood pressure are subject to homeostatic regulation to ensure that blood flow in the body is matched to each organ's needs.
6. Interstitial fluid is formed by ultrafiltration from capillary blood and flows through the tissues, eventually draining into the lymphatic system to become lymph. Lymph flows through lymph nodes before returning to the systemic circulation.

Test yourself! Go to *www.lanternpublishing.com/AandP* and try the questions to check your understanding.

CHAPTER 6
THE RESPIRATORY SYSTEM

It is possible to live for a few days without drinking and a few weeks without food, but only a few minutes without breathing because the body needs a continuous supply of oxygen for the release of energy. Breathing is also essential for the excretion of carbon dioxide to prevent its accumulation as too much in the body is harmful.

6.1 Structure of the respiratory system

The respiratory system is concerned with ventilation (breathing), which is the movement of air into and out of the lungs so that the blood can obtain oxygen and lose carbon dioxide (→ Fig. 6.1).

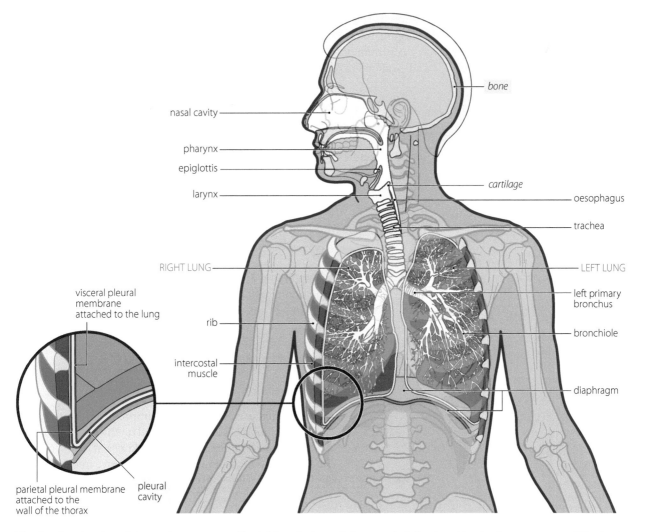

Fig. 6.1 Anterior view of the respiratory system. The left lung is shown fully expanded after breathing in; the areas coloured blue in the right lung indicate the reduction in lung volume after breathing out. Note that the person's organs in this figure are on the opposite side to the reader's.

6.2 Respiratory tract

The respiratory tract is the pathway along which air flows in and out of the body. It consists of nasal cavity, pharynx, larynx, trachea, bronchi, bronchioles and alveoli.

6.2.1 Nose

The space inside the nose is divided by a septum into two nasal cavities with each half having an opening – nostril – on the face and another into the pharynx (throat). The cavities are lined with ciliated mucosa which contains many blood vessels and chemorecepters (→ Box 6.1). As air is breathed in it is moistened by water from the mucous membrane, heated by warmth from the blood vessels in the lining, and dust particles in the air become trapped in the mucus. The cilia move the mucus along the nasal cavity to the pharynx, where it is swallowed. The nose is connected to the sinuses in the bones of the skull and face (→ Fig. 6.6).

6.2.2 Pharynx

The pharynx (throat) is a muscular cavity lined with mucosa that links the mouth and nasal passages with the oesophagus and trachea, which allows breathing to take place through the nose or the mouth (→ Fig. 6.2). It serves as a common pathway for air and food and is important for both breathing and swallowing (**deglutition**) (→ Box 6.2).

Box 6.1 As air passes through the nostrils, any odours it contains can be detected by chemoreceptors – specialised nerve endings that are part of the olfactory system (→ 10.5).

Box 6.2 Because swallowing depends on the precise timing and coordination of many muscles, it can be difficult for people affected by strokes, Alzheimer's disease or other disorders that involve the autonomic nervous system (→ 9.8). Swallowing is also affected by disorders of the nerves that control the muscles involved in swallowing, e.g. Parkinson's disease, myasthenia gravis and muscular dystrophy.

Taking it Further
Healthcare professionals are trained to observe and understand how and why respiratory function, swallowing and speech may change.

You can read more about physiological measurements in online Chapter 17.

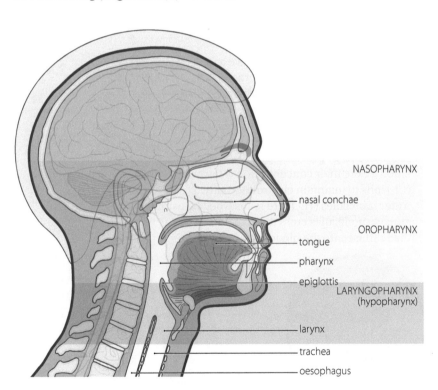

Fig. 6.2 Sagittal section through the head and neck.

NASOPHARYNX
nasal conchae
OROPHARYNX
tongue
pharynx
epiglottis
LARYNGOPHARYNX (hypopharynx)
larynx
trachea
oesophagus

Epiglottis

The epiglottis is a flap of cartilage located in the throat behind the tongue. It is usually upright at rest, allowing air to pass into the larynx and down to the lungs. When swallowing is taking place, the epiglottis folds down to cover the entrance of the larynx, which prevents food and liquid from entering the trachea and lungs, and breathing briefly stops (→ Box 6.3).

6.2.3 Larynx

The cartilages in the wall of the larynx form a rigid framework with the two ligaments – **the vocal cords** – stretched across the opening with a V-shaped space between them called the **glottis** (→ Fig. 6.3). When we breathe in, the cords are held apart and air flows freely through the opening. When the cords are brought closer together, air from the lungs is forced between them, which makes the cords vibrate and produce sounds (→ Box 6.4).

Speech depends on vibrations of the vocal cords, which are controlled by the speech centre in the left hemisphere of the brain (Broca's area → Fig. 9.7). The vibrations produce sounds which are converted into meaningful speech through movements of the muscles of the throat, tongue, lips, cheeks and jaws. Sounds are normally created on the outward breath (expiration).

6.2.4 Trachea

The trachea (windpipe) is the airway that extends from the larynx to the lungs. It is supported and kept open by incomplete rings of cartilage and is lined by ciliated mucosa (→ Fig. 6.4). The mucus keeps the surface moist and traps inhaled particles, and cilia waft the mucus upwards toward the larynx and into the pharynx, where it is swallowed or coughed out.

Box 6.3 Chewing, speaking, breathing, coughing and vomiting are automatic processes that must stop for the **deglutition** (swallowing) **reflex** to work properly. This reflex uses the epiglottis to cover the opening of the trachea during swallowing.

Box 6.4 During puberty the rising levels of testosterone in young men cause enlargement of the larynx. The vocal cords thicken, which makes them vibrate at a lower frequency than in women, and this is why men's voices usually have a deeper pitch. In men, the larynx is often known as 'Adam's apple'.

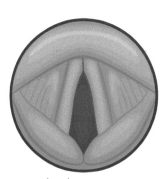

vocal cords open during breathing to allow air into lungs

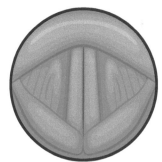

vocal cords close when speaking so air from the lungs presses between them to cause vibrations that produce sound

Fig. 6.3 Vocal cords.

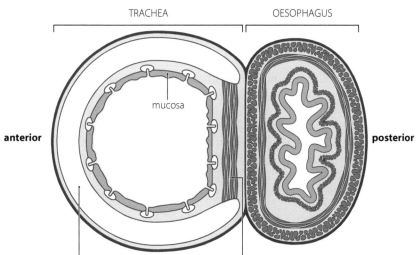

C-shaped cartilage are not complete rings but have a break in them adjacent to the oesophagus; this is occupied by muscle tissue which allows the oesophagus to extend when a bolus of food passes down to the stomach

muscle tissue forms the side of the trachea adjacent to the oesophagus; it folds inwards when the oesophagus expands to allow food to pass through to the stomach

Fig. 6.4 Cross-section of oesophagus and trachea.

6.3 Lungs

The right lung is divided into three lobes and the left lung into two lobes. Lung tissue is composed of a mass of airways and millions of **alveolar sacs** which enable them to carry out their function of gaseous exchange (→ Fig. 6.5). Gaseous exchange is the diffusion of gases from an area of higher concentration to an area of lower concentration. In the lungs this process takes place in the alveoli as oxygen diffuses from air to blood and carbon dioxide diffuses in the opposite direction.

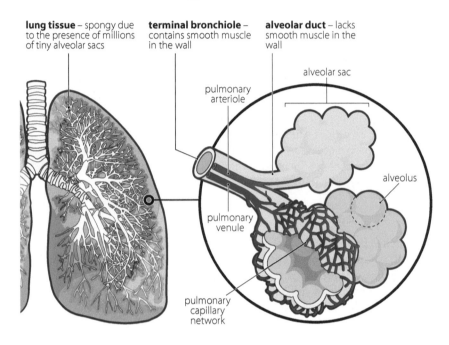

lung tissue – spongy due to the presence of millions of tiny alveolar sacs

terminal bronchiole – contains smooth muscle in the wall

alveolar duct – lacks smooth muscle in the wall

alveolar sac

pulmonary arteriole

alveolus

pulmonary venule

pulmonary capillary network

Fig. 6.5 Section through a lung.

6.3.1 Airways

The trachea divides into two **bronchi**, one to each lung, which are kept open by cartilage rings. Like the trachea, the bronchi are lined with mucous membrane and without muscle tissue in their walls. Each bronchus divides about 5–6 times before becoming bronchioles. **Bronchioles** are the narrower air tubes in which spirals of smooth muscle tissue gradually replace cartilage and makes them the site of bronchoconstriction (→ Box 6.5). They branch repeatedly into smaller and smaller tubes that eventually end in terminal bronchioles and alveolar sacs.

Alveolar sacs

Air fills the alveolar sacs with every intake of breath, and is forced out as the lungs deflate. The very thin walls of the alveolar sacs are prevented from collapsing when empty because some of the cells of the alveoli secrete **pulmonary surfactant** which decreases the surface tension of the moisture (mostly water) in the lungs to almost zero (→ Box 6.6).

Box 6.5 Bronchoconstriction occurs when the smooth muscle fibres in the bronchiole walls contract and narrow the airways, leading to coughing, wheezing and shortness of breath.

Bronchodilation is an increase in diameter of the bronchioles in response to autonomic nervous activity (→ 9.8) or medication.

Box 6.6 The ability to make surfactant begins before birth, from 32–34 weeks' gestation. Premature babies don't have this ability, which leads to lung stiffness and **respiratory distress syndrome**. The babies may require the support of a ventilator, and may also be given artificial surfactant.

6.3.2 Pleura

The pleura is a **serous** membrane which folds back onto itself to form a two-layered pleural sac – the **visceral pleura** attached to the outer surface of each lung and also attached to the diaphragm and the **parietal pleura** attached to the thorax wall (➔ Fig. 6.1). The thin layer of **pleural fluid** between them allows the layers to slide smoothly against each other as the lungs expand and recoil with each breath (➔ Box 6.7).

6.4 Mucus

Mucus is the clear, thin, viscous fluid produced by the goblet cells in the mucosa (➔ Fig. 2.10e) that lines the respiratory tract. It:
- forms a barrier over the surface to protect the delicate tissues underneath and prevent them from drying out
- is sticky, which helps to trap dust particles, bacteria and other inhaled debris
- contains substances that help to destroy inhaled bacteria (➔ Box 6.8).

In the nose, trachea and bronchi, the ciliated mucosa moves the mucus towards the pharynx where it is swallowed into the stomach and digested.

Phlegm is thick mucus secreted in the repiratory tract during inflammation and disease. It usually contains bacteria, debris, and sloughed-off inflammatory cells (➔ Box 6.9).

Sneezing

The nasal mucosa has many sensory nerve endings and, when irritated, a reflex action causes a violent expulsion of air through the nose and mouth – a sneeze – to expel the cause of the irritation.

Coughing

The cough reflex is a normal protective action to clear the airways of mucus or irritants such as dust or smoke. A **'chesty' cough** is usually caused by infection which produces excess phlegm, e.g. the common cold, flu or bronchitis. A **dry cough** starts as a tickle in the throat when the upper airways are inflamed, but does not produce phlegm. **Smoker's cough** occurs when the cilia of the mucous membrane are paralysed by smoke, which makes the removal of mucus more difficult.

6.4.1 Rhinitis

Rhinitis is inflammation of the nasal mucosa causing excess mucus to be produced that blocks the nose, e.g. hay fever or infection (➔ Box 6.10).

6.4.2 Sinusitis

Sinusitis is inflammation of the mucosa that lines the air-filled spaces (**sinuses**) in the bones of the face (➔ Fig. 6.6). Symptoms may include facial pain, discharge from the nose and a reduced sense of smell. Thickening of the mucus may produce nasal or sinus drainage problems and promote infection. Many cases are self-limiting, others need medical treatment, and a few cases need surgery.

Box 6.7 When air builds up between the pleura due to a fractured rib or other trauma, it puts pressure on the lung so that it cannot expand as much as normal. This condition is known as **pneumothorax** (collapsed lung), making breathing difficult, and pain that is worsened when coughing.

Box 6.8 The thin, delicate linings of the lungs are well protected by lysozyme, antibodies and phagocytes.

Box 6.9 Sputum is phlegm expelled by coughing. It can change colour to yellow or green when infected by bacteria or viruses; pink or red colour indicates the presence of blood. The colour, consistency, volume and smell of sputum and the appearance of any solid material it contains can provide information affecting the diagnosis and management of respiratory disease.

Box 6.10 In cold weather movement of the mucus slows and it sometimes gathers in the nose and drips or dribbles out, causing a **winter runny nose**. Excess nasal mucus can be removed by blowing the nose.

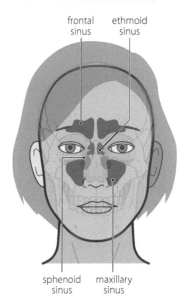

Fig. 6.6 Position of the sinuses in the bones of the cranium.

6.5 Ventilation

Box 6.11 Before birth, the foetus obtains oxygen from the mother's blood in the placenta and excretes carbon dioxide by the same route (→ 12.6.3). At the moment of birth, the baby's lungs are not inflated, but when the newborn's nervous system reacts to the sudden change in temperature and environment, the lungs inflate as the baby takes its first breath, usually within about 10 seconds of the delivery (→ 12.7.2).

Ventilation (breathing) is a regular and mainly automatic process in which air is alternately inhaled into the lungs (**inspiration**) and then exhaled (**expiration**). The movement of the lungs as they expand and contract during breathing depends on movements of the intercostal muscles of the ribcage and the diaphragm muscle. With each breath:

- the ribcage enlarges and the diaphragm flattens, allowing the lungs to expand, which lowers the pressure within the lungs and air rushes in to fill up the space (→ Fig. 6.7)
- gaseous exchange takes place in the alveoli where oxygen moves from the air into the blood and carbon dioxide moves in the opposite direction
- the ribcage reduces in size, the diaphragm relaxes, and air is forced out of the lungs (→ Box 6.11).

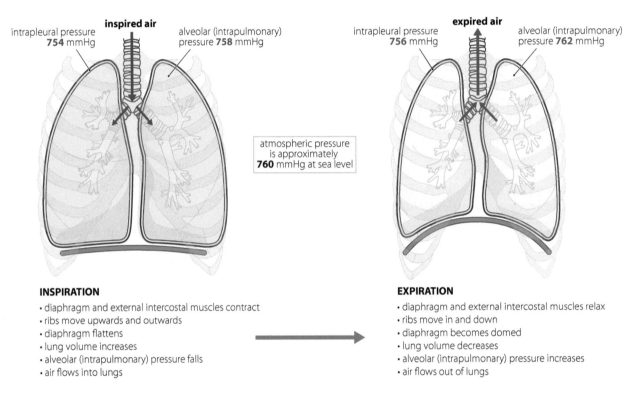

intrapleural pressure **754** mmHg — **inspired air** — alveolar (intrapulmonary) pressure **758** mmHg

intrapleural pressure **756** mmHg — **expired air** — alveolar (intrapulmonary) pressure **762** mmHg

atmospheric pressure is approximately **760** mmHg at sea level

INSPIRATION
- diaphragm and external intercostal muscles contract
- ribs move upwards and outwards
- diaphragm flattens
- lung volume increases
- alveolar (intrapulmonary) pressure falls
- air flows into lungs

EXPIRATION
- diaphragm and external intercostal muscles relax
- ribs move in and down
- diaphragm becomes domed
- lung volume decreases
- alveolar (intrapulmonary) pressure increases
- air flows out of lungs

Fig. 6.7 Inspiration and expiration.

Ways of breathing

Box 6.12 A number of factors can affect breathing, e.g. exercise, emotions, allergens and smoking. Recognition of what is 'normal' for an individual, and assessment of changes from that level, can provide health professionals with insight into that person's wellbeing.

Although breathing usually involves the intercostal and abdominal muscles, the extent to which each is used varies with individuals, with training, and with the demands made upon the lungs at any particular time:

- **thoracic breathing** uses the intercostal muscles – the chest can be seen to rise and fall
- **abdominal breathing** uses the diaphragm – as the diaphragm moves upwards and downwards, the abdomen moves in and out
- **eupnea** (quiet breathing) is mainly abdominal, with most of the work being done by the diaphragm muscle (→ Box 6.12).

6.5.1 Accessory muscles

Accessory muscles are those not normally used for breathing, but only when there is a high demand for gaseous exchange, e.g.:
- during exercise, forceful breathing can be assisted by contraction of **abdominal muscles** which push the abdominal organs upwards to help reduce the volume of air in the thoracic cavity
- when there is dysfunction of the respiratory system such as an asthma attack or in people with emphysema, the muscles in the neck (**scalene** and **sternocleidomastoid** (→ Fig. 4.20) can be recruited to assist with raising the ribcage to increase the flow of air into the lungs (→ Box 6.13).

Box 6.13 Use of accessory muscles during quiet breathing is usually taken as a sign of respiratory distress.

6.5.2 Respiration rate

The **respiration rate** is the number of breaths taken in one minute. The average number of respirations for an adult are 12–20 per minute. The number of respirations increases when undertaking physical activity, due to fever, or when feeling anxious or frightened. Breathing is slower when asleep, or feeling calm, or due to the effect of sedative drugs (→ Box 6.14).

Box 6.14 Assessing the **respiratory rate** (RR or 'Resps') and the depth, rhythm and sounds of a patient's breathing is an essential skill for all healthcare practitioners (→ 17.1.1). The continuous monitoring of depth and rate of breathing is more likely to happen in a hospital setting, e.g.: intensive care.

6.5.3 Lung function

Lung function describes how well a person is breathing, which is affected by gender, age and height. It is also affected by lifestyle and physical condition, being better than normal in athletes and worse in smokers and those who are unfit, overweight, or have lung disorders. Lung function can be measured using a **spirometer** – a device for measuring the air capacity of the lungs (→ Fig. 6.8a). The results are used in the diagnosis and classification of severity of lung disorders. A **peak flow meter** (→ Fig. 6.8b) is a device which measures peak expiratory flow rate (PEFR) and is used in the management of asthma and to monitor the effectiveness of treatment (→ Fig. 6.9).

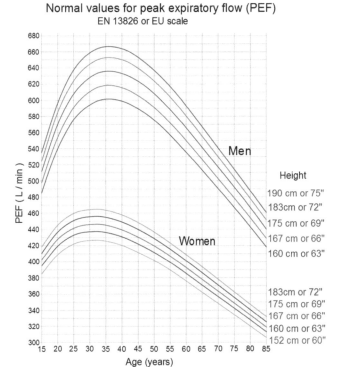

Fig. 6.9 (figure) Normal values for peak expiratory flow (PEF), EN 13826 or EU scale. PEF (L / min) versus Age (years).

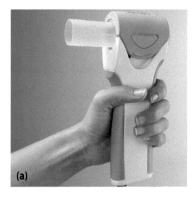

(a)

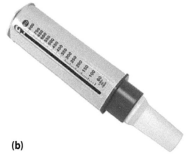

(b)

Fig. 6.8 (**a**) Digital spirometer; (**b**) peak flow meter.

Fig. 6.9 Normal range of values of peak flow expiratory flow rate (PEFR) in adults aged up to 85 years.

6.5.4 Lung capacity

Lung capacity describes the volume of air that an individual can hold in the lungs (→ Fig. 6.10). The average total lung capacity of an adult human male is about 6 litres of air (→ Box 6.15). **Tidal breathing** is normal, resting breathing; the **tidal volume** is the volume of air that is inhaled or exhaled in just one such breath (→ Table 6.1).

Dead space in the lungs is the area that is not involved in gas exchange. It can be:

- **anatomical dead space** (conducting zone) – the area that includes mouth, nose and all of the airways where air is present but no gaseous exchange is taking place
- **physiological dead space** represents alveolar sacs where gaseous exchange is reduced because:
  - **ventilation** (air flow to the alveoli) is restricted, e.g. in pneumonia where fluid is present in the air sacs, or in asthma when bronchoconstriction and mucus obstruct the bronchioles, and
  - **perfusion** (blood flow to the lungs) is restricted, e.g. when a clot blocks the supply of blood (perfusion) of pulmonary capillaries in pulmonary embolism (→ Box 6.16).

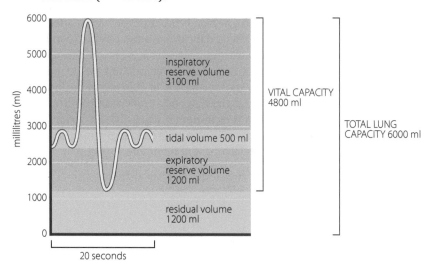

Fig. 6.10 Lung volume and capacities in an adult.

Table 6.1 Average lung volumes of an 80 kg man

	Description	Volume
Tidal volume (TV)	Amount of air that moves into and out of the lungs during normal, relaxed breathing	500 cm³
Inspiratory reserve volume (IRV)	Additional air that can be forcibly inhaled following inspiration	3100 cm³
Expiratory reserve volume (ERV)	Additional air that can be exhaled during a forced breath	1200 cm³
Residual volume (RV)	Amount of air still remaining in the lungs after the expiratory reserve volume is exhaled	1200 cm³
Vital capacity (VC)	Total amount of air that can be forcibly exhaled after fully inhaling	4800 cm³
Total lung capacity (TLC)	Maximum amount of air that can fill the lungs, calculated by adding vital capacity (VC) and reserve volume (RV)	6000 cm³
Functional residual capacity (FRC)	Amount of air remaining in the lungs after a normal expiration	2400 cm³
Dead space	The volume of air in the bronchi and bronchioles which does not participate in gas exchange	150 cm³

6.6 Respiration and gas transport

External, internal and cellular respiration are different processes. **External respiration** occurs in the alveoli where oxygen diffuses from the air into the blood, and carbon dioxide diffuses into the alveolar air. **Internal respiration** occurs in the tissues, where oxygen diffuses from the blood and into the tissue cells, and carbon dioxide diffuses from the cells and into the blood (→ Box 6.17). **Cellular respiration** takes place inside living cells to release energy from food in a form that can be used for all the cell's activities. It can take place in the presence of oxygen (**aerobic**) or in its absence (**anaerobic**) (→ 20.13).

6.6.1 Composition of air

Air is composed of the gases nitrogen and oxygen, with very small amounts of other gases, e.g. carbon dioxide, argon, methane and ozone, with water vapour present in variable amounts (→ Table 6.2).

Table 6.2 Approximate composition of inhaled and exhaled air

	Inhaled air	Exhaled air
Nitrogen	78%	78%
Oxygen	21%	17%
Carbon dioxide	0.03%	4%
Other gases	1%	1%
Water vapour	varies	saturated

6.6.2 Partial pressure

Each of the gases in air has its own **partial pressure**, which is its concentration in the mixture, measured in mmHg (→ Box 6.18):

P_{O_2} is the partial pressure of oxygen
P_{CO_2} is the partial pressure of carbon dioxide.

The movement of the respiratory gases both in the lungs and the tissues is along a pressure gradient, and the higher the concentration of the gas, the greater its partial pressure. For example, it is the higher partial pressure of oxygen in inhaled air than in the blood, that drives oxygen molecules to dissolve into the alveolar membrane and then move into the blood of the pulmonary capillaries where they bind to haemoglobin.

6.6.3 Gas exchange in the alveoli

The purpose of breathing is to maintain an optimum composition of the air in the alveoli where the process of gaseous exchange takes place (→ Box 6.19). Oxygen and carbon dioxide move rapidly between air and blood because the millions of **alveoli** have:

- **a large surface area** for gaseous exchange to take place
- **thin walls**; the air in the alveoli comes very close to the blood, being separated by only two layers of cells (the alveolus wall and the capillary wall), which allows rapid diffusion (→ 20.7.1)
- **excellent blood supply** due to the dense network of pulmonary capillaries surrounding the alveoli
- **moist surfaces** that allow oxygen and carbon dioxide to go into solution, which is necessary for diffusion to take place (→ Fig. 6.11).

Box 6.17 Internal respiration is the driving force for rapid diffusion of O_2 into the tissue and the removal of CO_2. Blood which is deoxygenated – with low P_{O_2} and high P_{CO_2} – flows from the tissue capillaries into veins and then back to the heart via the vena cava.

Box 6.18 mmHg = millimetres of mercury. Although mmHg is not an SI unit, it is still routinely used in medicine. The pascal (Pa) or kilopascal (kPa) is the SI unit of pressure measurement that is widely used across the globe and may also be used in clinical settings. However, when arterial blood samples are taken with the aim of determining the acid–base balance, the printouts include measurements of P_{O_2}, P_{CO_2}, pH and HCO_3^-.

Box 6.19 A change in cardiac output (→ 5.12.1) can affect gaseous exchange in the lungs because any fall in cardiac output tends to result in reduced perfusion of the lungs, reduced O_2 content of blood and increased CO_2 content.

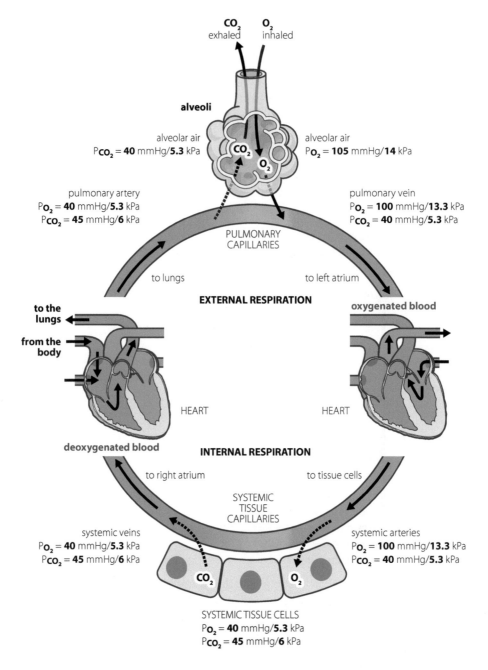

Fig. 6.11 Gaseous exchange, internal and external respiration and the role of the circulatory system.

Box 6.20 A pulse oximeter is a device that monitors the oxygen content of a patient's blood by determining the percentage of oxyhaemoglobin in blood pulsating through a capillary network. Typically, the device is attached to a finger, toe or ear, and is often used to monitor a patient's oxygen level during and after surgery to detect hypoxaemia (→ Fig. 17.2).

6.6.4 Transport of oxygen

Although oxygen dissolves in plasma, only a very small amount is transported in solution in the blood. Nearly all the oxygen – about 98.5% – becomes attached to haemoglobin molecules inside the red cells to form oxyhaemoglobin for transportation in the bloodstream to the tissues (→ Fig. 6.12) (→ Box 6.20).

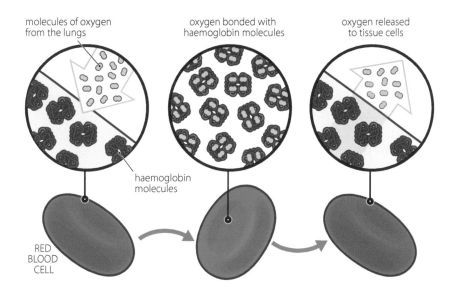

molecules of oxygen from the lungs

oxygen bonded with haemoglobin molecules

oxygen released to tissue cells

haemoglobin molecules

RED BLOOD CELL

Fig. 6.12 Transport of oxygen in the blood.

6.6.5 Use of oxygen by cells

Living cells need a continuous supply of oxygen to release energy from glucose by the process of aerobic respiration (→ 20.14), which can be summed up in the equation:

$$C_6H_{12}O_6 \quad + \quad 6O_2 \quad \longrightarrow \quad 6CO_2 \quad + \quad 6H_2O \quad + \quad energy$$

(glucose)　　　(oxygen)　　　(carbon dioxide)　(water)　　(ATP + heat)

During aerobic respiration, energy in the form of **adenosine triphosphate** (ATP) is released from glucose by three metabolic processes: glycolysis, the citric acid cycle and the electron transport chain (→ Box 6.21).

Glycolysis ('splitting sugar') takes place in the cytoplasm and is the stage during which a molecule of glucose is split enzymatically by hydrolysis to produce:
- two molecules of pyruvic acid ($C_3H_4O_3$)
- four atoms of hydrogen which are transported to the electron transfer chain by the hydrogen carriers NAD and FAD
- two molecules of ATP.

Citric acid cycle (Krebs cycle) takes place after glycolysis and occurs in the presence of oxygen in the mitochondria. It is a series of biochemical reactions that removes carbon and hydrogen from pyruvic acid. The carbon forms carbon dioxide for excretion, the hydrogen ions (protons) are attached to the coenzyme molecules $NADH_2$ and $FADH_2$. The cycle is repeated twice – once for each molecule of pyruvic acid – and results in:
- two molecules of ATP
- six molecules of CO_2, which are removed and exhaled
- ten pairs of hydrogen ions that go into the electron transfer chain.

Electron transfer (ET) chain (oxidative phosphorylation) is a system of carrier molecules that transfer hydrogen ions and electrons from one carrier to the next to generate ATP. Hydrogen ions are supplied to the chain from $NADH_2$ and $FADH_2$. When the energy is transferred to ATP, inhaled oxygen serves as the final hydrogen acceptor, combining to form water (→ Box 6.22).

Taking it Further
The energy required for living processes is supplied from cell respiration of carbohydrates and lipids.

You can find out more about these nutrients and energy balance in online Chapter 19 (→ 19.3, 19.8).

Box 6.21 If glucose is not available to make ATP, glycogen can be broken down to glucose by glycogenolysis. When there is no glycogen, fats in the body, then proteins, can enter the citric acid cycle to provide energy (gluconeogenesis).

Box 6.22 Summary of aerobic respiration
Glycolysis – each glucose molecule is split to produce:
- pyruvic acid → citric acid cycle
- two molecules of $NADH_2$ → ET chain
- small amount of ATP.

Citric acid cycle produces:
- CO_2 → excreted
- hydrogen ions → ET chain
- small amount of ATP.

Electron transfer chain produces:
- water which is excreted
- much more ATP.

Taking it Further
The energy required for living processes is supplied through metabolic reactions that take place either aerobically or anaerobically in every cell in the human body.

You can find out more about metabolism and cell respiration in online Chapter 20 (→ 20.11).

6.6.6 Anaerobic respiration

Anaerobic respiration is a type of respiration that does not require oxygen to release energy from glucose and takes place in the cytoplasm (not in the mitochondria). It is not nearly as energy-efficient as aerobic respiration, producing only a small amount of ATP because the glucose is partially, not completely, broken down (→ 20.14.1).

6.6.7 Lactic acid

Lactic acid is produced continuously in small amounts in all tissues but only accumulates when the rate of production exceeds the rate of removal during:
- strenuous exercise
- acute illness when oxygen delivery to the tissues is not adequate despite an increased rate of breathing, e.g. sepsis (→ 16.5.1).

The **oxygen debt** is the amount of oxygen needed to oxidise lactic acid to carbon dioxide and water after exercise has stopped. The debt is repaid by breathing quickly and deeply until the lactic acid has been oxidised (→ 20.14.2).

6.6.8 Transport of carbon dioxide in the blood

Some carbon dioxide is transported in solution in plasma, but most diffuses into the red cells where it becomes converted into hydrogen ions (H^+) and bicarbonate (HCO_3^-), with a small amount becoming attached to haemoglobin (→ Fig. 6.13).

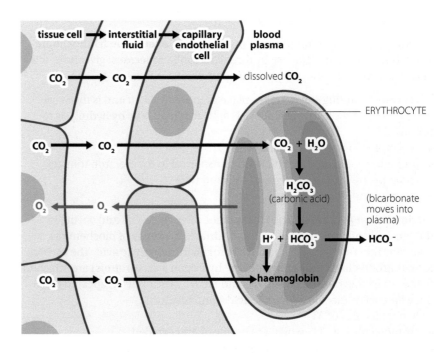

Fig. 6.13 Gaseous exchange between the tissues and blood.

6.6.9 Homeostatic control of breathing

Carbon dioxide levels in blood are a major driver of ventilation (→ Fig. 6.14). Regulation of carbon dioxide homeostasis is closely linked to the acid–base balance in the body. This is because H^+ is acidic while HCO_3^- is alkaline (base). Chemoreceptors which are located within the brainstem and in major arteries are responsive to changes in partial pressure of CO_2 and changing levels of H^+ (→ Box 6.23).

Box 6.23 Although H^+ and HCO_3^- are formed in equal amounts from CO_2, these chemical substances alter the pH of blood in different ways because H^+ is usually buffered by plasma proteins while HCO_3^- is not.

Buffers are fluids with special chemical properties which mean they are able to maintain a stable pH even when small amounts of acids or bases (alkali) are added to them.

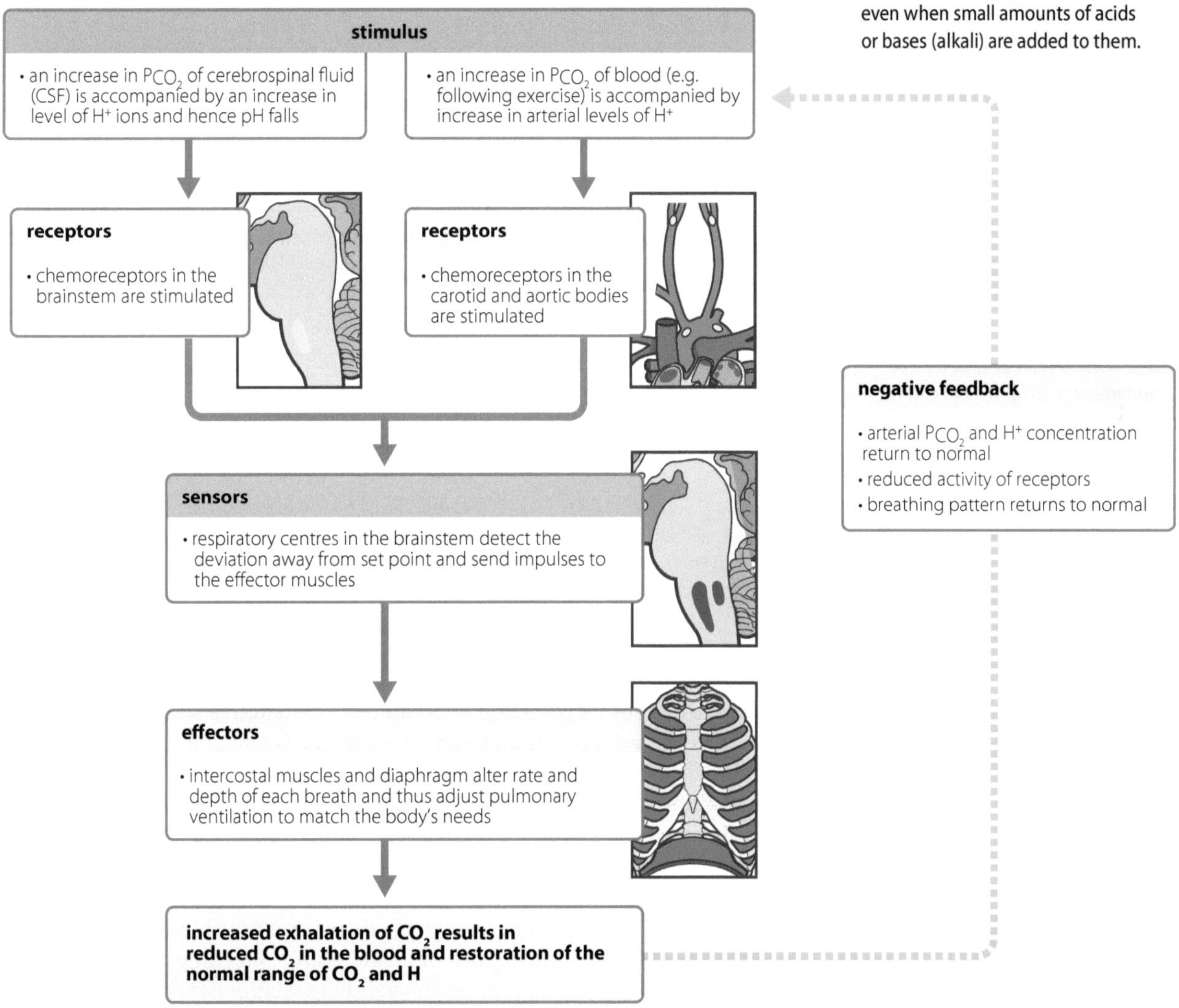

stimulus

- an increase in P_{CO_2} of cerebrospinal fluid (CSF) is accompanied by an increase in level of H^+ ions and hence pH falls

- an increase in P_{CO_2} of blood (e.g. following exercise) is accompanied by increase in arterial levels of H^+

receptors

- chemoreceptors in the brainstem are stimulated

receptors

- chemoreceptors in the carotid and aortic bodies are stimulated

negative feedback

- arterial P_{CO_2} and H^+ concentration return to normal
- reduced activity of receptors
- breathing pattern returns to normal

sensors

- respiratory centres in the brainstem detect the deviation away from set point and send impulses to the effector muscles

effectors

- intercostal muscles and diaphragm alter rate and depth of each breath and thus adjust pulmonary ventilation to match the body's needs

increased exhalation of CO_2 results in reduced CO_2 in the blood and restoration of the normal range of CO_2 and H

Fig. 6.14 Regulation of breathing based on the body's response to an increase in the partial pressure of carbon dioxide (P_{CO_2}).

6.6.10 Abnormal breathing

Abnormal breathing is usually an indicator of problems in the lungs, airways or elsewhere in the body.

Stridor

Stridor is a term used to describe noisy breathing in general, and refers specifically to a high-pitched crowing sound associated with croup, respiratory infection, and airway obstruction.

Hyperventilation

Hyperventilation (over-breathing) is unnaturally fast, deep breathing at times of extreme anxiety or during a panic attack or temper tantrum. It can be accompanied by dizziness or fainting, trembling, tingling and cramp in the hands. These symptoms are caused by exhaling too much carbon dioxide from the blood – a characteristic of disturbance of acid–base homeostasis known as **respiratory alkalosis**.

Hypoxia

Hypoxia is a reduced amount of oxygen in the blood caused by impaired breathing or gas exchange. Inadequate oxygenation of the blood or poor circulation results in **cyanosis** – blueish discolouration of the nails and skin (e.g. 'blue lips' in cold weather), blue baby syndrome (→ Box 6.24) and respiratory distress syndrome (→ 6.8.2). Cyanosis in dark-skinned people can be observed in the mucous membranes around the lips, gums and eyes. Hypoxia is a common complication of infections e.g. pneumonia, meningitis and sepsis (→ Box 6.25).

Box 6.24 Blue baby syndrome is a rare condition in babies born with a congenital heart defect that prevents circulating blood from becoming fully oxygenated.

Hyperoxia

Hyperoxia is excess oxygen in the body or a higher than normal partial pressure (→ 6.6.2), leading to toxicity, a condition that can damage the nervous system, respiratory system and vision.

Box 6.25 Oxygen therapy may be administered for acute and chronic hypoxia, low cardiac output states, lung conditions when gaseous exchange is poor or when patients are anaesthetised. It may also be used in aviation.

Snoring

Snoring occurs when the soft tissue at the back of the mouth, nose or throat vibrates when a person breathes in and out during sleep.

Apnoea

Apnoea is temporary cessation of breathing. **Obstructive sleep apnoea (OSA)** is a relatively common sleep disorder that is characterised by pauses in breathing and temporary stopping of airflow into the lungs due to relaxation of muscles around the upper airway. This leads to extremely loud, heavy snoring interrupted by gasps, snorts and sharp intakes of breath before the brain automatically wakes the affected person up – maybe 30 times an hour (→ Box 6.26).

Box 6.26 If OSA is not treated, the person will be excessively sleepy in the daytime, a condition associated with reduced quality of life and an increased risk of cardiovascular events.

Cheyne–Stokes respiration

Cheyne–Stokes respiration is an abnormal pattern of breathing characterised by progressively deeper and sometimes faster breathing, followed by a gradual decrease that results in a temporary stop in breathing (apnoea), usually preceding death of the person.

6.7 Respiratory disorders

6.7.1 Dyspnoea

Box 6.27 Sudden shortness of breath is a common reason for visiting a hospital A&E department, and one of the most common reasons for calling the emergency services. It can be a warning sign of a serious medical or surgical condition.

Dyspnoea (shortness of breath; breathlessness) can be caused by:
- a disorder of the respiratory system
- a disorder of the circulatory system (heart and blood vessels)
- other conditions, e.g. severe anaemia or high fever (→ Box 6.27).

Acute dyspnoea – sudden shortness of breath – can be:
- the normal response to exercise or altitude
- pulmonary embolism – blockage in a pulmonary artery
- bronchospasm – the sudden contraction of smooth muscle in the walls of bronchioles (→ Box 6.28).

Chronic dyspnoea – long-term shortness of breath – can result from:
- obesity
- anaemia due to insufficient red cells or haemoglobin
- asthma that is not properly controlled
- permanently damaged lungs due to chronic obstructive pulmonary disease (COPD) or emphysema
- heart disorders such as atrial fibrillation (irregular, fast heart rate), tachycardia (regular, fast heart rate) or heart failure.

Box 6.28 Allergic bronchospasm is sudden contraction of the muscles in the walls of bronchioles in response to an allergen, e.g. peanuts or insect bites.

6.7.2 Asthma

Asthma occurs when the airways in the lungs become constricted. It is caused by **bronchospasm**, inflammation of the lining of the bronchioles (→ Fig. 6.15) and a build-up of mucus and sputum (phlegm). The symptoms of asthma are cough, wheeze, shortness of breath and a feeling of tightness in the chest as a result of:
- infection of the respiratory tract
- physical and emotional factors including cold air, exercise, tobacco smoke and stress.

Asthma is regarded as a reversible disease because its symptoms can be managed and relieved by physiotherapy (breathing exercises) and medication, and some children 'grow out of it' (→ Box 6.29).

Box 6.29 Asthma can be difficult to diagnose in children because other conditions can cause similar symptoms such as coughs, colds and shortness of breath.

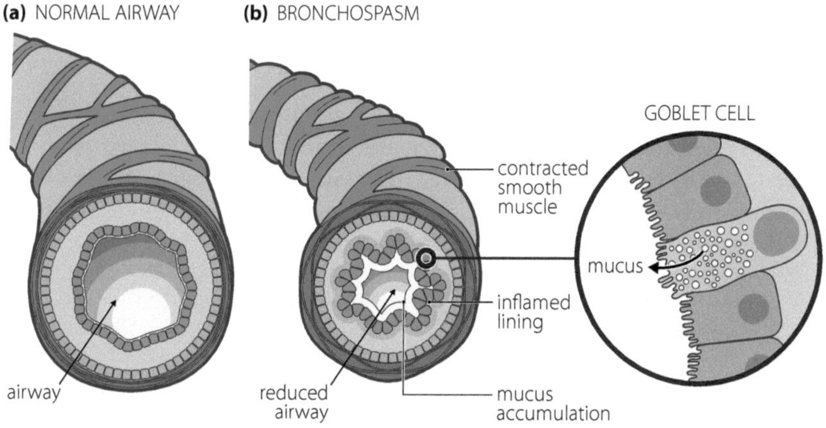

(a) NORMAL AIRWAY   **(b)** BRONCHOSPASM

GOBLET CELL

contracted smooth muscle

mucus

inflamed lining

airway

reduced airway

mucus accumulation

Fig. 6.15 Congested airways blocked by the constriction of the surrounding smooth muscle fibres, inflamed membranes lining the bronchioles and the accumulation of mucus.

Box 6.30 COPD is an inflammatory response to long-term exposure to noxious particles, particularly from cigarette smoke, so it mainly affects those over 40 with a history of smoking or the inhalation of airborne pollutants. In severe cases normal activities are impossible (→ Fig. 6.16).

6.7.3 Chronic obstructive pulmonary disease

Chronic obstructive pulmonary disease (COPD) has symptoms similar to asthma; it differs in being irreversible or only partly reversible because the air sacs become damaged (→ Box 6.30). Two forms of COPD are:
- **emphysema** – the air sacs in the lungs become permanently damaged, causing a decrease in respiratory function (→ Box 6.31)
- **chronic bronchitis** (→ 6.8.2).

Box 6.31 People with COPD have difficulty exhaling all the carbon dioxide they produce, so it accumulates in tissues. This leads to **respiratory acidosis** causing symptoms such as headaches, confusion and lethargy.

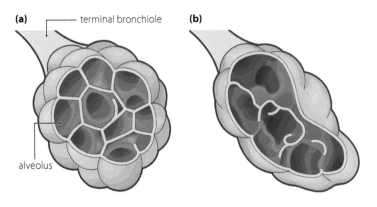

Fig 6.16 (**a**) Normal, and (**b**) damaged alveoli.

6.8 Respiratory tract infections

Respiratory tract infections (RTIs) are any infection of the sinuses, throat, airways or lungs. They are usually caused by viruses (→ Box 6.32), but sometimes by bacteria. For many, easing the symptoms is all that is necessary, allowing time for the immune system to fight off the infection. If necessary, bacterial infections may be treated with antibiotics which aim to destroy the bacteria and allow the symptoms to disappear. Antibiotics have no effect on viruses but antiviral drugs may be suitable.

6.8.1 Upper respiratory tract infections

Upper respiratory tract infections (URTIs) are among the most common acute illnesses and tend to be self-limiting syndromes with profuse nasal secretions and/or cough (→ Box 6.33).

Common cold

The common cold is a viral infection that causes inflammation of the mucous membranes of the nose, throat and bronchial tubes. The virus is transmitted by coughing and sneezing; the symptoms appear 1–2 days after infection and last about a week. Although usually mild, it can be serious in babies and in patients with a pre-existing respiratory disorder or low immunity (→ Box 6.34).

Influenza

Influenza is a highly contagious viral infection mainly spread by droplets, but also by touching a surface or object that has virus particles on it. Besides causing sore throat, cough and a runny or stuffy nose, other symptoms are fever, headache, aching muscles and fatigue. Most people recover completely in 1 to 2 weeks, but some develop serious complications, e.g. pneumonia. There are different strains of the influenza virus and infection rates around the world are influenced by the seasons. Flu vaccine is available to protect against the currently circulating influenza viruses.

Pertussis

Pertussis (whooping cough) is a highly contagious bacterial infection of the lungs and airways. It causes repeated coughing bouts that can last for two to three months, or occasionally even longer. The bacteria attached to the

Box 6.32 The most common virus infections are the rhinoviruses (the main cause of the common cold), respiratory syncytial virus (RSV) and influenza. These infections are so common that few people escape multiple infections in their lifetime. Since we generate antibodies (→ 14.6) each time we are infected, people tend to get fewer colds as they get older.

Box 6.33 Children tend to get more upper RTIs than adults because they have not built up immunity to the many viruses that can cause these infections.

Box 6.34 Coronaviruses are a large family of viruses that can cause illness. In humans, coronaviruses cause respiratory infections including the common cold and more severe diseases including severe acute respiratory syndrome (SARS). A recently emerged coronavirus is the cause of the pandemic infection COVID-19.

cilia in the trachea release toxins which increase resistance by narrowing the airways, causing the characteristic "whoop" on inspiration.

The pathogen only infects humans and people can be infected at any age although babies and young children, especially those under 6 months of age, are usually the most severely affected and at increased risk of serious medical complications (→ Box 6.35).

Sinusitis, **pharyngitis**, **tonsillitis**, **laryngitis** and **tracheitis** are other examples of infections of the upper respiratory tract.

6.8.2 Lower respiratory tract infections

Bronchitis

Bronchitis is obstructive inflammation of the lining of the bronchi – the main airways of the lungs. The inflammation leads to increased secretion of mucus with impaired activity of cilia to clear it, which leads to characteristic yellow phlegm, and coughing to clear it. It may take several weeks for the lining to repair and renew itself, so a cough may continue even after the infection has been cleared.

- **Acute bronchitis** – the infection usually clears up within two weeks.
- **Chronic bronchitis** – the infection is severe, long-lasting, and damages the lungs. Typically, mucus, neutrophils and **exudate** – the mass of cells and fluid that seeps out of inflamed blood vessels – accumulate in the small airways. These contribute to the obstruction of airflow, especially during expiration. It is often a complication that arises because of irritation and injury to the bronchial walls after many years of exposure to cigarette smoke. Also additional goblet cells are often present, making extra mucus which bacteria can adhere to and increasing the risk of infection (→ Box 6.36).

Pneumonia

Pneumonia is infection of lung tissue with bacteria or viruses that cause the alveoli and smaller bronchioles to become inflamed and filled with fluid. This reduces the area for gas exchange and makes breathing difficult. Other symptoms are fever, headaches, cough, chest pain and malaise. Elderly people, infants, and young children are at highest risk, as are people with reduced immunity such as those with human immunodeficiency virus (HIV) or those who have organ or tissue transplants.

Pneumonia is classified as:
- **lobar** – affecting one lobe of a lung
- **multifocal** (**bronchopneumonia**) – affecting more than one lung
- **interstitial** – affecting the areas between the alveoli.

The affected person will become increasingly deprived of oxygen (**hypoxaemia**) while retaining carbon dioxide (**hypercapnia**), so their breathing rate becomes very rapid (**tachypnoea**) and the accessory muscles (→ 6.5.1) are often recruited.

Cough will be the most persistent problem but people with pneumonia also usually show signs of fast heart rate (**tachycardia**), hyperthermia, altered level of consciousness and cyanosis.

Box 6.35 People who are at high risk of upper respiratory tract infections, e.g. babies, young children and the elderly, are offered vaccination against pertussis.

Box 6.36 Bronchiolitis is inflammation of the bronchioles that tends to affect babies and children under two years of age. It is often caused by the **respiratory syncytial virus (RSV)** which attacks the epithelium of their small, narrow airways and triggers an inflammatory response. This results in coughing, wheezing and shortness of breath which can cause difficulties in feeding.

Acute respiratory distress syndrome

Acute respiratory distress syndrome (ARDS) is trauma to the lung caused by pneumonia, septic shock or breathing in noxious chemicals. When this happens it can lead to major inflammation that results in a build-up of fluid in the alveoli which prevents gaseous exchange from taking place. The lungs become heavy, stiff and increasingly difficult to expand (reduced compliance). Typically, patients in whom ARDS develops will need to be cared for in an intensive care unit (→ Box 6.37).

Tuberculosis

Tuberculosis (TB) is a bacterial infection that mainly affects the lungs but can spread to many other parts of the body. It is caused by a bacterium (→ 15.2) belonging to the *Mycobacterium tuberculosis* complex, which includes *M. tuberculosis*, *M. africanum*, *M. bovis* and some rare bacteria such as *M. microti* and *M. pinnipedii*. The pathogen is caught through inhaling tiny droplets of fluid from the coughs or sneezes of an infected person. The disease develops slowly and symptoms may not appear for many months or years after a person is infected. Typical symptoms include a persistent cough, blood-tinged sputum, weight loss and night sweats. Treatment is with antibiotics and if resistance to one type of antibiotic develops, other types can be tried. If left untreated, damage to the lungs and breathlessness develop, and eventually death occurs (→ Box 6.38).

Pleurisy

Pleurisy is inflammation of the pleura – the double layer covering the lungs (→ 6.3.2). The pleural fluid becomes sticky, making deep breathing painful (→ Box 6.39).

Box 6.37 Diagnosis of specific pathogens by blood culture or nasopharyngeal specimens may happen if a person is acutely ill in hospital because this can help clinicians to target therapy.

Box 6.38 People at high risk of tuberculosis infection can be vaccinated against it.

Box 6.39 Medical treatment may not be needed for pleurisy caused by a viral infection. Bacterial infection of the pleura will usually need to be treated with antibiotics.

Key points

1. The respiratory tract is the pathway through which air is conducted between the atmosphere and the lungs.
2. The pharynx serves as a common conduit for air and food.
3. The trachea branches repeatedly into smaller and smaller tubes that eventually end in alveoli where gaseous exchange takes place between air and blood.
4. Breathing is homeostatically regulated by respiratory centres in the brain, which control the action of intercostal muscles, diaphragm and accessory muscles needed for ventilation.
5. Oxygen is carried in blood by haemoglobin and is consumed by cells in aerobic respiration which yields adenosine triphosphate (ATP).
6. Carbon dioxide is produced by cells and transported to the lungs where it is eliminated.

Test yourself! Go to *www.lanternpublishing.com/AandP* and try the questions to check your understanding.

CHAPTER 7
THE DIGESTIVE SYSTEM

The digestive system comprises the alimentary canal and accessory organs of digestion – the salivary glands, liver and pancreas. As food moves through the alimentary canal it is broken down into nutrient molecules that are small enough to be absorbed through the gut wall into the bloodstream. The nutrients are first taken to the liver for processing and then distributed around the body for use by the cells.

7.1 Alimentary canal

The **alimentary canal**, or **gut** (→ Fig. 7.1), is a food-processing tube about 9 m long in adults which extends from the mouth to the anus. The food inside the tube is not available to the body until it has been digested and absorbed through the gut wall. The undigested remains form faeces and are expelled from the body through the anus.

Taking it Further
There is more information about nutrition and dietary choices in online Chapter 19.

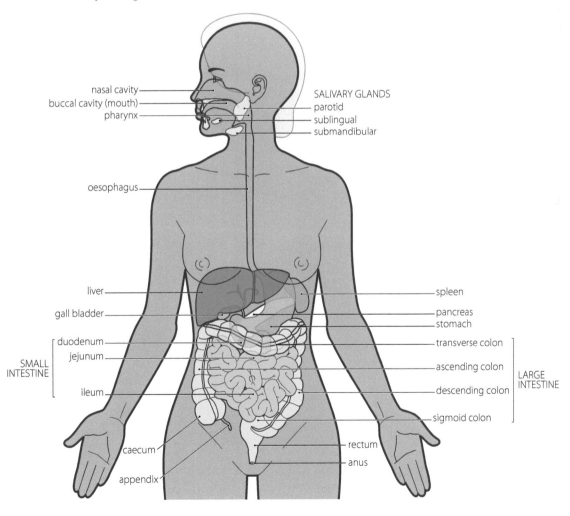

Fig. 7.1 The digestive system.

7.1.1 Peritoneum

The **peritoneum** is thin, tough, fibrous connective tissue that lines the abdominal cavity and covers all the organs inside the abdomen. It has a moist, slippery surface which allows easy movement of the organs against each other as food passes through the alimentary canal. The intestines are loosely attached to the back of the abdomen by the **mesentery** which is formed from a double layer of peritoneum, with arteries, veins, lymph vessels and nerves between the layers.

7.1.2 Gastrointestinal tract

The **gastrointestinal (GI) tract** is formed by the oesophagus, stomach and intestines (→ Box 7.1). Its wall is constructed to move food through the tract without itself being digested by the enzymes in the digestive juices, and has four layers (→ Fig. 7.2):
- **serosa** – a thin, tough outer layer which is smooth and moist and allows the parts of the GI tract to move smoothly against other organs as food material is pushed through (→ Box 7.2)
- **muscularis externa** – smooth muscle tissue responsible for peristalsis. The muscle fibres in the inner part of this layer are arranged in a circular manner, whereas in the outer part they are arranged lengthways

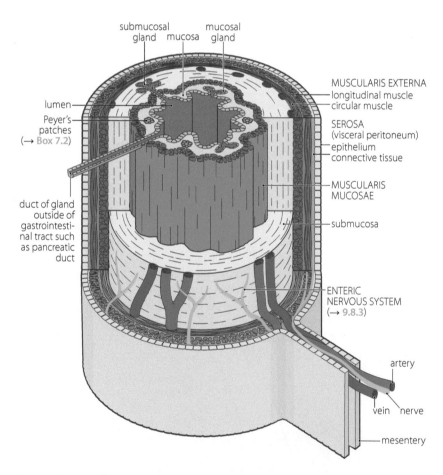

Fig. 7.2 Section of the gastrointestinal tract showing the different layers.

- **submucosa** – a layer of loose connective tissue; variations in the thickness of this layer create folds and ridges
- **muscularis mucosa** – a continuous sheet of smooth muscle tissue.
- **mucosa** – an inner layer of mucous membrane which lines the GI tract and continuously secretes mucus; this thick, sticky substance prevents the wall from being damaged by the digestive juices and, being slippery, facilitates the movement of food along the tract.

7.1.3 Gastrointestinal transit time

Gastrointestinal (GI) transit time is the length of time it takes for food to travel through the GI tract, and this varies according to factors such as diet, physical activity, medication and GI surgery. Roughly, it takes less than an hour after a meal for 50% of the contents of the stomach (called **chyme**) to empty into the intestines, with total emptying taking about 2 hours; 50% emptying of the small intestine takes 1–2 hours, and transit through the colon takes 12 to 50 hours.

7.1.4 Gastrointestinal motility

Gastrointestinal motility is a term used to describe the rhythmic contraction and relaxation of the smooth muscles that moves food through the GI tract, churning it up and mixing it with the digestive juices as it moves along to the rectum and anus. Two types of movement are involved – peristalsis and segmentation.

Peristalsis

Peristalsis is the rhythmic wave-like movements of the gut wall that normally push (squeeze) the contents forwards in one direction only (→ Fig. 7.3a). The squeezing movements are produced by the alternate contraction of circular and longitudinal muscles. When the circular muscles behind the bolus of food contract (❶), the longitudinal muscles relax and the bolus is pushed onwards (❷). **Vomiting** is reverse peristalsis (→ Box 7.3).

Box 7.3 Vomiting (**emesis**) is the result of forceful contractions of the diaphragm and abdominal muscles which increase gastric pressure. When the cardiac sphincter relaxes (→ Fig. 7.10), gastric contents are ejected. Vomiting is often accompanied by sweating and tachycardia (increased heart rate) because the sympathetic division is activated (→ 9.8.2), but the person often feels relieved when the pressure is reduced.

Stages of emesis
The first stage is usually the feeling of nausea, which may come in waves, and increased salivation, which helps to protect tooth enamel from the damaging effects of acid and enzymes.

Retching (dry heaving) is a series of spasmodic respiratory movements against a closed glottis which precedes vomiting. The upper segment of the stomach and lower oesophagus relax, and reverse peristalsis propels the contents of the intestine and stomach through the pyloric sphincter.

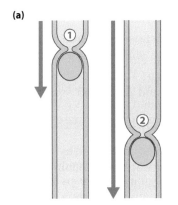
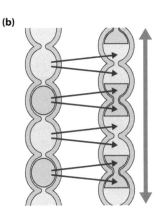

Fig. 7.3 (**a**) Peristalsis in the oesophagus; (**b**) segmentation in the small intestine.

Segmentation

Segmentation dominates in the intestines, especially the small intestine. The muscle tissue in the intestine wall contracts in segments, and as the food is squeezed it is pushed both backwards and forwards, churning it up at the same time (→ Fig. 7.3b). While peristalsis results in movement of food through the digestive system, segmentation slows the progress down, giving time for the digestive juices to act on the intestinal contents and the opportunity for the nutrients to be absorbed through the gut wall.

7.2 Principles of digestion

Digestion is a breaking down process which is either mechanical or chemical.

- **Mechanical digestion** includes the chewing of food in the mouth, churning it in the stomach and the processes of peristalsis and segmentation in the intestines.
- **Chemical digestion** depends on the use of digestive **enzymes** to break down the carbohydrates, fat and protein in food into simpler nutrients that can be absorbed into the body and used by the cells. The digestive enzymes act on food in the mouth, stomach and small intestine (→ Box 7.4).

Substances that remain unchanged by the digestive process are:

- small molecules such as water, glucose, vitamins and minerals
- fibre, which is resistant to digestion in the small intestine but is partly or completely broken down by the gut microbiota in the colon (→ 7.7.2).

7.2.1 Regulation of digestion

The digestive process starts by thinking about food or smelling it, which stimulates the salivary glands to secrete saliva. When a person is feeling relaxed and calm, the **parasympathetic division** of the autonomic nervous system is dominant and secretion of digestive juices and peristalsis are increased; when involved in exercising or feeling worried or frightened, the **sympathetic division** is dominant and the digestive process is inhibited (→ Box 7.5).

After food has been swallowed, digestion is an involuntary process regulated by the **enteric nervous system** (→ Box 7.6). In addition, hormones are produced by cells scattered among endocrine cells in the mucosal glands of the GI tract. For example:

- **gastrin** is secreted in the pyloric region of the stomach wall and circulates in the blood to the rest of the stomach wall where it stimulates the production of gastric juice
- **secretin** is secreted by cells in the duodenal wall when acidified chyme leaves the stomach. It stimulates the secretion of alkaline pancreatic juice to counteract the acid in the chyme, allowing the intestinal enzymes to act, and it also stimulates the secretion of bile
- **cholecystokinin** (**CCK**) is a signalling molecule secreted by cells of the duodenal wall; when the acidic chyme enters the duodenum it makes the gall bladder contract and squirt out bile containing CCK (→ Box 7.7)
- **incretins** are secreted by the gastrointestinal wall and signal to the pancreas to secrete insulin.

7.2.2 The need for water

Digestion can only take place in an aqueous medium, as water is required to turn solid food into a suspension that allows the many chemical reactions to take place and enables the absorption of nutrients. Between 7 and 9 litres

Box 7.4 Enzymes are **catalysts**, that is, they speed up chemical reactions and work best in optimal conditions of temperature and pH. The temperature inside the body is more or less constant, but the pH in the digestive tract varies according to the requirements of the enzymes in the mouth, stomach and small intestine (→ 20.8.3).

Box 7.5 Although the digestive system can operate independently of the brain and spinal cord, the nervous system exerts a very profound effect on the process of digestion through its involuntary division, which is known as the enteric nervous system (→ 9.8.3).

Box 7.6 The enteric nervous system (ENS) is a subset of the nervous system which contains extensive neural circuits that lie within the sheaths of tissue lining the alimentary canal. These circuits are essential for generating motility of the digestive system and for coordinating secretion of digestive juices.

Box 7.7 As well as acting within the digestive system, cholecystokinin (CCK) has an important role within the central nervous system. CCK acts on receptor proteins (→ 11.2.1) that are widely distributed in cell membranes and it is thought to suppress feelings of hunger.

of fluid pass in and out of the digestive tract each day. Approximately 1.5 litres is contained in ingested food and drink, the rest in the digestive juices secreted by the accessory organs of digestion – salivary glands, gastric glands, pancreas, liver and intestinal glands. Besides water, digestive juices contain varying proportions of enzymes, hormones, mucus, and electrolytes (e.g. H^+ HCO_3^-) (→ 20.8.2). Nearly all of the fluid is reabsorbed in the colon so that faeces normally contain only a small volume of water.

7.3 Accessory organs of digestion

7.3.1 Salivary glands

The three pairs of salivary glands open into the mouth near the tongue (→ Fig. 7.1). The saliva they produce is an alkaline fluid that:
- keeps the mouth moist, which aids chewing and swallowing (→ Box 7.8)
- enables dry food to be tasted
- contains the enzyme **amylase** that starts the digestion of starch
- has antibacterial properties; when the flow of saliva is poor, the mouth is more susceptible to infections, e.g. candidiasis (thrush)
- counteracts acidity in the mouth, making teeth less vulnerable to dental caries and the gums to gingivitis (→ Box 7.9).

7.3.2 Liver

The liver is the second largest organ in the body, with only the skin being larger and heavier. It is dark reddish-brown, situated beneath the diaphragm in the upper right side of the abdomen and protected by the ribcage. The liver consists of two main lobes, each with eight segments containing many lobules connected to small ducts (→ Fig. 7.4).

Box 7.8 Tasting food is quite a complex process (→ 10.5) and is under the control of the autonomic nervous system (→ 9.8) which can increase saliva production by up to 10-fold compared to baseline when chewing something with an intense taste.

Saliva contributes to oral homeostasis but its volume and composition can be affected by the person's psychological state, by a wide range of different disorders and by some medications.

Box 7.9 Patients with a dry mouth and who also have their own teeth should be given non-acidic, sugar-free saliva substitutes, mouth washes and dietary advice.

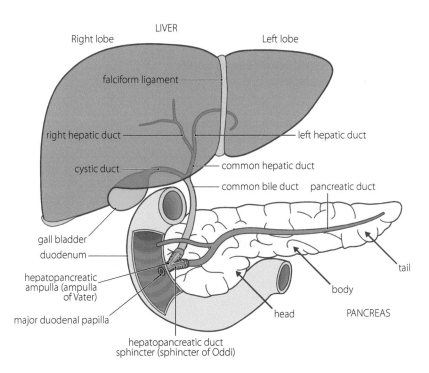

Fig. 7.4 Liver and pancreas arranged to show the hepatopancreatic duct.

Vessels connected to the liver

The liver is unusual because it receives blood from two sources – oxygenated blood from the hepatic artery and deoxygenated but nutrient-rich blood from the intestine via the hepatic portal vein. Blood then drains from the liver via one vessel – the hepatic vein – and is returned to the circulation via the inferior vena cava (→ Fig. 7.5).

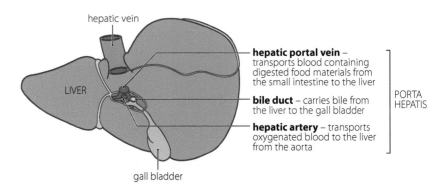

Fig. 7.5 Vessels connected to the undersurface of the liver (the hepatic vein is obscured from view).

Structure of the liver

The liver is composed of units called **lobules** (→ Fig. 7.6). Each lobule contains rows of **hepatocytes** (liver cells) which radiate out from a **central vein**. The hepatocytes are in close contact with blood-filled **sinusoids** (→ Box 7.10), and also lie adjacent to **canaliculi** into which bile is secreted. Branches of the hepatic artery, hepatic portal vein and bile duct are clustered together at the edge of the lobule, forming what is called the **portal triad**. Blood flows into the lobule through the hepatic portal venules and hepatic arterioles and mixes together before flowing through the sinusoids to the central vein and on to the hepatic vein.

Liver tissue

The two main types of cells in liver tissue are:
- **hepatocytes** – cuboidal epithelial cells that line the sinusoids and perform most of the liver's functions (→ Box 7.11)
- **Kupffer cells** – specialised macrophages that capture and break down old, worn-out red blood cells passing through the sinusoids.

Regeneration

The liver possesses the remarkable capacity to heal and regenerate quickly to its normal size and functions, either after surgical removal of a part or when damaged by disease (→ Box 7.12).

7.3.3 Pancreas

The pancreas is a whitish-coloured gland, about 15 cm long, situated at the back of the abdomen behind the lower part of the stomach (→ Fig. 7.4). Large amounts of pancreatic juice are rapidly secreted by the acinar cells soon after food is eaten, which drains into small ducts that open into the pancreatic duct (→ Fig. 7.7). The pancreatic duct unites with the bile duct before opening into the duodenum (→ Box 7.13).

Box 7.10 A liver sinusoid is a type of vessel in which oxygen-rich blood from the hepatic artery mixes with the nutrient-rich blood from the hepatic portal vein.

Box 7.11 The liver performs hundreds of functions that are essential to homeostasis. The hepatocytes are able to regulate nutrient levels and synthesise (make) substances that are needed elsewhere in the body from the raw materials delivered from the digestive tract.

Box 7.12 A healthy liver should contain few or no fat deposits, but if fat builds up in the liver cells it can cause **non-alcoholic fatty liver disease (NAFLD)**, a relatively common condition in people who are overweight or obese.

Box 7.13 Besides its role in the digestive system, the pancreas is also part of the endocrine system (→ 11.6). The two pancreatic hormones – insulin and glucagon – are produced in the islets of Langerhans and are carried around the body in the bloodstream. Their function is the homeostasis of blood sugar (→ 1.3.2).

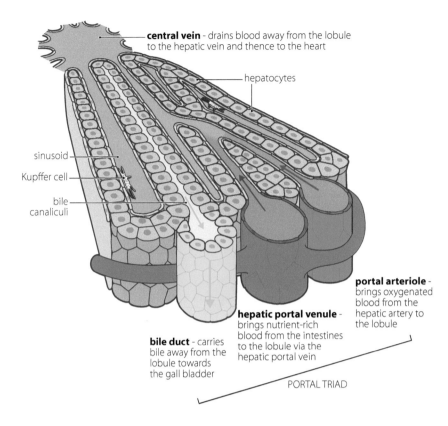

central vein - drains blood away from the lobule to the hepatic vein and thence to the heart

hepatocytes

sinusoid

Kupffer cell

bile canaliculi

portal arteriole - brings oxygenated blood from the hepatic artery to the lobule

hepatic portal venule - brings nutrient-rich blood from the intestines to the lobule via the hepatic portal vein

bile duct - carries bile away from the lobule towards the gall bladder

PORTAL TRIAD

Fig. 7.6 Microscopic structure of part of a lobule.

Pancreatic juice

Pancreatic juice is an alkaline mixture containing:

- **bicarbonate ions** (HCO_3^-) that neutralise the hydrochloric acid from the stomach, stop the action of pepsin (→ 7.5.1), and allow the pancreatic enzymes to act on the food in the small intestine
- three pancreatic enzymes – **lipase**, **amylase** and **trypsin**. Trypsin is a **protease** (protein-digesting enzyme) and is secreted by pancreatic cells in its inactive form called **zymogen** (→ Box 7.14).

Box 7.14 The zymogen molecules are only activated when they reach the lumen of the intestine – a process that requires a third enzyme called **enterokinase**. (Mucus protects the lumen wall from proteases.)

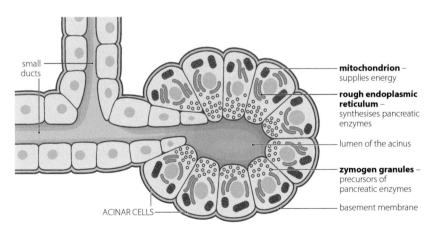

small ducts

mitochondrion – supplies energy

rough endoplasmic reticulum – synthesises pancreatic enzymes

lumen of the acinus

zymogen granules – precursors of pancreatic enzymes

basement membrane

ACINAR CELLS

Fig. 7.7 Acinar cells surrounding a duct.

7.4 Oral phase of digestion

7.4.1 Buccal cavity

The oral phase of digestion, also called the **cephalic phase** since it is a conscious process, takes place in the buccal cavity – the mouth (→ Fig. 7.8). Oral mucosa lines the buccal cavity and the oesophagus and protects the underlying tissues from mechanical damage and microorganisms. It consists of stratified squamous epithelium containing numerous minor salivary glands. These, together with the three pairs of much larger salivary glands, produce mucus that helps to keep the interior of the mouth moist (→ Box 7.15). **Saliva** contains the enzyme **amylase**, which begins the digestion of starch. Mouth ulcers may form, most often on the inside of the cheeks or lips (→ Box 7.16).

> **Box 7.15** Some medications including chemotherapy agents, antibiotics and diuretics (→ Chapter 18) may reduce salivary gland function. Since a dry mouth can cause swallowing and speech difficulties, an important aspect of healthcare practice is to ensure that water or other drinks are at hand. Some people may need artificial saliva or mouth gel, which helps to keep the interior of the mouth moist.

> **Box 7.16 Mouth ulcers** are small, painful sores that form in the mouth due to injuries, e.g. biting the cheek, or poorly fitting dentures.
>
> Mouth ulcers of unknown cause are known as **aphthous stomatitis** (canker sores) and these often cause discomfort and pain. They can be the result of infections (e.g. herpes) or immune defects (e.g. leukaemia or HIV), or chemotherapy.

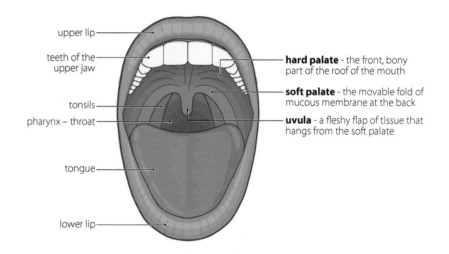

Fig. 7.8 Buccal cavity.

Lips

Lips surround the opening to the mouth. The skin is thinner here than elsewhere in the body and has fewer melanocytes, allowing the blood vessels to show through. The lips are usually a reddish colour, but bluish (cyanosed) when the body is cold. There are no hairs, sweat glands or sebaceous glands in the skin of the lips, and the lack of sebum to keep the skin moist means that it dries out faster and becomes chapped more easily than skin elsewhere on the body. Lips are muscular structures that play a key role in the formation of facial gestures, sounds and speech as well as in eating (→ Box 7.17).

> **Box 7.17** Lips are important sensory organs and are **erogenous zones** – parts of the body that excite sexual feelings when touched or stimulated, e.g. kissing and intimate activity.

Cheeks

Cheeks form the side walls and are lined with buccal mucosa composed of squamous epithelial cells that divide about once every 24 hours to replace the cells that are continually being worn away (→ Box 7.18).

> **Box 7.18** A buccal swab collects cells from the inside of the cheeks for DNA testing.

Tongue

The tongue covers the floor of the buccal cavity. It is a large mass of skeletal muscle covered by mucosa and can move in the many directions required for chewing, swallowing and speaking. The upper surface of the tongue is normally moist, pink and covered by small projections called papillae, some with taste buds on their sides that can taste dissolved substances (→ 10.5.2).

7.4.2 Teeth

The teeth are the hard structures in the mouth needed to bite, chew and grind up food, and to speak clearly. They also affect the appearance of the face.

There are two sets of teeth. The first set – the deciduous dentition – begin to erupt when a child is a few months old, with twenty milk teeth, ten in each jaw. From the age of five onwards the roots of the milk teeth are resorbed and the crown falls out, to be replaced by larger permanent teeth. When complete, the permanent set contains 32 teeth, sixteen in each jaw (→ Fig. 7.9).

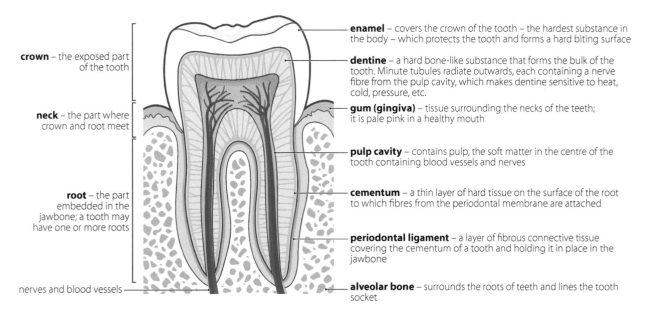

crown – the exposed part of the tooth

neck – the part where crown and root meet

root – the part embedded in the jawbone; a tooth may have one or more roots

nerves and blood vessels

enamel – covers the crown of the tooth – the hardest substance in the body – which protects the tooth and forms a hard biting surface

dentine – a hard bone-like substance that forms the bulk of the tooth. Minute tubules radiate outwards, each containing a nerve fibre from the pulp cavity, which makes dentine sensitive to heat, cold, pressure, etc.

gum (gingiva) – tissue surrounding the necks of the teeth; it is pale pink in a healthy mouth

pulp cavity – contains pulp, the soft matter in the centre of the tooth containing blood vessels and nerves

cementum – a thin layer of hard tissue on the surface of the root to which fibres from the periodontal membrane are attached

periodontal ligament – a layer of fibrous connective tissue covering the cementum of a tooth and holding it in place in the jawbone

alveolar bone – surrounds the roots of teeth and lines the tooth socket

Fig. 7.9 Section through a tooth with two roots.

Dental caries

Dental caries is tooth decay and is one of the most common causes of toothache (→ Box 7.19). Cavities develop when the bacteria in dental plaque on the teeth use sugar from the diet to produce acid, which dissolves the tooth surface (→ Chapter 19). If caries reaches the dental pulp it can cause infection that may lead to a dental abscess (→ Box 7.20).

Gingivitis

Gingivitis is inflammation of the superficial pink gums. The first sign is usually bleeding gums when the teeth are being brushed or sometimes spontaneously. The condition is common and associated with poor dental hygiene and retention of dental plaque on teeth (→ Box 7.21).

Periodontitis

Periodontitis – the most common cause of tooth loss in adults – is inflammation of the alveolar bone and periodontal ligament that support teeth and gums. Periodontitis is a complex inflammatory and immune

Box 7.19 Preventable tooth decay is the most common reason why 5–9-year-olds in England are admitted to hospital, some for multiple tooth extractions under general anaesthetic.

Box 7.20 Dry mouth increases the risk of dental decay because the protective layer of saliva is changed or reduced. People with dry mouth should take care to avoid sugary drinks and use high fluoride toothpaste. They are also prone to ulcers due to trauma on the unlubricated mucosal surface.

Box 7.21 People presenting with bleeding gums should be advised to see a dentist or a dental hygienist.

Box 7.22 Research shows associations between type 2 diabetes, cardiovascular disease, rheumatoid arthritis and adverse pregnancy outcomes. Links to other conditions are emerging.

Box 7.23 Something like 50 muscles are involved in swallowing, so people – including children – who have dysphagia (difficulty in swallowing) may gag or choke on their food or liquid when they are trying to swallow. The experience can cause people to lose their appetite, skip meals or avoid eating.

A wide range of different causes can lead to difficulty in swallowing, including developmental problems, learning disability, multiple sclerosis (MS), Parkinson's disease, oesophageal cancer and Alzheimer's disease.

Specialised imaging techniques (→ 17.2) can help with diagnosis. Treatment strategies vary, but helping people with dysphagia to swallow food often involves allied health professionals, e.g. dietitian, pharmacist/prescriber, occupational therapist and speech therapist.

Box 7.24 Dyspepsia (indigestion; heartburn) is pain or discomfort in the upper abdomen after eating. It is caused by stomach acid coming into contact with the mucosa that lines the wall of oesophagus and stomach. The acid breaks down the mucosa, leading to inflammation (redness and swelling).

disease mediated by dental plaque and is worse in people who are high risk. Risk factors include smoking, family history of early tooth loss, diabetes and stress (→ Box 7.22).

7.4.3 Digestion in the mouth and swallowing

When food is ingested it is mixed with saliva which moistens it, making the food easier to chew and swallow. The enzyme in saliva – **salivary amylase** – begins the digestion of starch by breaking it down into the sugar called maltose.

Deglutition (swallowing)

The swallow reflex is a complex neuromuscular activity. The muscular tongue helps to make the food into a **bolus** (rounded mass) and push it up against the hard palate and into the pharynx. Touch receptors in the palate and pharynx stimulate the reflex action that pushes the bolus to the back of the mouth and into the oesophagus.

During swallowing, the respiratory centre is inhibited and breathing stops while swallowing (**deglutition apnoea**). At the same time, the bolus is prevented from 'going the wrong way' because the soft palate closes the entrance to the nose and the epiglottis covers the entrance to the trachea.

In its resting state, the oesophagus is almost flat but opens up as the bolus is pushed by peristalsis along the tube and to the stomach. The **cardiac sphincter** (→ Fig. 7.10a) is the ring of muscle that acts as a valve. When the muscle relaxes, the sphincter opens and allows food into the stomach, then contracts and closes to prevent the stomach contents from moving back into the oesophagus.

Dysphagia is difficulty in swallowing and passing food from mouth to stomach which may include coughing or choking when eating or drinking. It can be due to abnormal nerve or muscle control that can occur, e.g. after a stroke or head injury, or in people with dementia or cancer (→ Box 7.23).

7.5 Gastric phase of digestion

The gastric phase of digestion takes place in the stomach, which is situated below the diaphragm and partly under the liver. The stomach is a muscular bag in which food is stored, mixed with gastric juice and partly digested. When empty it is almost flat but swells as it fills up with food, then gradually collapses as it empties. The **pyloric sphincter** controls the passage of chyme (the partly digested food) from the stomach into the duodenum – the first part of the small intestine. The sphincter relaxes at intervals allowing a small quantity of food to pass from the stomach into the duodenum.

7.5.1 Gastric juice

The stomach is lined with **gastric mucosa** – a much-folded and highly specialised layer of epithelium. The goblet cells secrete a thick layer of mucus that protects the stomach wall from the corrosive effects of gastric juice produced by the numerous **gastric glands** at the base of the **gastric pits** (→ Box 7.24). The several million gastric pits are tubular exocrine glands in the mucosa that secrete gastric juice into the lumen of the stomach (→ Fig. 7.10).

Gastric juice contains:

- **hydrochloric acid**, which provides an acid medium that allows the stomach enzymes to work effectively. The hydrochloric acid in the stomach has a pH of 1–2 which is lethal to many pathogens and helps to protect the body against pathogens ingested in food and water. An exception is ***Helicobacter pylori*** – a bacterium that can thrive in acid conditions and can cause peptic ulcers (→ Box 7.25)
- protein-digesting enzymes – rennin and pepsin. **Pepsin** starts the digestion of protein by splitting it into peptides; **rennin** curdles milk and is important in infancy (→ Box 7.26)
- **intrinsic factor** – necessary for the absorption of vitamin B_{12} in the ileum of the small intestine.

> **Box 7.25 Peptic ulcers** are open sores that develop on the lining of the stomach (gastric ulcers) or the duodenum (duodenal ulcers), commonly causing severe pain in the centre of the abdomen. The two main causes are *Helicobacter pylori* (*H. pylori*) bacteria and **non-steroidal anti-inflammatory drugs** (**NSAIDs**) such as ibuprofen or aspirin which are used to relieve pain.

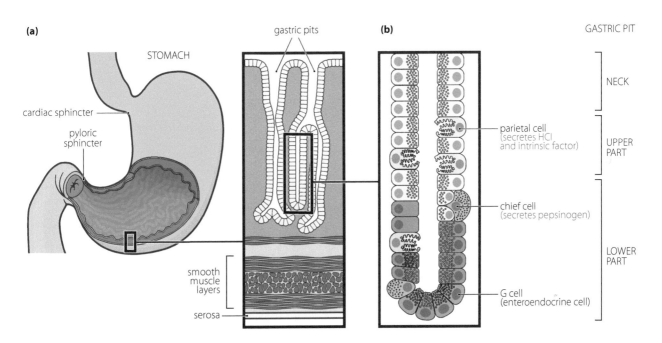

Fig. 7.10 (**a**) Stomach; (**b**) gastric pits in the stomach lining.

Gastric motility

Gastric motility results from strong peristaltic waves that travel from the cardiac sphincter towards the pyloric region at about three times a minute. These contractions of the smooth muscle tissue in the stomach wall crush the ingested food into smaller particles and mix it with gastric juice to form a liquified mixture called **chyme**.

Gastric emptying is the process of using the peristalsis contractions to push small amounts of chyme through the pyloric sphincter into the duodenum, at intervals.

> **Box 7.26** Rennin (also known as chymosin) assists the digestion of milk in infants by preventing the rapid passage of the liquid through the digestive system. Because curdled milk is lumpy, it stays longer in the digestive tract, which gives time for digestion and absorption.

7.6 Intestinal phase of digestion

The function of the small intestine is digestion of food and absorption of nutrients. It is basically a long tube coiled into loops and filling most of the abdominal cavity (→ Fig. 7.1). It has three regions:

- **duodenum** – the first part which receives bile from the gall bladder and pancreatic juice from the pancreas
- **jejunum** – the middle section
- **ileum** – the last part which connects with the colon and is where most absorption of nutrients takes place. It also contains **mucosa-associated lymphoid tissue** (**MALT**). MALT contains lymphatic tissue that identifies and destroys potentially harmful substances passing through the gut (→ Box 7.27).

7.6.1 Glands of the small intestine

Brunner's glands

Brunner's glands are found in the first section of duodenum (→ Fig. 7.11). Their main function is to produce alkaline secretions which protect the lining of the duodenum from acid chyme from the stomach, and neutralise the chyme. They also provide the optimal environment for chemical digestion by intestinal enzymes, and secrete the hormone secretin (→ 7.2.1).

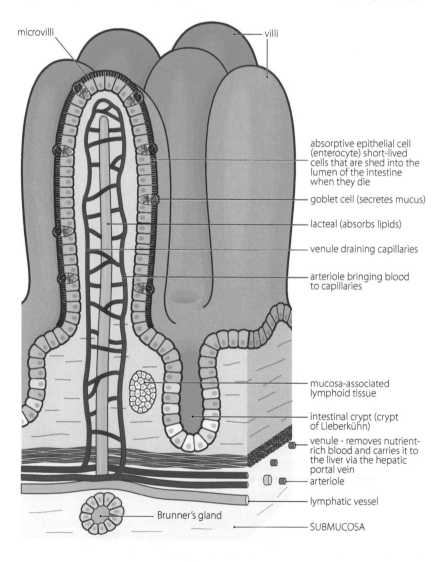

Fig. 7.11 Structure of the intestine wall showing the villi.

Crypts of Lieberkühn

Crypts of Lieberkühn are invaginations shaped like narrow tubes containing stem cells and Paneth cells.
- **Stem cells** at the base of the crypts divide to form new epithelial cells which migrate up the walls of the crypts to become part of the absorption epithelium of the villus. Loss of control of the rate of proliferation of these cells contributes to colon cancer.
- **Paneth cells** are found within the crypts close to the stem cells. Their function is not entirely understood but one theory is that they are important in protecting the stem cells from damage by secreting antimicrobial intestinal juice.

7.6.2 Chemical digestion in the small intestine

When chyme enters the small intestine, the hydrochloric acid it contains is neutralised by sodium bicarbonate ($NaHCO_3$) secreted from glands in the intestine wall, which also stops the action of pepsin. As the chyme is slowly pushed through the small intestine by the rhythmic movements of peristalsis, it is churned up by the segmentation contractions and mixed with the digestive juices – bile, pancreatic juice and intestinal juice.

Bile is made in the liver and stored in the gall bladder. It contains:
- bile acids containing cholesterol which helps to emulsify fats, breaking them down into tiny globules with a large surface area on which lipase, the fat-digesting enzyme, can act
- bilirubin – the yellow pigment from the breakdown of red cells, which is mostly excreted in the faeces, with a small amount excreted in urine.

Pancreatic juice contains the following enzymes for chemical digestion:
- lipase splits up the globules of fat into fatty acids and glycerol (→ Box 7.28)
- amylase splits up starch to maltose
- trypsin splits up protein to peptides.

Intestinal juice contains sodium bicarbonate ($NaHCO_3$), which makes it alkaline, and the following enzymes:
- erepsin splits up peptides to amino acids
- amylase continues the digestion of starch to maltose
- maltase splits up maltose to glucose
- sucrase splits up sucrose to glucose and fructose
- lactase splits up lactose to glucose and galactose (→ Box 7.29).

7.6.3 Absorption in the small intestine

Absorption is the diffusion of nutrients and water from the gut into the bloodstream. Although most of the absorption takes place in the **ileum**, a small amount of water, glucose, alcohol and other substances which do not need to be broken down further may be absorbed in the stomach. The wall of the ileum provides a very large surface area through which rapid absorption can take place because:
- it is very long – about 5 m in an adult
- the inner surface has many finger-like folds called **villi** (singular = villus)
- the cells of the villus wall have **microvilli** (→ Fig. 7.11) which are the numerous microscopic projections of the epithelial cell membranes which increase the surface area for absorption.

Box 7.28 Fat is hydrophobic, meaning that it cannot dissolve in water, but the enzyme that digests fat – lipase – is hydrophilic and functions only in an aqueous environment. To solve this problem, fat is emulsified by bile into small globules, which increases the surface area, allowing lipase to act.

Box 7.29 Lactose intolerance occurs when the body does not produce enough lactase – the enzyme that digests lactose (milk sugar) into its constituent parts (glucose and galactose). When the undigested lactose reaches the colon it is fermented by the gut microbiota (→ 7.7.2), producing symptoms that include a bloated abdomen, flatulence and diarrhoea.

Absorption of nutrients

Each villus has a very thin epithelial wall containing a blind-ended lymphatic vessel – **lacteal** – surrounded by capillaries (→ Fig. 7.11). This means that the contents of the small intestine come very close to the bloodstream so that:

- **lipids** (fats) can be absorbed through the intestine wall into the lacteals in the form of fatty acids and glycerol. Lacteals are part of the lymphatic system and the lipids are carried away in lymph vessels that join the bloodstream near the heart (→ Box 7.30)
- other **nutrient** molecules such as simple sugars, amino acids, vitamins and minerals can be absorbed through the villus wall and into the capillaries to be carried away by the **hepatic portal vein** which takes them to the liver.

Box 7.30 After a meal, lymph flowing back from the digestive tract has a milky appearance because of its high fat content and is known as chyle.

7.6.4 Processing nutrients in the liver

After nutrients in the **hepatic portal vein** reach the liver they are converted into substances that the body can use immediately or store until they are needed. This process is called **assimilation**. The liver:

- regulates the amount of glucose in the blood by converting excess glucose to glycogen for storage until required
- converts excess carbohydrates into fatty acids and triglycerides which are then transported for storage in adipose tissue
- synthesises essential amino acids from non-essential ones
- uses amino acids to synthesise proteins like albumin and clotting factors
- converts amino acids to glucose or lipids (gluconeogenesis) during periods of fasting, starvation, low-carbohydrate diets, or intense exercise
- removes excess amino acids by breaking them down into ammonia and finally urea for release into the blood and excretion by the kidneys
- synthesises cholesterol, phospholipids and lipoproteins
- stores vitamins (A, D and K) and minerals (iron and copper)
- removes alcohol, medicines and other drugs from the blood
- produces heat that helps maintain body temperature.

7.7 Large intestine

Box 7.31 The large intestine is much wider than the small intestine and has longitudinal ribbons of smooth muscle on the outside called taeniae coli. Its lining has more crypts and goblet cells than other sections of the intestine.

The large intestine (large bowel) (→ Fig. 7.12) is the final section of the alimentary canal and it has three parts – **colon**, **rectum** and **anus** (→ Box 7.31). It is attached to the abdominal wall and held in place by the mesentery which is formed by the double fold of peritoneum. The mesentery contains blood vessels, lymphatics, and nerves that supply the intestines, and it also stores fat.

7.7.1 Colon

Box 7.32 Until recently the micro-organisms in the gut microbiota were difficult to grow in culture, but the situation is changing and it is now known that each person has 500–1000 different species of bacteria amongst the trillion bacterial cells.

The waste material that passes from the small intestine into the colon is mainly water and undigested matter such as fibre. As it is moved slowly through by peristalsis and segmentation, most of the water is absorbed back into the body leaving the **faeces** – a mass of solid or semi-solid undigested food remains mixed with bacteria and other microorganisms, mucus, bilirubin and water. The distinctive smell of faeces is due to bacterial action (→ Box 7.32).

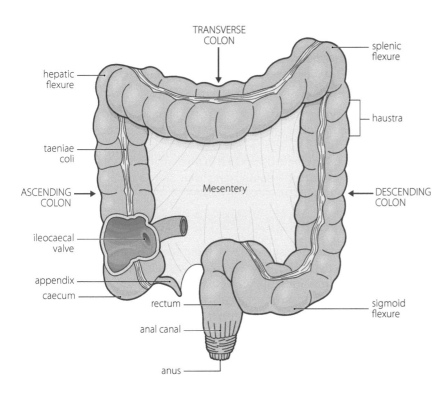

Fig. 7.12 Large intestine.

Haustra

Haustra are small pouches that are repeated along the length of the colon. They swell and distend as they fill with undigested food and contract about every 25 minutes, pushing the contents on to the next pouch. The loss of the haustral folds is characteristic in people who have ulcerative colitis.

7.7.2 Gut microbiota

The **gut microbiota** (gut flora) refers to the vast numbers of micro-organisms that live in the colon, mainly different species of bacteria with some microscopic fungi and other types of microbes (→ Box 7.33). They feed on the undigested matter in the colon and are useful to the body in a number of ways. For example, they:

- ferment some of the undigested fibre, releasing energy and nutrients for use in the body
- synthesise vitamins K and (B$_7$) biotin
- prevent the growth of harmful, pathogenic bacteria; in a healthy gut, the useful bacteria predominate and keep the harmful ones under control.

Flatulence

Flatulence is excessive gas – **flatus** – in the digestive tract. Flatus is composed partly of air that has been swallowed and partly of gas produced by the activity of the microbiota, and it is released through the anus about twelve times a day. On average, about half a litre of flatus is produced every day, the amount varing widely depending on the diet and the efficiency of the digestive system. When faeces stay too long in the colon, the contents have time to putrefy and produce larger quantities of foul-smelling gas. As there will be more time to remove water, the faeces will be drier and harder.

Taking it Further
You can find out more about common investigations of gastrointestinal function in online Chapter 17.

Box 7.33 A wide range of factors in the environment affect an individual's gut microbiota and can reveal details about that person's health, diet or ethnicity. Microbes in the gut therefore carry a unique **bacterial signature** of the human body that they colonise.

Current research is showing that the gut microbiota plays many important roles in ensuring its host's metabolic health. Sustained interactions between the host's gastrointestinal tract and the microbiota appear to contribute to co-adaptation and maturation of the adaptive immune system (→ 14.5) and the hypothalamic–pituitary–adrenal axis (→ Fig. 11.10). Translocation of gut bacteria, e.g. following intestinal surgery, can be a cause of peritonitis.

7.7.3 Rectum and anus

The **rectum** is the terminal part of the large intestine, about 12 cm long and the place where waste matter (**faeces**) from the colon are stored until leaving the body through the anus (→ Box 7.34).

The **anus** is the opening at the lower end of the alimentary canal. It is controlled by two sphincters which are kept closed except during defecation. The:
- **internal anal sphincter** is composed of involuntary muscle
- **external anal sphincter** is composed of voluntary muscle and is the muscle that young children learn to control.

7.8 Defecation

Defecation is a bowel movement in which the faeces are eliminated through the anus. The urge to empty the bowel comes when it is stretched by the presence of a stool, and muscular movements of the rectum push the faeces through the anus and outside the body. The normal range of frequency for emptying the bowel ranges from three per week to three per day.

Defecation is controlled by the action of two sphincters. The **internal sphincter** is smooth muscle that is continuous with the colon and regulated by the autonomic nervous system The **external sphincter** is skeletal muscle of the pelvic floor which is under voluntary control (→ Fig. 7.13).

7.8.1 Stools

A stool is faeces eliminated from the anus containing the waste products of digestion together with biota and mucus from the colon. Normally the stool is semi-solid with a mucus coating and is brown in colour. However, it varies in appearance according to the state of the digestive system, diet and general health (→ Box 7.35).

Diarrhoea is the frequent passing of loose, watery stools. Most acute diarrhoea is due to a bacterial or viral infection. Chronic diarrhoea needs to be investigated by a health professional (→ Box 7.36).

Constipation is the infrequent passing of hard, dry stools. It occurs when faeces are being held too long in the rectum, allowing water to continue to be absorbed. Constipation can be due to:
- ignoring the signals to empty the bowel
- lack of food or exercise
- a diet lacking fibre
- repeated use of laxatives (→ Box 7.37)
- repeated use of some medications.

Blood in the stools

Blood in the stool can come from any part of the digestive system:
- **bright-red blood on the toilet paper** is a typical sign of haemorrhoids (→ Box 7.38) or a small tear (anal fissure) in the anal membrane caused by straining when stools are hard to pass
- **bright red or maroon-coloured stools** may indicate a problem in the lower part of the digestive tract, such as diverticulitis
- **dark red blood in the stools**, which may appear as streaks of black or like coffee grounds, can indicate bleeding further up in the digestive tract, possibly the stomach or duodenum

Box 7.34 When disease of the colon or rectum is suspected, **colorectal screening** can be carried out to detect inflammation, ulcers, polyps, cancer and other conditions.

Box 7.35 When bilirubin (→ 7.6.2) reaches the colon, it is converted by bacteria into a substance called **urobilinogen**. This is converted to **stercobilin**, which gives stools their characteristic brown colour.

Box 7.36 A **stool test** may be carried out to help diagnose disease of the digestive tract, liver and pancreas that is causing symptoms such as prolonged diarrhoea, bloody diarrhoea, an increased amount of flatus, nausea, vomiting, loss of appetite, bloating or abdominal pain.

Box 7.37 An **enema** is the procedure that introduces liquid into the rectum through a tube passed into the anus. The liquid causes the rapid expansion of the rectum and stimulates powerful peristaltic movements that push the stools out through the anus. The advantage of an enema over a laxative is its speed and certainty of action.

Box 7.38 Haemorrhoids (piles) are swollen blood vessels inside the rectum. They arise as a result of straining due to constipation. Sometimes they protrude from the anus during a bowel movement. They may go back naturally, or can be pushed back, but occasionally they stay down, become inflamed and painful. The main symptom of piles is bleeding. Haemorrhoid creams reduce pain and itching.

- **occult blood** (blood not apparent to the naked eye) is present in very small quantities and can only be detected by a stool test (→ Box 7.36). It can result from any disorder affecting the GI tract or be caused by drugs that irritate the lining. The chronic loss of occult blood can result in anaemia.

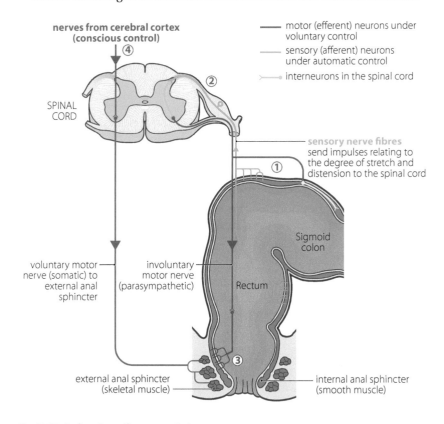

Fig. 7.13 Defecation reflex stages 1–4.

Defecation reflex stages

① The defecation reflex is initiated by distension of the rectal wall which occurs several times a day when propulsive movements of the colon move faecal contents forwards.
② Impulses from the stretch receptors in the sigmoid colon arrive in the spinal cord.
③ The involuntary response is to send signals via parasympathetic neurons to the colon, sigmoid colon, rectum and anus to increase peristaltic movements and relax the internal sphincter.
④ If defecation is not appropriate, the cerebral cortex of the brain sends nerve impulses to inhibit the involuntary response.

7.8.2 Bowel incontinence

Bowel incontinence is the inability to control bowel movements and results in the involuntary passing of stools. It is a symptom of an underlying problem or medical condition but not a disease in itself, many cases being caused by diarrhoea, constipation or weakening of the anal sphincter. Other causes include long-term conditions such as diabetes, multiple sclerosis, dementia and spinal injury. Bowel incontinence is relatively common, with about one in ten people affected at some point in their life, either on a daily basis or only occasionally. The problem is more common in elderly people, and in more women than men, but it can affect people of any age (→ Box 7.39).

Box 7.39 Healthcare professionals in all clinical settings will come across people who have a stoma (Greek = 'mouth' or 'opening') which is an opening on the surface of the abdomen which has been surgically created to divert the flow of faeces (or urine). The most common reasons for surgery to create a stoma are birth defects, trauma or disease including cancer, diverticular disease or inflammatory bowel disease (→ 7.9).

- colostomy is a stoma formed by bringing part of the large bowel to the surface of the abdomen;
- ileostomy is a stoma formed by bringing a loop of the ileum (small intestine) to the surface of the abdomen;
- urostomy is a stoma formed when the ureters are diverted away from the bladder (→ Fig. 8.1)

Faeces or urine will pass through the stoma, depending on the type of surgery and is collected in a soft, external pouch.

Although urostomy is a permanent stoma, some colostomies and ileostomies may be temporary, allowing the bowel to heal before the stoma is reversed.

Box 7.40 One theory about IBD is that the immune system mistakes bacteria inside the colon for a threat and attacks the tissues lining the colon and rectum, causing them to become inflamed.

Box 7.41 IBD is often accompanied by bloating, nausea, feelings of urgency, alternating between diarrhoea and constipation. It may be eased by adjustments to the diet, and there are various medicines that may help.

Box 7.42 Crohn's disease and ulcerative colitis are more common in urban, industrialised areas and northern climates. Genetic and immunological profiling suggests that some people may have a genetic predisposition to an abnormal response to gut microbiota.

It has also been suggested that people with sedentary lifestyles may have a delayed GI transit time, resulting in increased contact between antigens (→ 14.5) in food and the mucosal lining.

Box 7.43 Bowel obstruction is a common surgical emergency across the globe because of the associated risk of **ischaemia** (inadequate blood supply leading to **necrosis** (death of tissue)).

About 20% of hospital admissions for acute abdominal pain are due to a bowel obstruction and the majority of these occur in the small intestine.

Box 7.44 A **hernia** is the protrusion that pushes through a weakness in the surrounding tissues, e.g.:
- **inguinal hernia** – part of the bowel squeezes through the lower abdominal wall into the groin
- **hiatus hernia** – part of the stomach pushes up into the chest through an opening in the diaphragm
- **strangulated hernia** – the blood supply to the protrusion is cut off.

7.9 Disorders of the colon

7.9.1 Inflammatory bowel disease

Inflammatory bowel disease (IBD) is inflammation and ulceration of the lining of the colon and rectum and is thought to be an autoimmune disease (→ Box 7.40). These are complicated, uncontrolled inflammatory conditions that can affect any part of the digestive tract from mouth to anus, but are predominantly seen in later portions of the ileum or in the colon (→ Box 7.41). Crohn's disease and ulcerative colitis are subcategories of IBD (→ Box 7.42).

Crohn's disease

Crohn's disease is a chronic inflammatory disorder that affects the lining of the digestive tract from mouth to rectum, commonly occurring in the ileum and colon. Symptoms include abdominal pain, diarrhoea, fever, weight loss or blood in the stools. The condition can be mild or severe, last for a few months or disappear for a long time. There is currently no cure, but medication can help improve the symptoms.

Ulcerative colitis

Ulcerative colitis (UC) is a long-term condition that results in inflammation and ulcers of the colon and rectum, the primary symptoms being abdominal pain and diarrhoea mixed with blood.

7.9.2 Other disorders of the colon

Irritable bowel syndrome

Irritable bowel syndrome (IBS) is a disorder in which the muscles of the colon wall go into spasm (tighten) and their peristaltic movements fail to coordinate. The result is pain in the lower left side of the abdomen, with diarrhoea or constipation. The condition is painful but not a sign of a more serious disorder, and is often associated with stress or anxiety.

Diverticular disease

In diverticular disease small bulges (diverticuli) develop in the lining of the intestine. Diverticulitis develops when these bulges become inflamed or infected.

Bowel obstruction

A partial or complete bowel obstruction can occur anywhere in the small or large intestine. The bowel contents accumulate above the blockage, distending the bowel wall and inhibiting its normal functions. A completely blocked large intestine is a medical emergency (→ Box 7.43).

There are various causes for bowel obstruction including:
- **adhesions** – fibrous bands of scar tissue that form between tissues and organs that can form after abdominal surgery and trap a section of the bowel
- **hernia** – when part of the small intestine protrudes through a weak point in the abdominal wall (→ Box 7.44)
- **inflammatory bowel disease**
- **impacted stools** from severe constipation.

7.10 Diseases of the liver

Liver disease does not usually cause any obvious signs or symptoms until it is fairly advanced and the liver is damaged (→ 17.5.7). Hundreds of diseases can affect the liver, a few of them being described below (→ Box 7.45).

7.10.1 Gallstones

Gallstones are small hard stones composed mainly of cholesterol that commonly form in the gall bladder and usually cause no symptoms. They only become troublesome when:

- a stone becomes trapped in the bile duct and triggers sudden severe abdominal pain (**biliary colic**) which usually lasts from one to five hours
- the stones irritate the gall bladder lining, causing inflammation, persistent pain and fever (**cholecystitis**)
- a stone completely blocks the bile duct and stops bile from leaving the liver; the yellow pigment bilirubin that is normally excreted in bile enters the bloodstream, causing **jaundice** (→ Box 7.46).

7.10.2 Cirrhosis

Cirrhosis is a progressive disease in which healthy liver tissue is replaced by abnormal, lumpy, fibrous tissue, and the liver gradually shrinks and becomes stiffer (→ Fig. 7.14). The build-up of fibrous tissue cannot be reversed, and it may become so extensive that the liver stops functioning – a condition called liver failure (→ Box 7.47).

People at greatest risk of cirrhosis include those who:

- misuse alcohol
- are clinically obese and have a fatty liver
- have long-term contact with poisons and some medications
- have a chronic liver infection, e.g. primary biliary cirrhosis that causes the small bile ducts in the liver to become inflamed, damaged and destroyed
- have an immune problem that increases their risk, e.g. autoimmune primary biliary cholangitis which attacks biliary epithelium and damages it
- have an inherited disease, e.g. **haemochromatosis**, that causes the body to retain excessive amounts of iron, which overloads the liver.

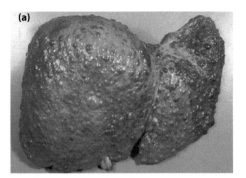
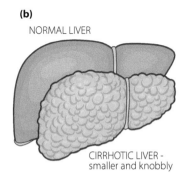

Fig. 7.14 (**a**) A cirrhotic (fatty) liver; the yellowish patches indicate the presence of oil; (**b**) comparison between a normal and cirrhotic liver in terms of size and appearance.

7.10.3 Hepatitis

Hepatitis is inflammation (swelling) of the liver that interferes with the secretion of bile, causing jaundice. It can be due to poisoning with harmful chemicals and alcohol, or to autoimmune hepatitis (→ Box 7.48), but it

Box 7.45 Cholestatic pruritus is an intense sensation of itching that is associated with many forms of liver disease. Bile salts are not cleared effectively from the liver and end up being deposited in the skin, making it itch.

Box 7.46 Treatment for gallstone disease:
- medication can be prescribed to break up the stones, but more stones often form again, or
- keyhole surgery can be performed to remove the gallbladder.

Box 7.47 The stage of cirrhosis can be estimated by using a FibroScan to measure how quickly vibration waves pass through the liver. The more stiff the liver, the more rapidly the waves will pass through it. The scan is painless, takes less than ten minutes and provides immediate results.

Taking it Further
There is more information about liver function tests in online Chapter 17.

Box 7.48 Autoimmune hepatitis occurs when white blood cells attack the liver and damage it, causing chronic inflammation.

is usually **viral hepatitis** caused by one of the types of the hepatitis virus (→ Box 7.49).

Viral hepatitis

The initial (acute) phase of the infection may include symptoms of fatigue, nausea, lack of appetite, vague abdominal discomfort, mild fever or occasionally jaundice. The symptoms are insidious, in that they develop gradually without being noticed but are causing harm. Normally the disease resolves (clears up) with the production of protective antibodies. But when the disease is not recognised until it has becomes chronic, the liver may already be damaged by one or more of the different types of viral hepatitis (→ Table 7.1).

Table 7.1 Different forms of the hepatitis virus

Type	Description	Source	Vaccine	Chronic illness
Hepatitis A	Acute illness lasting 3 weeks–6 months	Water contaminated with faeces from an infected person	Yes	No
Hepatitis B	Most recover fully in 2 months	Inoculation with body fluids from an infected person	Yes	Yes in 5–10% of all people who are infected
Hepatitis C	Slowly progressing disease	Blood of people who are infected	No vaccine available	Yes in 75–85% of people who are infected
Hepatitis D	Only acquired by those who have existing hepatitis B	Blood of people who are co-infected with hepatitis B and hepatitis D	HBV vaccine	Yes
Hepatitis E	3–8 weeks	Food and water contaminated by faeces from infected person	Vaccine available but not widely used	No
Hepatitis G	Most people clear the virus within 2 years	Blood and body fluids from infected people	Inconclusive evidence that HGV causes liver disease	No

Hepatitis C

Hepatitis C virus (HCV) was discovered in the 1980s and so far, six different genotypes (→ 13.6.1) are known, and it is possible to be infected by more than one at the same time. This virus persists in the liver of 80% of people who are infected and can often recur. It predominantly affects the liver but can also affect the lymphatic system, digestive system, brain and immune system.

The hepatitis C virus slowly damages the liver over many years, often progressing from inflammation to permanent, irreversible scarring (cirrhosis). Often, people have no signs or symptoms of liver disease or have only mild symptoms for many years until they have cirrhosis. End-stage hepatitis C means the liver has been severely damaged by the hepatitis C virus, and is the most common reason for adult liver transplantation.

There is a rising prevalence of end-stage liver disease and liver cancer amongst marginalised and under-represented groups, including people who inject drugs and those in prison. HCV is known to spread by:

- needle-stick injuries – wounds caused by needles that accidentally puncture the skin
- poorly sterilised equipment, e.g. tattoo needles
- sharing needles, razors and toothbrushes.

Key points

1. The alimentary canal and its accessory organs process the nutrients in food and drink, making them available for distribution and use by the body through the process of enzymatic (chemical) and mechanical digestion.
2. The oral phase of digestion is under conscious control and ensures that ingested food is moistened by saliva, chewed and formed into a bolus in the mouth, and then swallowed.
3. Rhythmic muscular activity, called peristalsis, moves the swallowed bolus along the oesophagus to the stomach where it is mixed with acidic gastric juice.
4. The small intestine is a long, coiled organ in which enzymes complete the digestive process and simple nutrient molecules are absorbed across its extensively folded lining.
5. The large intestine (colon) absorbs vitamins, minerals and water and eliminates faeces via the rectum and anus.

Test yourself! Go to *www.lanternpublishing.com/AandP* and try the questions to check your understanding.

CHAPTER 8
THE URINARY SYSTEM

The urinary system consists of the organs involved in the production and elimination of urine from the body. By regulating the composition of the blood and body fluids, and removing waste substances from them, the urinary system is the body's most important mechanism for maintaining homeostasis of the internal environment.

8.1 Urinary system

The **urinary system** (renal system) excretes water, salt, urea, alcohol, drugs, hormones and many other substances in urine (→ Box 8.1). **Urine** is made in the kidneys and contains many waste products which become poisonous if not eliminated from the body. The **urinary tract** is the system of ducts and channels that conduct urine from the kidneys to the exterior and it consists of two kidneys, two ureters, a bladder and a urethra (→ Fig. 8.1).

Box 8.1 Excretion is the removal of the waste products of metabolism – the chemical processes that occur in living cells. It takes place mainly through the urinary system but also includes the loss of water, salts and urea through the sweat glands, and carbon dioxide and water from the lungs.

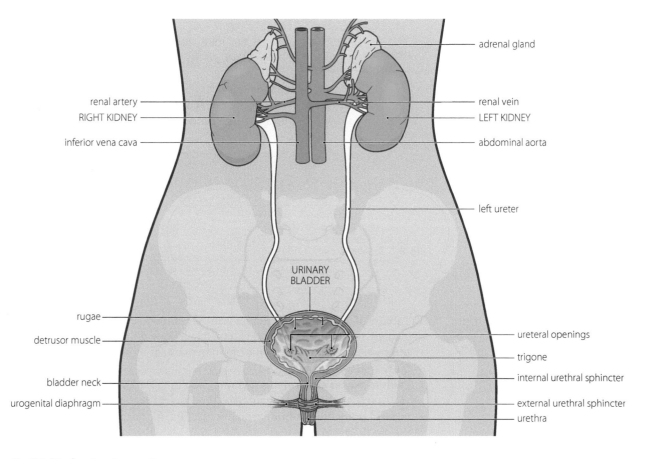

Fig. 8.1 The female urinary system.

8.1.1 Kidneys

The kidneys are two bean-shaped organs, the size of the fist, located on either side of the body, just beneath the ribcage and attached to the back wall of the abdomen above the level of the waist, one each side of the spine. They are delicate organs and are surrounded and protected from damage by the bones of the lower ribs and spine, the bulky skeletal muscles of the back, abdominal wall and intestines, a tough membrane – **capsule** – and the layer of fat that encloses each kidney.

When a kidney is dissected, different areas can be seen (→ Fig. 8.2):
- **renal cortex** – the outer region
- **renal medulla** – the middle region with pyramid-shaped areas
- **renal pelvis** – the central cavity which narrows into the ureter
- **blood vessels** (→ Box 8.2)
- **ureter** – the tube which drains urine to the bladder.

Box 8.2 The **renal arteries** carry about 1/5th of the cardiac output, which means that about 600 cm³ of blood passes through the adult kidneys every minute. Kidneys are so efficient at removing the waste products that it is possible for the body to function normally with only one. An individual might be born with only one kidney, or a kidney might have been removed because of disease, an accident or for transplanting to another person.

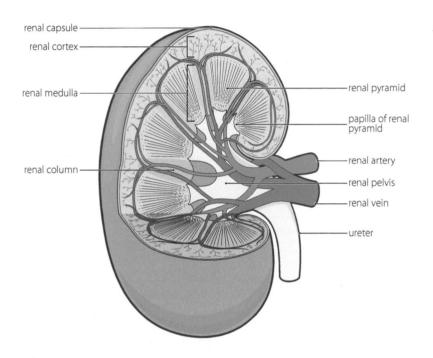

Labels: renal capsule, renal cortex, renal medulla, renal column, renal pyramid, papilla of renal pyramid, renal artery, renal pelvis, renal vein, ureter

Fig. 8.2 Section through a kidney.

8.1.2 Functions of the kidneys

The ability of the kidneys to excrete urine is central to their function, which is to regulate the composition and volume of all body fluids. They:
- **filter waste products** from the blood to maintain homeostasis of body fluids and form urine
- **excrete excess electrolytes** including sodium (Na^+), potassium (K^+), calcium (Ca^{2+}) and phosphate (PO_4^{3-})
- **control body fluid volume** which is essential for normal functioning of the cardiovascular system
- **monitor blood pressure** and take corrective action if it drops below a set level by secreting **renin** – an enzyme that helps to maintain fluid balance (→ 8.7)
- **activate vitamin D** (calcitriol) obtained from synthesis in the skin or from the diet, which is inactive and needs to be activated in the kidneys and liver

Taking it Further
You can find more information about electrolytes in blood in online Chapter 17.

- **secrete erythropoietin** – a hormone essential for the production of red blood cells in the bone marrow
- **excrete foreign substances**, e.g. drugs, pesticides and toxins.

8.2 Nephrons

Nephrons (**renal tubules**) are the microscopic functional units of the kidneys, and each kidney contains over a million of them (→ Fig. 8.3). The beginning of the tubule lies in the renal cortex and is expanded into a cup-shaped capsule – **Bowman's capsule** – which encloses a small network of capillaries called the **glomerulus**. Bowman's capsule extends into the proximal convoluted tubule, which dips down into the renal medulla as the loop of Henle, then back to the distal convoluted tubule to the collecting duct. Capillaries surround the tubule until it joins the collecting duct which leads to the renal pelvis (centre) of the kidney (→ Box 8.3).

Box 8.3 A normal aspect of ageing is the loss of up to 30% of nephrons by the age of 80 years. The kidneys retain their capacity to maintain normal function except at times of stress, e.g. infection.

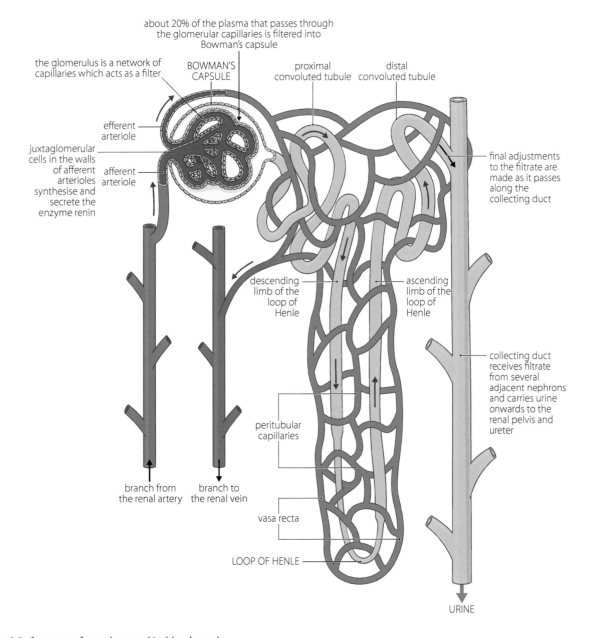

Fig. 8.3 Structure of a nephron and its blood supply.

Box 8.4 Ultrafiltration is high pressure filtration of liquids using a semipermeable membrane – in this case the glomerular capillary membrane – that allows only the smallest particles to pass through it. The ultrafiltrate is therefore devoid of proteins, blood cells or platelets. In adults, the **glomerular filtration rate (GFR) is 90–140 ml/min** which means that up to 180 litres of filtrate are made by the glomeruli every day. Less than 1% of the water and solutes in filtrate are excreted because of reabsorption by other segments of the nephron.

Reductions in GFR are a common sign of renal disease.

Box 8.5 The glomerular filter allows small particles like water, nutrients and electrolytes to pass through but large particles including cells, platelets and proteins are held back. This is the reason why urine should not normally contain any significant amounts of protein. **Proteinuria** is therefore a sign that there may be a problem with kidney function.

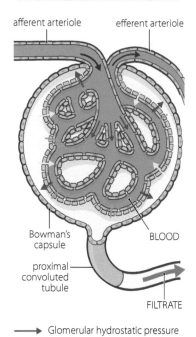

afferent arteriole   efferent arteriole

Bowman's capsule   BLOOD

proximal convoluted tubule

FILTRATE

→ Glomerular hydrostatic pressure
→ Blood colloid osmotic pressure
→ Filtrate hydrostatic pressure

Fig. 8.4 Forces that determine the rate of glomerular filtration.

Functions of the nephrons

As blood passes through the kidneys, three key processes take place in the nephrons that result in urine:
- **ultrafiltration** of the blood in the glomerulus that filters out urea, salt, water, glucose and other small particles from the blood (→ Box 8.4)
- **reabsorption** of essential substances back into the blood in the capillaries surrounding the tubule, e.g. water, glucose, electrolytes
- **secretion** of substances such as acid or drugs into the filtrate.

8.2.1 Ultrafiltration

Ultrafiltration (**glomerular filtration**) occurs in the glomerular capillaries, which act as a semipermeable membrane (→ Box 8.5). The **efferent arteriole** carrying blood away from Bowman's capsule has a smaller diameter than the **afferent arteriole**, making the resistance in the efferent arteriole higher than that in the afferent arteriole (→ Fig. 8.4). The pressure difference forces small molecules from the blood, e.g. water, glucose, amino acids, sodium chloride and urea, through the filter into Bowman's capsule. The fluid filtered in this way is called **glomerular filtrate**.

Glomerular filtration rate

The rate of filtration from blood depends on the strength of opposing forces, one forcing substances from the capillaries into Bowman's capsule, the other forcing them back again.
- **Hydrostatic pressure in glomerular capillaries** tends to push water and solutes into Bowman's capsule (→ Fig. 8.4: red arrows)
- Forces that oppose glomerular filtration are:
  - **colloid osmotic pressure of blood** which tends to attract fluid back into blood (→ Fig. 8.4: blue arrows)
  - **hydrostatic pressure of the filtrate** already in Bowman's capsule (→ Fig. 8.4: yellow arrows).

The net effect of filtration in the glomerulus is that small particles pass through the glomerular capillaries into the nephron while large particles, the cells and proteins, remain in blood and flow through the efferent arteriole and onwards through the network of capillaries surrounding the nephron to join the renal vein. There is a natural decline in glomerular filtration as people get older.

8.2.2 Reabsorption

Reabsorption allows many useful solutes that have been filtered out from the blood in Bowman's capsule, to return to the blood in different segments of the nephron (→ Fig. 8.5).
① The **proximal convoluted tubule** is responsible for reabsorbing most of the water and solutes in the filtrate (→ Fig. 8.6).
② The **descending limb** of the loop of Henle is permeable to water but impermeable to sodium chloride. This means that the filtrate becomes more concentrated and its osmolality reaches the maximum of about 1200 milliosmoles/litre of solution (mOsm/L).
③ The **ascending limb of the loop of Henle** actively transports sodium chloride back into the blood. However, this segment is impermeable to water so it does not follow the sodium chloride. Overall, relatively more sodium chloride than water has been reabsorbed by the loop, making the filtrate very dilute when it enters the distal convoluted tubule.

④ The **distal convoluted tubule** and **collecting duct** adjust the final composition and volume of the filtrate to match the needs of the body, depending on the action of the hormones ADH (antidiuretic hormone) and aldosterone.

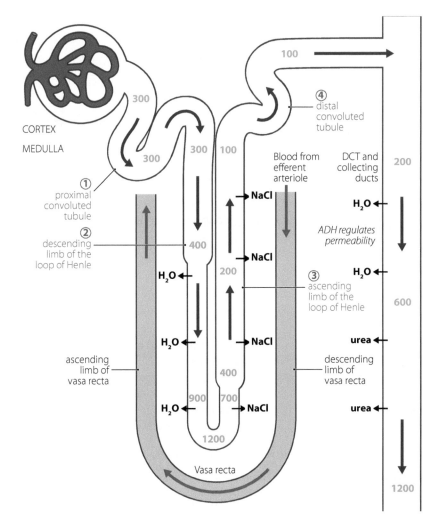

Fig. 8.5 Variation in reabsorption of solutes from filtrate in different segments of the nephron. The numbers in blue indicate the osmolality (mOsm/L) of the filtrate, which changes as it flows along the nephron (→ Box 8.6).

Box 8.6 Osmolality is the concentration of a solution expressed as the total number of solute particles per kilogram (1 kilogram = 1 litre), e.g. the reference value for bloods is 275–295 mOsm/L.

The process of reabsorption in the proximal convoluted tubule

The cells of the proximal tubule have a folded **luminal membrane** (plasma membrane) with **microvilli** (microscopic finger-like processes) which are in contact with the filtrate and provide a very large surface area for reabsorption (→ Fig. 8.6). The luminal membrane is selectively permeable and determines which substances from the filtrate are reabsorbed and by what method:

- **sodium ions** (Na⁺) are actively transported (→ Fig. 2.3), a process which requires energy provided by ATP. The sodium ions then diffuse into the blood where their concentration is lower, and are followed by chloride (Cl⁻) ions to maintain electroneutrality
- **water** molecules (H_2O) are reabsorbed by **osmosis** (→ 20.5.2)
- **glucose** molecules cross the proximal tubule cells by **facilitated diffusion** then diffuse into the blood (→ 2.2.2).

The epithelium of the proximal tubule and loop of Henle is impermeable to the nitrogenous waste molecule urea so it becomes increasingly more concentrated as it flows along towards the distal tubule (→ Box 8.7). Some urea is reabsorbed from the collecting ducts.

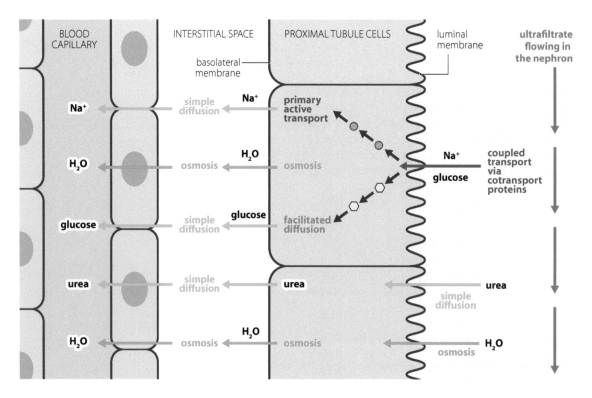

Fig. 8.6 Reabsorption in the proximal convoluted tubule.

Process of reabsorption in the loop of Henle

By the time filtrate enters the loop of Henle, it is reduced in volume when compared with the filtrate in Bowman's capsule. The cell membrane of the epithelium in the loop of Henle is also selectively permeable but the ways in which solutes and water are reabsorbed in this segment change (→ Fig. 8.5). Since the kidney contains millions of nephrons, the net effect of selective permeability in this segment is to create an **osmotic gradient** from the cortical region to the medullary region of the kidney (→ Box 8.7).

Processes of reabsorption in the distal convoluted tubule and collecting duct

The function of the distal tubule is to adjust the composition and volume of final urine to match the body's needs. The permeability of the distal tubule to:

- water depends on the action of **antidiuretic hormone** (ADH) (→ 8.2.4)
- sodium and potassium ions depends on the activity of the hormone **aldosterone** (→ 8.7); aldosterone stimulates the active transport of sodium ions (Na⁺) out of the filtrate in the distal tubule and into the bloodstream in exchange for potassium ions (K⁺)
- calcium ions (Ca²⁺) depend on the levels of **parathyroid hormone** (→ 11.5)
- urea is excreted in urine but some diffuses passively back into the bloodstream.

Box 8.7 Diffusion into and out of cells occurs along a concentration gradient from an area of high concentration to areas of lower concentration.

Taking it Further
Find out more about movement of substances across membranes in online Chapter 20.

8.2.3 Secretion into the nephrons

Secretion into the nephrons is the transport of substances in the opposite direction to reabsorption so that they can be excreted in urine. Normally only a few substances are added to the final urine in this way – hydrogen and potassium ions, nitrogenous wastes (ammonia, urea, uric acid and creatinine) and some drugs, e.g. penicillin.

Secretion of hydrogen ions and ammonium

Secretion of hydrogen ions (H^+) and the nitrogenous waste ammonium (NH_4^+) are both closely linked to reabsorption of bicarbonate ions (HCO_3^-). This process is part of the mechanism that homeostatically regulates the pH of blood. In collaboration with respiratory excretion of CO_2, acid–base balance is determined by conservation of plasma HCO_3^- and secretion of excess acid via the distal tubule (→ Box 8.8).

Box 8.8 Acid–base homeostasis. Both the kidneys and lungs play an important part in making sure that the relative amounts of acids and bases in the body are maintained within the homeostatic range.

Secretion of potassium ions

Potassium ions (K^+) are normally in low concentrations in plasma, and are secreted into final urine under the influence of the hormone aldosterone (→ 8.7). They are actively transported from blood into filtrate in the distal tubule and collecting duct in exchange for sodium ions (Na^+).

Secretion of drugs

Drugs, pesticides and toxins with relatively small molecular weights can filter through the glomerulus wall and into the tubule, but as they are not reabsorbed by tubular cells, they are eliminated in the urine. However, the majority of drugs and medications in blood are bound to plasma proteins, so active secretion against a concentration gradient takes place in the distal part of the nephron (→ Fig. 8.5) (→ Box 8.9).

Box 8.9 A range of factors affect the rate of the secretion of drugs into urine, e.g. plasma concentration of the substance, pH of urine, presence or absence of kidney disease. Drug elimination also takes place in bile, saliva, tears, sweat and breastmilk.

8.2.4 Antidiuretic hormone and water excretion

When the amount of water in the blood falls below a set level, e.g. dehydration, vomiting or excessive sweating, the hypothalamus sends a message to the pituitary gland which releases ADH (→ 11.3.1).

Antidiuretic hormone (ADH; vasopressin (→ 11.3.1)) controls the amount of water reabsorbed by the kidneys in order to keep the concentration of water in the blood more or less constant – a process known as **osmoregulation**. The osmolarity difference that was set up in the the loop of Henle (→ Fig. 8.5) means that, in the presence of ADH, more water is reabsorbed into the collecting duct and a small volume of very concentrated urine is excreted.

When the amount of water in the blood rises above a set level, e.g. due to increased drinking or reduced sweating, the hypothalamus detects the change, sends a message to the pituitary, and the release of ADH into the blood is slowed down or even stopped. Without ADH the kidney tubules do not reabsorb as much water, and large volumes of dilute urine are produced. The process continues until the level of water in the blood falls back to the normal range and ADH levels begin to rise again (→ Box 8.10).

Box 8.10 Both alcohol and Ecstasy interfere with the normal regulation of water by ADH and may have harmful long-term effects.

Alcohol can decrease the amount of ADH produced, which results in a greater volume of more dilute urine, and can lead to dehydration.

Ecstasy has the opposite effect. It increases the amount of ADH which reduces the amount of urine produced, so fluid does not leave the body. If the Ecstasy user drinks too much water, there is a risk of dilution of plasma – a condition known as **hyponatraemia** – which in rare cases, more commonly in females, leads to organ damage and possible death.

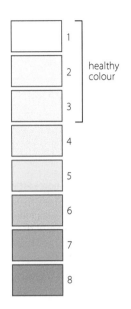

Fig. 8.7 Urine colour chart.

Taking it Further
You can find out more about urinalysis in online Chapter 17.

Box 8.11 Beetroot or red sweets can result in pink urine and carrots can tint it orange.

Box 8.12 Excess nitrogen is removed from the body by the process of deamination (→ 19.3.2) and converted to ammonia (NH_3). Ammonia is toxic to the human system, and enzymes convert it to **urea** or **uric acid** to be excreted by the kidneys. These **nitrogenous wastes** may not be excreted effectively if the kidneys are diseased or damaged.

Diabetes insipidus

Diabetes insipidus is a clinical condition caused by a deficiency of ADH (central DI) or a lack of renal response to ADH (nephrogenic DI) which results in the production of large volumes of urine and causes excessive thirst. This condition is not related to diabetes mellitus although it does share some of the same symptoms (→ 16.3).

8.3 Urine

Urine is the final product that leaves the kidney and has a very different composition to the filtrate at the start of the nephrons.

Smell

Fresh urine is normally sterile and has little smell. A strong smell develops when it is contaminated with bacteria and the urea in the urine is converted to ammonia. Cystitis may cause urine to have a strong unpleasant smell (→ 8.5.3).

Colour

The colour of urine depends mainly on its concentration of the pigment **urochrome** which is the end product of haemoglobin breakdown and is excreted through the kidneys. Urine is normally pale in colour, which is regarded as a healthy colour as it indicates a sufficient intake of fluid (→ Fig. 8.7).

Variations in colour

- Pale-coloured urine can be a result of taking **diuretics** – drugs that force the body to get rid of excess water.
- A darker colour is usually a sign of dehydration because enough water is not being consumed.
- Jaundice and other disorders of the liver can result in the excretion of bile pigments, making urine a dark yellow or orange colour.
- Red may be a sign of blood in the urine possibly due to an infection of the kidneys, bladder or ureters (→ Box 8.11).

Appearance

Urine should normally be clear; cloudiness can indicate dehydration or infection; protein tends to make it frothy.

8.3.1 Composition of urine

The main substances in urine and the approximate quantities are:
- **water** – about 1.5 litres per day. When less water is excreted, the urine is more concentrated and darker in colour
- **urea** – about 30 g. Urea is a breakdown product of protein metabolism in the liver and, being soluble in plasma, is transported to the kidney for excretion. It is filtered at the glomerulus and some is reabsorbed in the collecting ducts (→ Box 8.12)
- **salt** – about 15 g as sodium and chloride ions. Usually more salt is eaten than is lost in sweat or faeces, and the excess is excreted in the urine. When the body is short of salt, then almost complete reabsorption of the salt takes place in the nephrons and very little or none is present in the urine.

Small amounts of many other substances are normally found in urine, for example:

- **uric acid** and **creatinine** are the by-products of metabolism (→ Boxes 8.12 and 8.13)
- **hormones**, e.g. pregnancy hormones
- **minerals** such as ions of **potassium**, **calcium** and **magnesium**
- **ketones** are the waste product of fat metabolism and can be present in poorly managed diabetes or semi-starvation
- traces of **alcohol**, **steroids** or certain **drugs** or **medicines** appear in the urine if these substances are taken.

Box 8.13 High levels of uric acid can cause urate crystals to form in the joints. When this occurs, people may suffer from painful **gout** – a form of arthritis, especially in the smaller bones of the feet.

8.4 Micturition

Micturition (urination; voiding) is the process of emptying the bladder and involves both the urinary and nervous systems.

8.4.1 Bladder

The bladder is a hollow muscular sac that sits on the pelvic floor and varies in size according to the volume of urine it contains (→ Fig. 8.8). **Rugae** are folds in the bladder lining that allow the bladder to expand as it fills with urine.

The bladder wall contains three involuntary smooth muscles:

- **trigone** – a triangular area on the floor of the bladder which is very sensitive to stretch; when the bladder is full, nerve endings detect the stretch and transmit the information to the spinal cord
- **detrusor muscle** contracts and expels urine
- **internal urethral sphincter** must relax in order to allow urine to be expelled.

The **bladder neck muscles** connect the bladder to the urethra. One is voluntary, the other involuntary, and both function as **sphincters** (rings of muscle tissue).

The **external urethral sphincter** forms part of the pelvic floor muscles. It is composed of skeletal muscle and therefore under voluntary control, and must relax to allow voiding of urine.

Contraction of the **pelvic floor muscles** tightens the openings of the anus and urethra; relaxing them allows passage of urine and faeces.

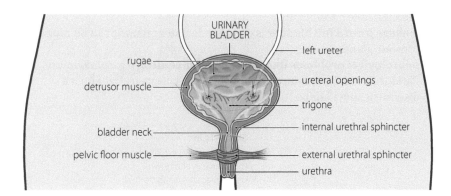

Fig. 8.8 Section through the bladder of a female.

8.4.2 Uncontrolled voiding

Voiding is uncontrolled in infants and young children until they have learnt to control the bladder sphincters, which is a complex process and requires coordination within different parts of the nervous system – brain, brainstem, spinal cord and nerves of the sympathetic and parasympathetic divisions of the autonomic nervous system (➜ 9.8).

Some diseases and injuries to the central nervous system can lead to incontinence – a major health issue, particularly for people who have neurological impairments.

8.4.3 Voluntary control of voiding

The urge to empty the bladder is perceived as an uncomfortable **sensation** that is correlated with the level of filling of the bladder. The brain begins the process of voiding urine by sending motor nerve impulses from the brainstem to the spinal cord. Impulses from spinal neurons stimulate the contraction of the detrusor muscle until the pressure of urine is high enough to empty the bladder. When voiding takes place:

- the external sphincter relaxes
- urine flows through the urethra to the exterior until the bladder is emptied, partly helped by gravity in women and contraction of the muscle that closes the vas deferens in men
- the process takes about 20 seconds (➜ Fig. 8.9).

However, if the bladder has become too full, or if a person is very frightened, then sphincters can relax involuntarily, allowing urine to be voided.

8.4.4 Urinary incontinence

Urinary incontinence is the involuntary passing of urine due to loss of voluntary control of the bladder (➜ Box 8.14). It can be due to:

- **stress incontinence** – a leak of urine when the bladder is under pressure, e.g. when coughing, sneezing or laughing. This is usually due to weakening of the muscles used to prevent urination such as the pelvic floor muscles and urethral sphincter. Stress incontinence is common in women when the pelvic floor muscles have been weakened by childbirth (➜ Box 8.15)
- **urge incontinence** is a sudden, intense urge to pass urine. This is usually the result of over-activity of the detrusor muscles which control the bladder. It is possible to have a mixture of both stress and urge incontinence (➜ Box 8.16)
- **leakage from a full bladder** is common in older men with an enlarged prostate gland
- **neurological problems that affect bladder control**, e.g. spinal injury, Parkinson's disease, motor neurone disease, late stage Alzheimer's disease or spina bifida.

Box 8.14 The chances of developing urinary incontinence are increased by pregnancy and vaginal birth, obesity, a family history of incontinence, lifting and handling, and increasing age – although incontinence is not an inevitable part of ageing.

Box 8.15 Pelvic floor exercises can help to strengthen the muscles and improve their tone with continuous and passive, partial muscle contraction.

Box 8.16 Urge incontinence (overactive bladder) is common. Symptoms include an urgent feeling to urinate or urinating frequently. Pelvic floor exercises and bladder training often cures the problem, sometimes with medication to relax the bladder.

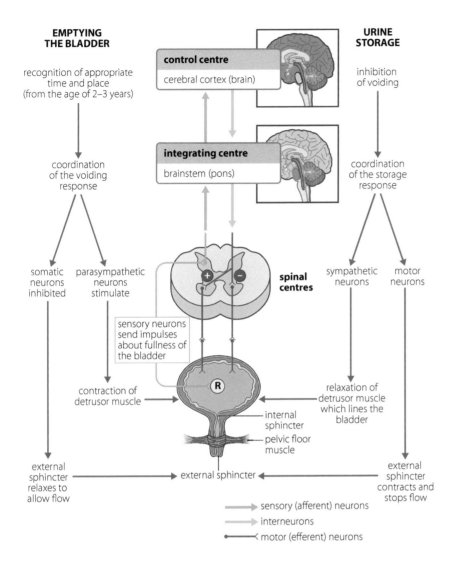

EMPTYING THE BLADDER

URINE STORAGE

control centre
cerebral cortex (brain)

integrating centre
brainstem (pons)

recognition of appropriate time and place (from the age of 2–3 years)

inhibition of voiding

coordination of the voiding response

coordination of the storage response

somatic neurons inhibited

parasympathetic neurons stimulate

spinal centres

sympathetic neurons

motor neurons

sensory neurons send impulses about fullness of the bladder

contraction of detrusor muscle

relaxation of detrusor muscle which lines the bladder

internal sphincter

pelvic floor muscle

external sphincter relaxes to allow flow

external sphincter

external sphincter contracts and stops flow

→ sensory (afferent) neurons
→ interneurons
→ motor (efferent) neurons

Fig. 8.9 The urinary bladder stores urine, allowing it to be emptied at infrequent intervals.

8.5 Urinary tract disorders

8.5.1 Kidney stones

These are hard stones that form in the kidney from calcium deposits (→ Fig. 8.10). Small stones can usually leave the body in the urine stream without causing any symptoms. If stones grow larger, usually to at least 3 mm, they can block the ureter and cause severe pain (**renal colic**) in the abdomen or groin, and sometimes a urinary tract infection. Kidney stones which are troublesome can be broken up by **lithotripsy** (the use of shock waves) into smaller pieces and passed in the urine or removed by surgery.

8.5.2 Prostate gland enlargement

The prostate gland is part of the male reproductive system (→ Fig. 12.2) and not the urinary system; it is discussed here because of its position surrounding the urethra – the tube through which urine is released from the bladder (→ Fig. 12.2). The prostate gland is normally about the size

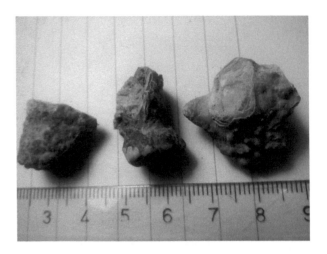

Fig. 8.10 Kidney stones with centimetre rule for scale.

of a walnut but if it enlarges and presses on the urethra, this may cause difficulties in starting urination or in fully emptying the bladder, resulting in the frequent need to urinate (➔ Box 8.17).

8.5.3 Urinary tract infections

Urinary tract infections (UTI) affect different parts of the urinary system.

Cystitis

Cystitis is inflammation of the bladder lining, sometimes caused by infection. Symptoms are the frequent passing of small amounts of urine that stings as it goes through the urethra.

This disorder is more common in women than men because the female urethra is much shorter and there are more bacteria in the outlet area which can more easily reach the bladder. Drinking large quantities of water may help to relieve the symptoms, but antibiotics may be needed.

Urethritis

Urethritis is inflammation of the urethra, making urination painful or difficult. It may be due to a sexually transmitted infection or to the presence of a catheter.

8.6 Renal failure

Renal failure (kidney failure) occurs when the kidneys lose most or all of their ability to filter waste products from the blood, usually due to an underlying injury to the kidneys. The two main forms are:
- **acute kidney injury (AKI)** – the sudden loss of kidney function, and often reversible with appropriate treatment
- **chronic kidney disease (CKD)** – a long-term condition that develops slowly and rarely causes symptoms until it reaches an advanced stage and is often irreversible. The two major underlying causes of CKD are **diabetes** and **hypertension** as both these disorders can damage the nephrons if they are not well controlled.

8.6.1 Kidney dialysis

Dialysis is the artificial process of eliminating waste substances and unwanted water from the blood by ultrafiltration. It is used when a person's kidneys are no longer able to meet the body's needs to remove excess fluids and waste products.

Haemodialysis

Haemodialysis uses a machine called an 'artificial kidney' to filter the blood (→ Fig. 8.11). Blood from a **fistula** – created by joining an artery to a vein – is pumped to a machine which performs the role of the kidney (shown on Fig. 8.11 as a dialysis filter). As the blood passes through the machine, unwanted substances are filtered out, and the blood is then returned to a nearby vein in the patient's arm. The process usually takes about four hours three times a week, perhaps in the patient's home if a machine is available for personal use.

Peritoneal dialysis

Dialysis fluid flows by gravity from a bag into the patient's abdominal cavity, using the lining of the abdomen as a filter. It is left there for a few hours to give time for waste substances to move from the blood into the fluid. The fluid is then drained off and the process is repeated three or four times a day. The direction in which the fluid flows is controlled by valves (→ Fig. 8.12).

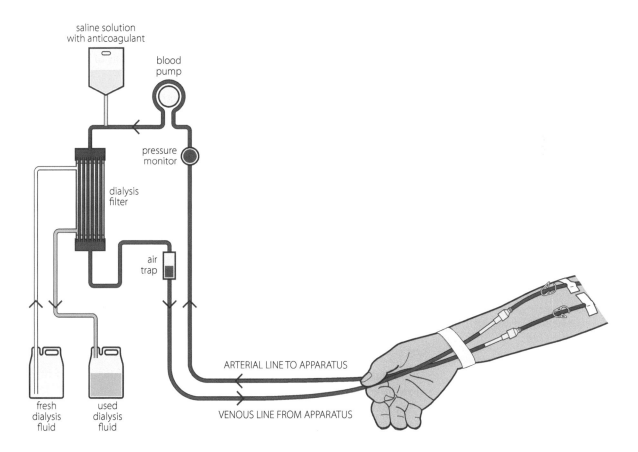

Fig. 8.11 Haemodialysis usually takes place in a specialist dialysis unit and requires the patient to sit in a recliner or lie on a bed for about four hours.

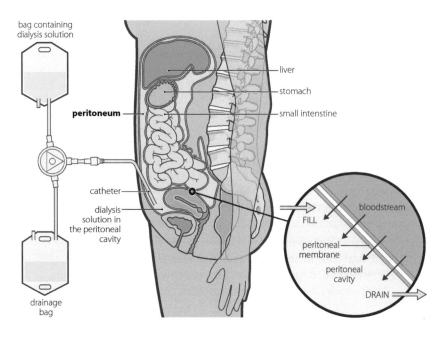

Fig. 8.12 Peritoneal dialysis can be done at home and may enable people to maintain their working life.

8.7 Renin–angiotensin–aldosterone system

The renin–angiotensin–aldosterone system (RAAS) regulates long-term **blood pressure** by means of a chain reaction that involves the kidneys, hormones and enzymes that work together for homeostasis of blood pressure.

Renin is an enzyme made by the juxtaglomerular cells in the kidneys (→ Fig. 8.3). The cells that secrete renin detect changes in blood pressure to the kidneys. Whenever blood pressure falls, blood flow to the kidneys is reduced and the output of renin increases, triggering the RAAS cascade that restores blood pressure to its original level (→ Fig. 8.13). When blood pressure returns to the normal range, the kidneys reduce their output of renin – an example of negative feedback.

8.7.1 RAAS cascade

The RAAS cascade is activated when **renin** encounters **angiotensinogen** – an inactive plasma protein (from the liver) – and the biochemical reaction produces **angiotensin I** which is a relatively inactive substance. In turn, angiotensin I must be converted to a much more powerful form, **angiotensin II**, to have its effect (→ Box 8.18). This is achieved when blood reaches the lungs because they contain another enzyme, called **angiotensin-converting enzyme (ACE)**.

Angiotensin II is a very powerful physiological agent which increases blood pressure by:
- stimulating smooth muscle cells in the walls of arteries and arterioles to contract, which increases vascular resistance (vasoconstriction)
- stimulating the adrenal glands to release the hormone **aldosterone**. This hormone increases reabsorption of sodium and water by the distal tubule of nephrons in the kidney.

Box 8.18 Disturbance and imbalance between renin and angiotensin II can result in a very large number of diseases, in part because this physiological cascade is influenced by other signalling pathways of the body and by diet. Understanding the hormone-producing capability of the renin–angiotensin–aldosterone system (RAAS) has been key to advancements in drug therapy for hypertension (→ 18.9).

The renin–angiotensin–aldosterone system is now a major target for many drugs that are routinely prescribed. Medications that alter the function of RAAS are used to treat hypertension, heart failure and kidney disease, high risk of cardiovascular disease, diabetes or renal failure.

Renin therefore plays a key role in blood pressure homeostasis because it determines the levels of angiotensin II that circulate at a given time. After renin levels fall, angiotensin I, angiotensin II and aldosterone are broken down by the body.

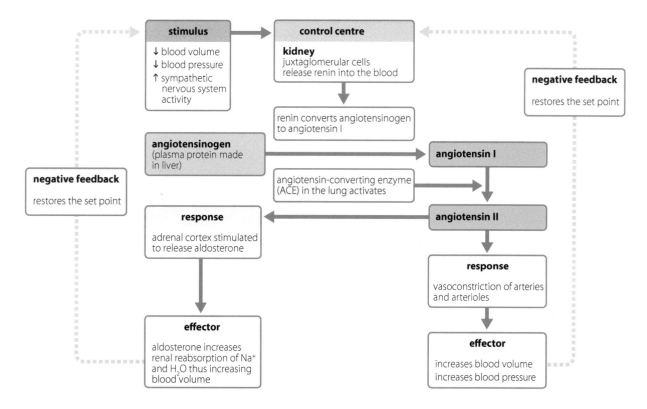

Fig. 8.13 Renin–angiotensin–aldosterone system (RAAS) cascade.

Key points

1. The urinary system comprises kidneys, ureters, bladder and urethra, all of which play a part in the elimination of body waste.
2. Nephrons are the functional unit of the kidneys which maintain fluid and electrolyte homeostasis and eliminate waste as urine.
3. Three processes are involved in the production of urine – ultrafiltration of blood, reabsorption of water and solutes, and secretion of solutes into urine.
4. Excretion of water in urine is homeostatically regulated by the hypothalamus and antidiuretic hormone (ADH) to match the body's needs.
5. The renin–angiotensin–aldosterone system regulates excretion of sodium and water by the kidneys and plays a key role in homeostasis of blood pressure.

Test yourself! Go to *www.lanternpublishing.com/AandP* and try the questions to check your understanding.

CHAPTER 9
THE NERVOUS SYSTEM

The nervous system is concerned with the fast transmission of signals – nerve impulses – from one part of the body to another. The brain coordinates the voluntary and involuntary actions of daily life, and the autonomic nervous system works with the endocrine system to maintain homeostasis (stability) of the internal environment. Damage to the nervous system can cause loss of wellbeing and affect a person's capacity to fully enjoy family and social life.

9.1 Structure of the nervous system

The nervous system is a vast network of nerve cells called **neurons** (→ 2.5.4) that are specialised to carry information rapidly along nerves to, and from, all parts of the body in the form of **nerve impulses**. Specialised tissue called **glia** (→ 2.5.5) forms a network of spidery cells that support the neurons. **Nerves** are bundles of parallel nerve fibres that connect with the different organs and tissues (→ Fig. 9.1).

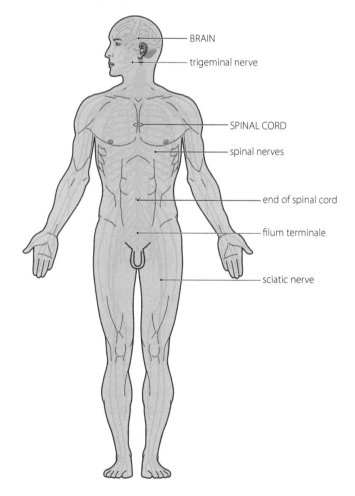

BRAIN

trigeminal nerve

SPINAL CORD

spinal nerves

end of spinal cord

filum terminale

sciatic nerve

Fig. 9.1 The spinal cord extends from the brain to the lumbar region with a thin thread – the filum terminale – continuing to the coccygeal region.

9.1.1 Divisions of the nervous system

The two main divisions of the nervous system are the **central nervous system (CNS)** composed of brain and spinal cord, and the **peripheral nervous system (PNS)** that contains all the nerves outside the CNS (→ Fig. 9.2). Nerves of the PNS are either:

- **motor nerves** exerting control of the voluntary movements of skeletal muscles (→ 9.7)
- nerves of the **autonomic nervous system** that regulate the involuntary muscles including the cardiac muscle, urinary bladder and glands (→ 9.8)
- **sensory nerves** connected to the sense organs and other tissues (→ 9.9 and *Chapter 10*).

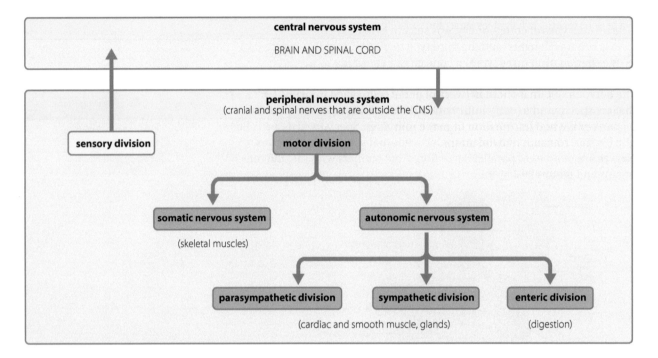

Fig. 9.2 Divisions of the nervous system.

Functions of the nervous system

The different divisions of the nervous system coordinate in carrying out its functions, namely to:

- **receive** information from the external environment through the sense organs – eyes, ears, skin, nose and tongue
- **monitor** conditions inside the body by means of internal sensors including baroreceptors and chemoreceptors
- **make constant adjustments** in response to the continuously changing internal and external environments
- **coordinate** muscles, movements and endocrine functions
- **carry out cognitive functions** – learning, reasoning, memory, language and decision making.

9.2 Central nervous system

The two parts of the central nervous system (CNS) are the brain and the spinal cord, and they carry out different functions.

The brain:

- receives information directly from the ears, eyes, nose and mouth, and indirectly from the rest of the body via the spinal cord
- uses this information to help learn, think, plan, remember and send out instructions for movement, speech and other responses (→ Box 9.1).

The spinal cord:

- receives information from the skin and the internal organs
- transmits information in the form of impulses to and from the brain
- carries the motor nerves that control movements and regulate the activity of the internal organs
- plays a key role in spinal reflexes (→ 9.6.2).

9.2.1 Protection of the CNS

The brain and spinal cord are delicate structures surrounded and protected by an outer covering of skin and bone (cranium and vertebrae), by layers of connective tissue called meninges, and by cerebrospinal fluid (→ Fig. 9.3).

Box 9.1 The human brain can learn because it is an extensive network of neurons connected by synapses with the property of **synaptic plasticity**. Interconnections at synapses strengthen or weaken over time in response to increases or decreases in their activity. The physiological basis for learning and memory is the strengthening of synaptic networks that are continually being used.

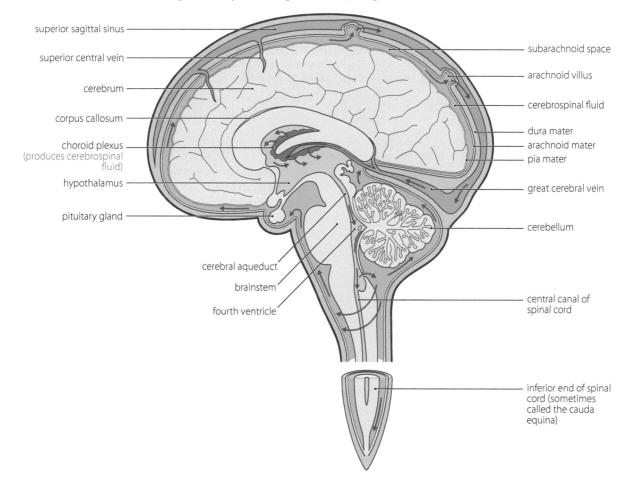

Fig. 9.3 Circulation of cerebrospinal fluid from its origin in the choroid plexus to all parts of the CNS. The red arrows indicate direction of flow.

Meninges

The meninges are three layers of different types of connective tissue that cover and protect the brain and spinal cord:
- **dura mater** is the tough, strong outer sac that encloses the brain, spinal cord and the cerebrospinal fluid (→ Box 9.2)
- **arachnoid mater** – a delicate cobweb-like layer lying beneath the dura mater that contains most of the blood vessels. The **sub-arachnoid space** separates the arachnoid and the pia mater. It contains delicate connective tissue through which cerebrospinal fluid circulates around the brain and spinal cord (→ Box 9.3)
- **pia mater** – the innermost layer that follows the contours of the brain and spinal cord and adheres tightly to the highly folded surface.

The meninges continue down within the spinal cavity for some distance below the spinal cord, with the pia mater forming the slender, tapering filament called the **filum terminale**. **Meningitis** is inflammation of the meninges (→ 15.7.1).

Cerebrospinal fluid

About 600–700 cm^3 of cerebrospinal fluid (CSF) is produced per day in the **choroid plexus** (→ Fig. 9.3) and circulates through a communicating network of **ventricles** (cavities) before being absorbed by the **arachnoid villi**. Important functions of the CSF are to:
- maintain a uniform pressure around the brain
- CSF cushions the brain from contact with the skull when sudden movements of the head occur (→ Box 9.4)
- provide the brain with the nutrients it needs to function properly
- remove waste products from the brain.

9.2.2 Blood–brain barrier

The capillaries in the brain develop differently from capillaries elsewhere in the body. The endothelium of the capillary walls has a thick basement membrane (→ 2.5.1) and is lined with astrocytes (→ 2.5.5) to form a unique structure – the blood–brain barrier (→ Box 9.5). The junctions between the cells of the blood–brain barrier are tightly fused and leakproof, which separates the blood from the cerebrospinal fluid to a much greater extent than elsewhere in the body. Small molecules in solution such as oxygen, glucose and alcohol can pass rapidly through the blood–brain barrier, but larger particles cannot because their movement is highly regulated. This protects brain tissue from toxic substances and pathogens, but may also be a barrier to some potentially useful medicines (→ Box 9.6).

9.2.3 Grey and white matter of the CNS

The central nervous system consists of two types of matter – grey and white:
- **grey matter** contains the **neuron cell bodies** (the part containing the nucleus) supported by glia (specialised connective tissue (→ 2.5.2)), with glia outnumbering the neurons by about nine to one
- **white matter** consists of nerve fibres; its white colour comes from **myelin** – a fatty, lipid-based substance that surrounds and insulates the neuron fibres.

Most parts of the brain have a layer of grey matter on the outside with white matter inside (→ Fig. 9.4a). The situation is reversed in the spinal cord, where grey matter in the central portion is shaped rather like a butterfly, with white matter surrounding it (→ Fig. 9.4b).

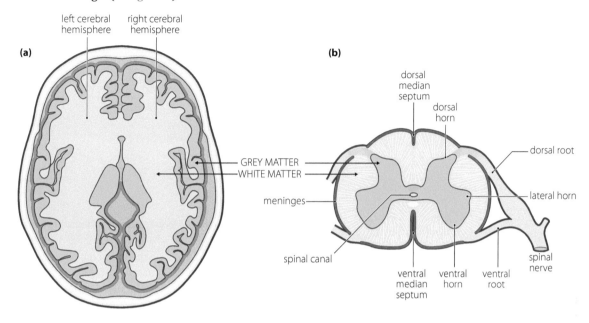

Fig. 9.4 Section through (**a**) the brain, (**b**) the spinal cord to show the distribution of the grey and white matter.

9.3 Brain

The brain is a complex organ that enables interaction with both the internal and external environment through electrical communication in the form of nerve impulses. It weighs about 1400 g in an adult and contains about 100 billion **neurons** and 900 billion glia (neuroglia (→ 2.5.4)). Neurons can only multiply before birth and during the early years of life (→ Box 9.7). After that, they grow in size and make more connections with other neurons, but they do not increase in number and, if damaged, cannot be renewed. During the first nine years of life the brain grows rapidly and full size is attained by about the age of eighteen.

The brain has three main parts:
- **forebrain,** most of which is cerebrum
- **midbrain,** a small but important part of the brain that includes the tectum, cerebral aqueduct and cerebral peduncles
- **hindbrain,** containing the cerebellum and brainstem.

9.3.1 Cerebrum

The cerebrum is the largest part of the brain and responsible for consciousness and cognitive (executive) functions, e.g. memory, reasoning, language and problem solving (→ Box 9.8). It is divided into two halves – the right and left **cerebral hemispheres** (→ Fig. 9.5). The two cerebral hemispheres are connected by the corpus callosum (→ Fig. 9.8). Each hemisphere has four lobes containing areas specialised for different functions (→ Fig. 9.6).

Box 9.7 Nutrients and growth factors regulate brain development during foetal and early post-natal life – the time that neurons are multiplying. Long chain fatty acids are especially important for the **development of the brain**, particularly during the first year of life. The brain doubles in size in the first year, and by age three has reached 80% of its adult volume. This growth is due mostly to increase in the size of the neurons and the number of nerve fibres.

Box 9.8 One of the five vital signs is the person's level of consciousness – alert and able to speak, or drowsy and confused. The rigid structure of the cranium normally protects soft tissues of the brain – cells, blood supply and CSF – which lie beneath it. Injury to the brain, e.g. trauma or stroke, can lead to swelling and a rise in intracranial pressure within the cranial vault which will change the individual's level of consciousness (→ Glasgow Coma Scale 17.1).

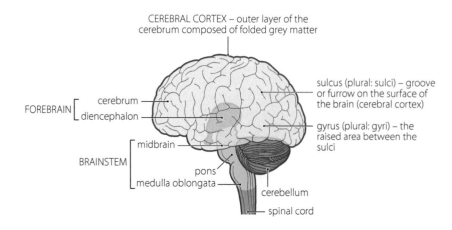

CEREBRAL CORTEX – outer layer of the cerebrum composed of folded grey matter

FOREBRAIN [cerebrum
           [diencephalon

sulcus (plural: sulci) – groove or furrow on the surface of the brain (cerebral cortex)

gyrus (plural: gyri) – the raised area between the sulci

BRAINSTEM [midbrain
          [pons
          [medulla oblongata

cerebellum

spinal cord

Fig. 9.5 Lateral view of the left cerebral hemisphere showing some of its parts.

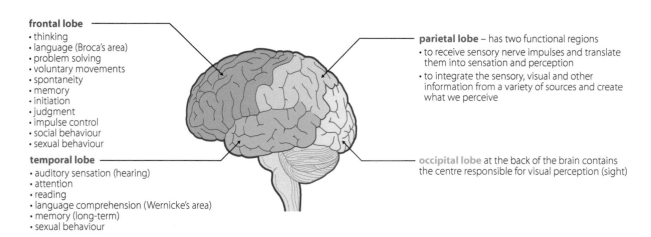

frontal lobe
- thinking
- language (Broca's area)
- problem solving
- voluntary movements
- spontaneity
- memory
- initiation
- judgment
- impulse control
- social behaviour
- sexual behaviour

temporal lobe
- auditory sensation (hearing)
- attention
- reading
- language comprehension (Wernicke's area)
- memory (long-term)
- sexual behaviour

parietal lobe – has two functional regions
- to receive sensory nerve impulses and translate them into sensation and perception
- to integrate the sensory, visual and other information from a variety of sources and create what we perceive

occipital lobe at the back of the brain contains the centre responsible for visual perception (sight)

Fig. 9.6 Lateral view of the left cerebral hemisphere showing the four lobes and their functions.

A layer of grey matter called the **cerebral cortex** includes many folds (**gyri**) and crevices (**sulci**) that allow the number of nerve cells in the cortex to be much increased. Each nerve cell connects with many others and the billions of nerve cells form an elaborate and complex network. The **prefrontal cortex** (PFC) is the part of the cerebral cortex which makes up the foremost part of the frontal lobe (→ Box 9.9).

Brain lateralisation refers to the fact that the two hemispheres of the human brain are not exactly alike. In most people, the left side of the brain has greater responsibility for speech, language and handedness while the right side is more musical, more artistically creative and better at interpreting faces and spaces.

Localisation of function

The different areas of the cerebrum are associated with specific functions (→ Fig. 9.7):

- the **prefrontal cortex** is responsible for executive functions, e.g. planning for the future, problem solving and organising multiple tasks
- the **motor cortex** is involved in the movement of skeletal muscles
- the **sensory cortex** receives and processes all the information received from the sense organs and from sensory cells, e.g. those that produce sensations of pressure, pain and warmth

Box 9.9 The cerebral cortex is highly active and requires approximately one-fifth of cardiac output. The blood supply to the brain comes from the carotid and vertebral arteries. At the base of the brain is a small interconnected structure (anastomosis) called the **circle of Willis** that distributes blood to all parts of the brain.

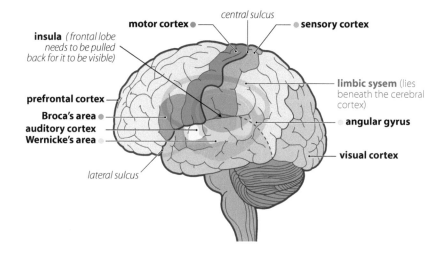

Fig. 9.7 Localisation of functions within the cerebral cortex.

- **visual cortex** processes information received from the retina of the eyes
- the **angular gyrus** is involved in processes related to language, number processing and spatial cognition and memory retrieval
- the **auditory cortex** processes auditory information (sounds)
- the **limbic cortex** lies beneath the cerebrum and includes important structures such as the thalamus, hypothalamus and amygdala. Together these make up the 'emotional' brain that provides drive, e.g. hunger, thirst, fear, sex drive and other motivations
- the **insula** (insular cortex) is a distinct but hidden part of the cerebral cortex folded deep within the lateral sulcus; it is believed to have diverse functions linked to consciousness, memory, learning and emotional response
- **Wernicke's area** is located in the left side of the brain and is responsible for the comprehension of speech
- **Broca's area** is a region in the frontal lobe of the dominant hemisphere (usually the left) involved in putting thoughts into words and speech production.

> **Taking it Further**
> To find out more about assessment of consciousness see online Chapter 17.

9.3.2 Neural tracts of the CNS

Neural tracts and pathways connect distant parts of the nervous system with each other by means of bundles of nerve fibres in the white matter (→ Fig. 9.8):

- **ascending tracts** (**somatosensory pathways**) are bundles of afferent nerve fibres that carry sensory impulses from the peripheral nerves to the brain, e.g. relating to touch, heat and pain
- the **thalamus** acts as a relay centre, directing sensory impulses (pink arrows in Fig. 9.8) to the appropriate part of the cerebral cortex for processing
- **descending tracts** are bundles of efferent nerve fibres that carry impulses from the motor cortex, via the spinal cord, to control movements of the body below the head
- the **reticular activating system** (RAS) comprises bundles of neurons in the brainstem that are responsible for sleep, wakefulness and the level of alertness
- the **corpus callosum** is a bundle of nerve fibres that cross the midline of the cerebrum, enabling the transfer of information between the two cerebral hemispheres.

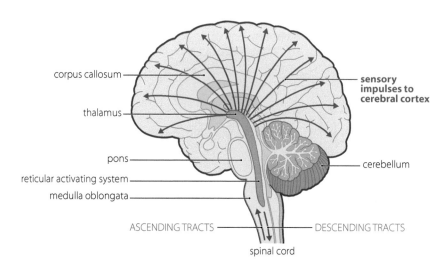

Fig. 9.8 Longitudinal section through the brain, showing the inner surface of the right cerebral hemisphere and the position of the reticular activating system.

9.3.3 Diencephalon

This part of the forebrain connects the cerebrum to the midbrain (→ Fig. 9.5). It consists of several distinct areas including the thalamus, hypothalamus and median forebrain bundle.

9.3.4 Limbic cortex

The word limbic comes from the Latin word *limbus*, which roughly means 'belt' or 'border', so the term 'limbic cortex' is used to describe a complex set of interconnected brain structures that lies beneath the cerebrum (→ Fig. 9.9). The limbic cortex:

- is responsible for instinctive feelings and **motivations** such as thirst, hunger, anger, fear and sex drive (→ Box 9.10)
- is under the control of the part of the cerebrum involved in executive functions such as memory and learning
- **regulates** the autonomic nervous system and the endocrine system via the hypothalamus (→ Box 9.11).

Box 9.10 In evolutionary terms, the **limbic cortex** is one of the most ancient regions of the brain. It has sometimes been described as 'the reacting and feeling' part of the brain, to distinguish it from the 'thinking' cerebral cortex.

Box 9.11 Disorders involving the limbic cortex include epilepsy, dementia and anxiety disorders. Neuroimaging and other studies show that people who have anxiety disorders have high levels of activity in this area and are particularly sensitive to emotional stimuli.

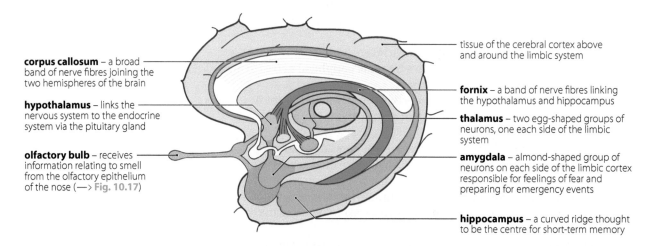

Fig. 9.9 The limbic cortex is involved in emotions, short-term memory and learning.

Thalamus

There are two thalami in the lower part of the cerebrum (→ Fig. 9.9). Each thalamus is an egg-shaped mass of grey matter containing many **nuclei** (clusters of neurons) that provide important relay functions transmitting sensory information to the appropriate part of the sensory cortex. Motor information is also relayed between parts of the cerebral cortex, the cerebellum and other centres.

Hypothalamus

The hypothalamus is situated in the floor of the cerebrum below the thalamus and above the pituitary gland, which is attached to it by a stalk (→ Fig. 11.1). Although only about the size of a pea, it is an extremely complex part of the brain and its primary function is **homeostasis**. To keep the body in a stable, constant state, the hypothalamus:

- receives sensory (afferent) information from the thalamus and cranial nerves about the external and internal environment
- detects changes in the state of the blood that flows through it, e.g. body temperature, fluid balance and thirst, using a set point to regulate each condition
- detects deviation from **homeostatic set points**, which triggers changes to compensate for disturbance by activating the autonomic nervous system and the endocrine system.

Median forebrain bundle

The median forebrain bundle (MFB) is a bundle of nerve fibres that links the forebrain with the limbic system and hypothalamus. Dopaminergic neurons in the MFB are an important source of **dopamine** which is released by pleasurable feelings of desire and craving, e.g. for food, sex and drugs, and acts as a reward system that encourages the learning of many specific behaviours (→ Box 9.12).

9.3.5 Cerebellum

The cerebellum is situated below and at the back of the cerebrum and, like the cerebrum, it is divided into two hemispheres which are linked together. Each cerebellar hemisphere has a ridged and folded outer layer of grey matter enclosing white matter arranged so that, in section, it resembles a tree with branches (→ Fig. 9.3). The function of the cerebellum is to coordinate smooth movement of the skeletal muscles, which includes:

- **maintaining muscle tone** that enables an upright posture and the ability to stand and walk (→ 4.7.2)
- **smoothness and accuracy of actions**, e.g. walking, talking, writing, feeding (→ Boxes 9.13 & 9.14) and the ability to learn patterns of coordinated movements, e.g. learning to walk.

9.3.6 Brainstem

The brainstem is the enlarged extension of the spinal cord in the skull with three parts: midbrain, medulla oblongata and pons (→ Fig. 9.5) (→ Box 9.15). The midbrain is the part that connects the pons and cerebellum with the cerebral hemispheres and is involved in many body functions including **consciousness**, sleep, vision, hearing and regulation of breathing.

Box 9.12 Dopamine is an important neurotransmitter in the brain (→ 9.4.3). It enables communication between centres involved in mood, pleasure and movement. Excessive dopamine has been associated with schizophrenia. Loss of dopaminergic neurons in parts of the brain which plan voluntary movements are responsible for Parkinson's disease.

Box 9.13 Cerebral palsy is the general term for a number of neurological conditions that affect movement and coordination. **Ataxic cerebral palsy** is caused by damage to the cerebellum.

Box 9.14 Dyspraxia affects coordination of movements and can cause a child to perform less well in daily activities for their age than expected.

Box 9.15 Brainstem death occurs when a person no longer has any activity in the brainstem and no potential for consciousness or independent breathing. A diagnosis of brainstem death requires that:
- the person must be unconscious and fail to respond to stimulation
- heartbeat and breathing can only be maintained using a ventilator
- there is clear evidence that serious brain damage has occurred and that function cannot be restored.

Reticular activating system

The reticular activating system (RAS) is a network of neurons in the brainstem that links with the hypothalamus and is responsible for transitions between sleep, **wakefulness** and high levels of attention.

Medulla oblongata

The medulla oblongata is continuous with the spinal cord and composed of white matter forming a network of nerve pathways. It contains the **vital centres** that control the involuntary reflex actions of:

- breathing, heart rate and blood pressure
- level of alertness as indicated by sight and sound reflexes via cranial nerves and the autonomic nervous system, e.g. blinking and startle reflexes
- maintenance of body temperature
- swallowing and vomiting (→ Box 9.16).

Pons variola

The pons bulges forward in front of the cerebellum and is part of the brainstem that links the medulla oblongata with the thalamus. It is responsible for many **reflexes** in the body, e.g. breathing, coughing, swallowing, vomiting and elimination through the bladder and bowel.

9.4 Nerves

A nerve is a bundle of nerve fibres that varies in thickness from those that contain thousands of neurons or very thin threads containing one or two neurons. The body contains 43 pairs of nerves which together form the **peripheral nervous system** (**PNS**) and they branch to connect the CNS with all parts of the body (→ Box 9.17). There is a huge variety of neuron types (→ 2.5.4).

9.4.1 Nerve impulses

A nerve impulse is a short burst of electrochemical change, called an **action potential**, that travels along the axon of a neuron. Neurons are excitable cells, which means that they can generate impulses in response to a stimulus. The stimulus can take a variety of forms – chemical neurotransmitter, heat, light, touch, etc. If the stimulus is intense enough, the response – an impulse – travels in a wave-like fashion until it reaches the terminal region of the neuron (→ Box 9.18).

Conduction velocity is the speed nerve impulses travel, which depends on the width of the nerve fibre and the presence or absence of a myelin sheath. Impulses travel most quickly – at a rate of 130 m/sec – in wide fibres (axons or dendrites) with myelin sheaths (→ Fig. 9.10), but only travel at about 0.5 m/sec in fibres which conduct slowly – thin fibres without myelin sheaths.

When an impulse reaches a terminal it triggers a cascade of events that lead to the release of **neurotransmitter** molecules. These diffuse across the gap (synapse) and bring about a response in the next muscle or gland (→ 9.4.4).

Direction of travel. Impulses travel along sensory neurons from a sense organ to the CNS (→ Fig. 9.10a). Impulses travel along motor neurons from the central nervous system to muscles or glands (→ Fig. 9.10b).

Box 9.16 The **Chemoreceptor trigger zone (CTZ)** is an area of the medulla oblongata that receives inputs from bloodborne drugs or hormones and communicates with the vomiting centre to initiate vomiting (→ Box 7.3).

Box 9.17 Neurons (→ Fig. 9.10) are the cells which make up nerve fibres and they can be:

- **sensory or afferent** when they carry nerve impulses from sense organs to the CNS
- **motor or efferent** – when they carry nerve impulses from the CNS to muscles or glands
- **enteric** – those that control the digestive system.

Box 9.18 Impulses always pass along a neuron in the **same direction** and are always of the **same strength**.

- An intense stimulus causes impulses to be sent at a high rate per second.
- A weak stimulus results in only a few impulses per second.
- If the stimulus does not reach a certain level – threshold level – there is no impulse.

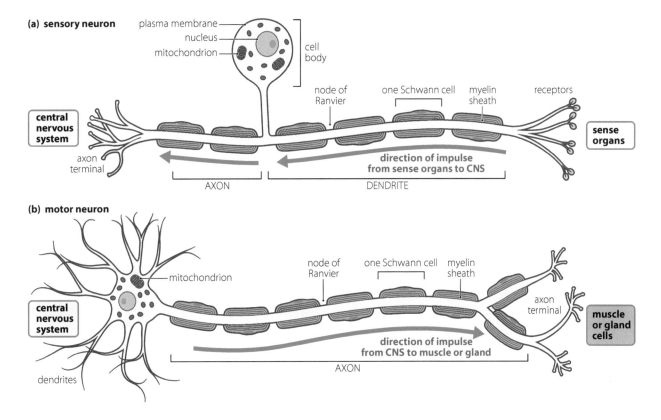

Fig. 9.10 (**a**) Sensory neurons; (**b**) motor neurons.

Resting potential

The resting potential is the potential difference between the two sides of the plasma membrane of a neuron when the cell is not conducting an impulse (→ Box 9.19). Several important processes contribute to the resting potential of cells:

- the negatively charged, large particles inside the cell cannot exit through the cell's semipermeable plasma membrane, e.g. proteins
- **permeability** of the plasma membrane to sodium (Na^+) and potassium (K^+) is different (→ 20.8.2)
- an energy-demanding **active transport** sodium/potassium ion exchange 'pump' (**Na^+/K^+-ATPase**) excludes sodium from the cell while accumulating potassium inside.

At rest, there are relatively more sodium ions outside the neuron and relatively more potassium ions inside, so the net effect of the chemical and electrical gradients is to make the interior of the neuron negatively charged (→ Box 9.20).

Action potential

Action potential is the change in electrical potential associated with the passage of an impulse along the plasma membrane of a muscle cell or neuron. The change in voltage occurs across the membrane of the cell when a nerve impulse is triggered by a stimulus. The passage of the nerve impulse is a rapid wave of depolarisation along the membrane of a nerve fibre (→ Fig. 9.11a (ii)–(iv)).

Box 9.19 All cells, including neurons, expend a relatively large amount of **energy** maintaining an electrochemical gradient between the cytoplasm which is negatively charged and the outside of the cell which is positively charged.

Taking it Further
To find out more about electrophysiological measurement please look in online Chapter 17.

Box 9.20 The **resting membrane potential** of a neuron is about **−70 mV** (mV = millivolt) – this means that the inside of the neuron is 70 mV less than the outside.

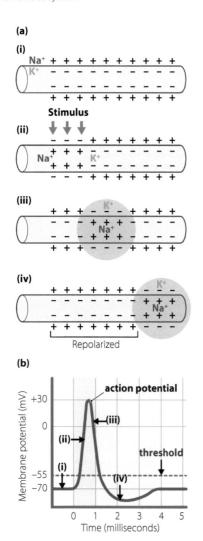

(a)

(i)

(i) **Resting potential** – the cell is expending energy to maintain electrochemical difference, so the inside of the membrane is relatively negative compared to the outside.

ACTION POTENTIAL

(ii) **Depolarisation** – the sudden surge of charged sodium ions (Na⁺) across the plasma membrane of a nerve cell or muscle cell due to the opening of the Na⁺ channels in the membrane. This reverses the cell's resting potential to produce an action potential.

(iii) **Repolarisation** – at the peak of the action potential, sodium channels close and voltage-gated potassium channels open. This allows potassium ions to leave the cell, and the membrane potential becomes negative once more.

(iv) **Hyperpolarisation** – there is a certain amount of 'overshoot' because the plasma membrane is very permeable to potassium so the membrane potential briefly becomes more negative than at rest. The neuron's plasma membrane is not responsive (**is refractory**) to further stimulation until after the resting stage has been restored.

Fig. 9.11 **(a)** Action potential that occurs as an impulse travels along the plasma membrane of an unmyelinated nerve fibre or muscle cell; **(b)** graph showing changes in voltage associated with the event.

9.4.2 Saltatory conduction

Saltatory conduction (from the Latin *saltare*, to hop or leap) is the movement of an action potential along a **myelinated** nerve fibre as it jumps from one node of Ranvier to the next, increasing the speed of conduction of the action potential (➔ Fig. 9.12).

Saltatory conduction occurs in axons which are wrapped in a myelin sheath by the Schwann cells because:
- the layers of myelin act as electrical insulation
- the myelin sheath is not continuous but has microscopic gaps (nodes of Ranvier) between neighbouring Schwann cells (➔ Fig. 9.10). At these nodes the intracellular and extracellular fluid are only separated by a single layer of membrane, and the action potential 'leaps' from one node to the next. This enables much more rapid conduction of impulses along the axon, while reducing demands for energy (➔ Box 9.21).

Box 9.21 Demyelinating disorders
Myelination is essential for the efficient functioning of neurons and the conduction of impulses; diseases that adversely affect myelination and cause muscle weakness include multiple sclerosis and Guillain–Barré syndrome.

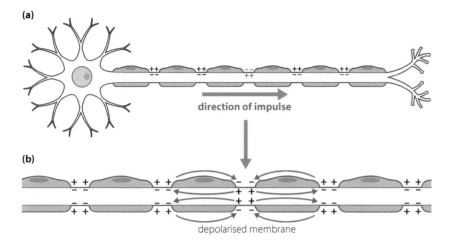

Fig. 9.12 Saltatory conduction of a nerve impulse along myelinated neurons showing (**a**) direction of travel and (**b**) local currents that flow to depolarise adjacent areas of the membrane to allow conduction of depolarisation.

9.4.3 Neurotransmitters

A **neurotransmitter** is a signal molecule that is released from a presynaptic neuron and diffuses across the synaptic cleft to either excite or inhibit the target cell, which will be either another neuron, a muscle cell or a gland cell. Neurotransmitters have special characteristics:

- they are made in the neuron and stored in vesicles in the axon terminal on the presynaptic side of a synapse (→ Fig. 9.13)
- when the neuron is stimulated, they are released and produce a specific response in the neighbouring target cell (postsynaptic cell)
- they are then degraded and removed, or taken back into the axon terminal for reuse.

Over 100 neurotransmitters have been identified and they:

- play a major role in many of the body's activities, e.g. mood, sleep, appetite, concentration and memory
- work best when present at their optimum level, and adverse symptoms may result when they are out of balance
- can be depleted in many ways, e.g. by stress, poor diet, genetic predisposition, drugs (prescription and illicit) and neurotoxins (→ 9.3.6).

Most neurotransmitters are either excitatory or inhibitory:

- **excitatory neurotransmitters** increase the likelihood that the target cell will produce an action potential and transmit an impulse, e.g. acetylcholine
- **inhibitory neurotransmitters** act by reducing the membrane potential so it is further away from threshold, making an action potential less likely, e.g. gamma-amino butyric acid (GABA).

9.4.4 Synapse

A synapse is the junction between two neurons (→ Fig. 9.13). Although coming very close together, axons and dendrites do not quite touch each other and there is a gap between them. When an impulse reaches a synapse, it stimulates the release of neurotransmitters from the axon terminal, e.g. acetylcholine or dopamine. These chemicals cross the gap (synaptic cleft) and cause a response in the adjacent cell (→ Box 9.22).

Box 9.22 Some neurotransmitters can be both excitatory and inhibitory depending on:
a) the amount that is released and
b) the response of target postsynaptic cells.

For example:
- Acetylcholine has an excitatory effect at neuromuscular junctions (→ 4.6.4) but is an inhibitory neurotransmitter when acting on the sinoatrial node of the heart (→ 5.11).
- Dopamine can have an excitatory effect on neurons in the medial forebrain bundle of the brain (→ 9.3.4), but is inhibitory in other parts, e.g. the regulation of prolactin release from the pituitary gland (→ 11.3.1).

Taking it Further
Many drugs affect transmission processes across synapses. For more information see online Chapter 18.

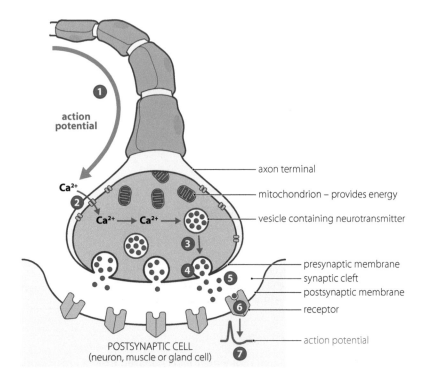

Fig. 9.13 Close-up of a synapse and the mechanism of transmitting a signal across the synaptic cleft.

Crossing the synapse (→ Fig. 9.13)
❶ An action potential (nerve impulse) arrives at the axon terminal.
❷ It triggers calcium ions to move into the axon terminal.
❸ Calcium ions trigger movement of neurotransmitter vesicles to fuse with the presynaptic membrane.
❹ The vesicles release their cargo of neurotransmitter molecules.
❺ The neurotransmitter molecules diffuse across the synaptic cleft.
❻ They bind with receptors on the postsynaptic membrane.
❼ The binding of the neurotransmitter molecules triggers a change in the membrane potential and may stimulate an action potential. The neurotransmitter is then broken down by enzymes and the breakdown products may be absorbed by the presynaptic neuron to make more neurotransmitter (→ Box 9.23).

9.4.5 Cranial nerves

Twelve pairs of cranial nerves arise directly from the brain and brainstem and pass through apertures in the skull, primarily to regions of the head and neck, the exception being the vagus nerve (→ Fig. 9.14). **Afferent** (sensory) **nerves** transmit nerve impulses towards the CNS; **efferent** (motor) **nerves** transmit nerve impulses away from the CNS.

Box 9.23 Psychoactive drugs act at synapses in the brain where they alter brain function, bringing about temporary changes in perception, mood, consciousness and behaviour. These drugs include medications and alcohol, and also illicit drugs, e.g. cannabis and cocaine. Some psychoactive drugs enhance the action of neurotransmitter systems, while others inhibit their action.

9.4.6 Spinal nerves

The 31 pairs of **spinal nerves** are connected to the spinal cord and pass outwards from the spinal column through openings between adjacent vertebrae. They are formed from the combination of nerve fibres from both dorsal and ventral roots (→ Fig. 9.4b) and are grouped according to the part of the vertebral column from which they emerge (→ Fig. 9.15).

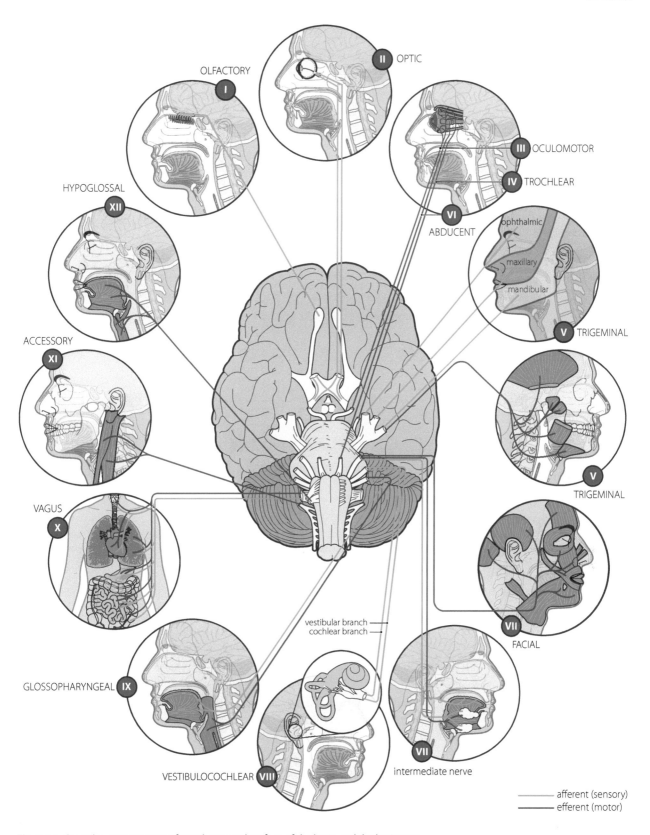

Fig. 9.14 Cranial nerves emerging from the ventral surface of the brain and the brainstem.

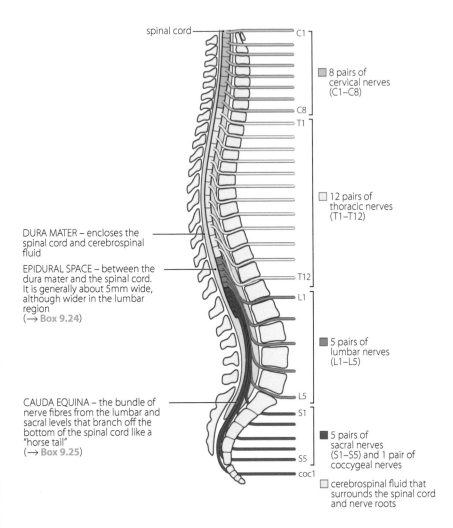

spinal cord

8 pairs of
cervical nerves
(C1–C8)

C1

C8

T1

12 pairs of
thoracic nerves
(T1–T12)

DURA MATER – encloses the
spinal cord and cerebrospinal
fluid

EPIDURAL SPACE – between the
dura mater and the spinal cord.
It is generally about 5mm wide,
although wider in the lumbar
region
(→ Box 9.24)

T12

L1

5 pairs of
lumbar nerves
(L1–L5)

CAUDA EQUINA – the bundle of
nerve fibres from the lumbar and
sacral levels that branch off the
bottom of the spinal cord like a
"horse tail"
(→ Box 9.25)

L5

S1

5 pairs of
sacral nerves
(S1–S5) and 1 pair of
coccygeal nerves

S5

coc1

cerebrospinal fluid that
surrounds the spinal cord
and nerve roots

Fig. 9.15 Arrangement of the spinal nerves arising from the spinal cord; the horizontal markings
on the spinal cord indicate the vertical segments through which the spinal nerve roots exit.

Box 9.24 Epidural anaesthesia,
often referred to as an **epidural**, is
an injection of a local anaesthetic
into the epidural space in the lower
back region to produce loss of
sensation, especially in the abdomen
or pelvic region.

Box 9.25 Cauda equina syndrome
can occur when the nerves of the
cauda equina become compressed.
Symptoms include pain in the lower
back, thighs and groin, numbness
in the groin, paralysis of one or
both legs, and bladder and bowel
incontinence. This condition needs
immediate medical assistance to
prevent permanent incontinence
and paralysis.

9.5 Voluntary actions

Humans are able to do many things. Most actions and behaviours occur
because of thoughts which have been generated in the mind. The human
brain is not 'hardwired' but is highly plastic, which means it is capable
of making new synaptic connections, even though it can be difficult for
neurons to regenerate (→ Box 9.1).

Cognition is a term used to describe the thinking and learning processes of
the brain and requires both sensory input to the brain as well as access to
information and experiences already stored there as memories.

Planning for future events is based on learned knowledge and experience,
and is a powerful and important aspect of human abilities and behaviours
that makes us distinct from other mammals. Planning skills are based on
the ability to encode the knowledge, retain it and recall it when necessary,
as well as converting ideas and concepts into language and physical action
and activity. All of these aspects require neuronal firing activity in different
networks of the brain.

9.5.1 Memory

Memory is about the ability to encode, store and recall words, concepts, facts and experiences within the neuronal circuits of the brain. The amygdala is part of the system that processes experiences and emotional responses, while the hippocampus is a part of the brain that is essential for short-term memory and the encoding to long-term memory.

Memories are not stored like files in a cabinet or videos in a computer. Instead of being a discrete entity, the recall of events, skills, habits and impressions depends on the synchronised firing of neurons within various neural networks scattered in different parts of the brain.

9.5.2 Emotions

Emotions are subjective feelings – happiness, hunger, thirst, anger, disgust, fear or sadness – so awareness of them is part of the cognition process. Emotions originate in the limbic system of the brain, can be positive or negative, and are important for determining behaviour, autonomic responses (→ 9.6.4) and the urge to take action(s). Emotions can create a stirred-up state of arousal which allows a rapid response that is specific to the altered situation, e.g. an episode of anxiety, the response to hearing music, suspense in a movie, feeling fearful or meeting a lover. The experience can be pleasurable or otherwise, depending on the trigger for the emotion (→ Box 9.26).

Box 9.26 People in all cultures have an understanding of the way **emotions** are accompanied by facial expressions. However, different cultures vary in the ways facial expressions are used to express different emotions.

9.6 Reflex actions

A **reflex action** is a rapid, involuntary response to a stimulus, and many have a protective or survival function (→ Box 9.27). Examples of reflex actions:
- **pupil reflex** – reducing the size of the pupil in bright light protects the retina
- **coughing** prevents asphyxiation
- **blinking** protects the eyes by keeping the surface moist
- **withdrawal reflex**, e.g. jerking the hand away when touching a hot surface.

Box 9.27 Newborn babies show a number of inborn reflex actions, including the:
- **rooting reflex.** When touched on the cheek, the baby turns its head and searches for the nipple or teat.
- **sucking reflex.** When the roof of the baby's mouth is touched, the baby will begin to suck. This reflex does not begin until about the 32nd week of pregnancy and is not fully developed until about 36 weeks, which accounts for the feeding difficulties of premature babies.

Other reflexes present at birth are the Moro reflex, grasp reflex, Babinski reflex, step reflex and tonic neck reflex.

9.6.1 Reflex arc

Reflex actions follow a specific nerve pathway known as a **reflex arc** which typically involves three types of neuron:
- **sensory receptors** detect the stimulus and convert it into impulses transmitted along **sensory** (afferent) **neurons** to the CNS
- **interneurons** receive the impulses and transmit them to motor neurons
- **motor neurons** transmit the impulses along efferent nerves to a muscle or gland which responds by producing the right reaction.

9.6.2 Spinal reflexes

A simple spinal reflex action involves only a few neurons and uses the spinal cord as a relay centre (integration centre) which functions without involving the brain. A simple spinal reflex involves only three neurons and is the reason why it still functions in a person with spinal cord injury (→ Fig. 9.16). Other spinal reflexes may involve more interneurons.

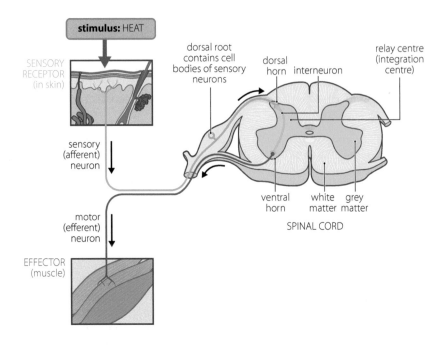

Fig. 9.16 Withdrawal reflex – an example of a spinal reflex. This spinal reflex arc starts when thermoreceptors in the skin are stimulated to send nerve impulses along sensory neurons to the spinal cord; these are relayed by interneurons to motor neurons that stimulate muscles to contract to move that part of the body away from the heat.

Box 9.28 The knee-jerk reflex is used as part of a neurological assessment. An exaggerated or slow or absent response is an aid to the diagnosis of certain diseases linked to nervous tissue between L2 and L4 segments of the spinal cord (→ Fig. 9.15).

Box 9.29 When a bright light shines through the pupil, the sensory information is carried by the optic nerve (cranial nerve II) to the brain. The oculomotor nerve (cranial nerve III) is activated and both pupils should respond to the stimulus by constricting. The pupillary reflex is commonly used as a neurological assessment by checking if the response is brisk or sluggish.

Box 9.30 When holding the breath, the level of carbon dioxide (PCO_2) in the blood rises, making it more acid. Chemoreceptors in the respiratory centres of the brainstem and the major arteries detect rising levels of acid (a fall in pH) that stimulate a reflex action and increase the rate and depth of breathing.

Knee-jerk reflex

The knee-jerk reflex (patellar reflex) is another example of a spinal reflex. A sharp tap on the patellar tendon just below the kneecap stretches the quadriceps muscles at the front of the thigh. The stimulus is detected by **proprioceptors** (→ 10.7) and transmitted to the spinal cord. The response is relayed along a motor nerve to the quadriceps muscle, making it contract and causing the lower leg to suddenly jerk forwards and upwards (→ Box 9.28).

9.6.3 Cranial reflexes

A cranial reflex action involves the cranial nerves and uses the brainstem as an integration centre. These reflexes tend to take place in the head area, e.g. the gag reflex and pupillary reflex (→ Box 9.29).

9.6.4 Autonomic reflexes

Many of the functions of the body are controlled by reflex actions of the autonomic nervous system (→ 9.8). The **autonomic neurons** originate in the brainstem and regulate the internal organs (viscera) without conscious awareness, e.g. heartbeat, digestion, blood pressure control (baroreflex). Some of these reflexes can be temporarily under voluntary control, e.g. breathing – it is possible to hold the breath for a short while until the reflex takes over again (→ Box 9.30).

9.6.5 Learned reflexes

Learned reflexes (**conditioned reflexes**) are actions that have to be learnt before they become automatic. Every time the action is repeated, the impulses involved pass along the same pathway in the nervous system, and eventually the action becomes automatic. Examples are walking, talking, reading, writing, bladder control, riding a bicycle, driving a car and playing a musical instrument (→ Box 9.31).

Habits are a type of learned reflex. They are actions which have been repeated so often that they become automatic, e.g. nail-biting, swearing and smoking after a meal. Once these reflexes have been learnt they are often difficult to unlearn and change.

9.7 Voluntary movements

The intention to make any voluntary movement, e.g. pointing a finger, chewing food, wiggling toes, dancing, speaking or playing a musical instrument, is known as a **central motor programme** and has its origin within the brain's motor cortex. A decision to move is swiftly followed by nerve impulses travelling to the appropriate muscles to make that movement by following the appropriate pathway.

9.7.1 Voluntary movement pathways in the CNS

Motor pathways control posture and balance, and coordinate the head, neck and eye movements. Motor commands from cells in the grey matter of the motor cortex initiate all voluntary movements and are modulated by pathways from other regions, including basal ganglia and cerebellum.

Descending motor pathways from the brain

- Impulses from upper motor neurons in the cerebrum and cerebellum descend via tracts (bundles of nerve fibres) through the **internal capsule** – the point where descending nerve fibres collect on their way to the spinal cord (→ Fig. 9.17)
- **Decussation** (crossing over the midline to the opposite side) takes place in most pathways but the level at which this happens can vary
- The impulses descend to synapse with lower motor neurons which exit via spinal nerves to appropriate muscles in the limbs.

Box 9.31 Walking involves more than the simple contraction and relaxation of antagonistic pairs of muscles. Complex actions are learned and require the coordination of many muscles and joints, a sense of balance, the ability to maintain an upright posture, and the activation of appropriate pattern-generating networks to produce the required gait and pace.

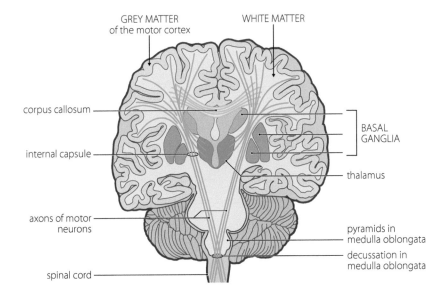

Fig. 9.17 Coronal section of the brain showing how motor pathways descend towards the spinal cord.

177

Pathway of the corticospinal tract (pyramidal tract)

- Nerve impulses originate in the motor cortex, are transmitted along motor nerve fibres and pass through the **pyramids** of the medulla to the cervical region of the spinal cord (→ Fig. 9.18)
- Decussation (crossing over) takes place to some of the fibres before they reach the spinal cord, while other fibres continue down to the spinal cord
- Synapses in the ventral horns of the lumbar spinal cord transmit impulses to the spinal nerve that supplies skeletal muscles.

Pathway of the rubrospinal tract

- The red nucleus in the midbrain integrates information from the cerebellum, eyes, ears and proprioceptors about posture and balance
- Impulses from the red nucleus travel along the rubrospinal tract through the medulla to the spinal cord (→ Fig. 9.19)
- Spinal nerves then transmit impulses to the skeletal muscles to help maintain balance and restore upright posture
- The rubrospinal tracts are responsible for large muscle movements of the upper limbs.

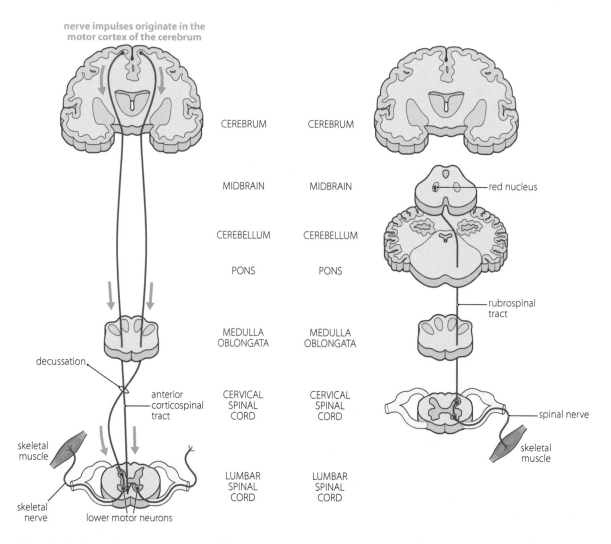

Fig. 9.18 Sections of the nervous system at different levels to show the pathway of the corticospinal tract.

Fig. 9.19 Sections of the nervous system at different levels to show the pathway of the rubrospinal tract.

9.8 Autonomic nervous system

The autonomic nervous system (ANS) is the part of the nervous system that:

- connects the brain and spinal cord to the **viscera** (internal organs of thorax, abdomen and pelvis) (→ Fig. 9.20)
- regulates the internal organs of the body by controlling the activities of smooth muscle, cardiac muscle, endocrine glands and secretory glands
- uses reflex actions to regulate the involuntary responses that maintain homeostasis, e.g. circulation, breathing, digestion, sweating, excretion and hormone production (→ Box 9.32).

Box 9.32 People are not normally aware of the homeostatic activity of the autonomic nervous system because its activities are instinctive and not under conscious control. But occasionally, we might be aware of some of the effects of ANS activity, e.g. when the brain receives impulses from the stretch receptors in the stomach and bladder, which indicate a feeling of fullness.

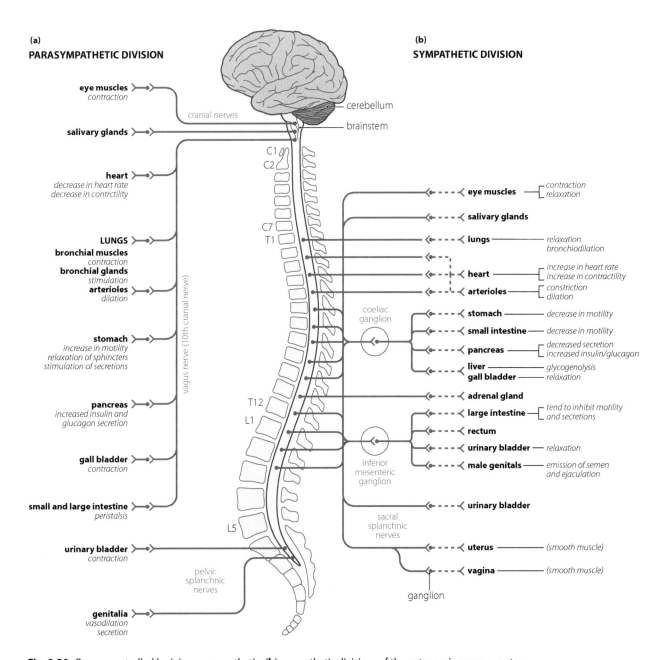

Fig. 9.20 Organs controlled by (**a**) parasympathetic; (**b**) sympathetic divisions of the autonomic nervous system.

Two subdivisions of the autonomic nervous system are the **parasympathetic division** and **sympathetic division**. The actions of these subdivisions are **reciprocal** because the effects of one system often, but not always, counteract the effects of the other (→ Fig. 9.20). A third subdivision – the **enteric nervous system** – governs the functioning of the gastrointestinal (GI) tract.

9.8.1 Parasympathetic division

The parasympathetic division prepares the body for rest, excretion and reproduction. One of the important parasympathetic nerves – the vagus (cranial nerve X) – emerges from the base of the brain and controls many thoracic and abdominal organs. The other parasympathetic nerves emerge from the cranial and sacral roots of the spinal cord. Parasympathetic nerves act by releasing **acetylcholine** at the synapses.

9.8.2 Sympathetic division

The sympathetic division prepares the body for action (fight, flight or freeze). The nerves emerge from the thoracic and lumbar regions of the spinal cord and innervate most body organs. Sympathetic neurons maintain homeostasis by releasing **noradrenaline** at the synapses. Sympathetic responses enable people to adapt quickly to changing or threatening circumstances and are important for survival. When the (potentially) dangerous situation has passed, activity of the sympathetic nervous system is reduced and parasympathetic activity increases – an example of homeostatic regulation. (N.B. noradrenaline is also sometimes known as norepinephrine).

9.8.3 Enteric division

The enteric division (**enteric nervous system**) consists of a network of neurons that control GI motility and secretions. It is embedded within the layers of the GI tract, starting in the oesophagus and extending to the anus. The nerves of the ENS are connected to two key ganglia – **coeliac ganglion** and **inferior mesenteric ganglion** (→ Fig. 9.20). Nerves of the ENS secrete a very wide range of neurotransmitters at the synapses which enable it to carry out its function of controlling the digestive process (→ Box 9.33).

9.8.4 Reciprocal innervation

Reciprocal innervation describes the dual supply of nerves to organs in the body, one set being supplied by the **parasympathetic division**, the other set by the **sympathetic** or **enteric division**. The interplay between the reciprocal nerves to an organ maintains the steady state of homeostasis which is achieved because at any one time, one tends to be more active while the other is less active, e.g. erection/ejaculation response (→ 12.3.2) and stage 1/stage 2 of labour (→ 12.7).

Example of reciprocal innervation

Regulation of cardiac output: stimulation of sympathetic nerves to the heart has an excitatory effect with increased heart rate and cardiac output. In contrast, stimulation of the parasympathetic nerves to the heart has an inhibitory effect by acting as a 'brake' and reducing the heart rate and cardiac output.

Box 9.33 A **ganglion** (plural = ganglia) is a cluster of nerve cell bodies along the course of a nerve which acts as a relay station for nerve impulses.

The ganglia are the sites where the sympathetic and parasympathetic divisions strongly influence the enteric division which is located within the digestive system itself.

Parasympathetic nerves tend to increase digestive secretions, promote peristalsis and enable digestive processes; sympathetic nerves tend to do the opposite, inhibiting digestion.

9.8.5 Neurotransmitters in the autonomic nervous system

Neurotransmitters are chemicals that relay signals between neurons at synapses. **Acetylcholine** is the neurotransmitter released in the ganglia (→ Fig. 9.21), but the parasympathetic and sympathetic divisions are mediated by different neurotransmitters with opposing effects on the organs and glands they affect (→ 11.1.1):

- the parasympathetic division releases **acetylcholine** in effector tissues. Acetylcholine tends to have an inhibiting effect on smooth muscle and glands, e.g. when danger has passed, it slows the heart rate, breathing becomes slower and shallower, the pupils constrict, the digestive processes are activated and the body relaxes (→ Fig. 9.21a)
- the sympathetic division releases **noradrenaline** (norepinephrine) in effector tissues. Noradrenaline is an excitatory neurotransmitter producing diverse effects, e.g. increase in heart rate, increased depth and rate of breathing, dilatation of the pupils, increased blood flow to skeletal muscles and inhibition of activity of smooth muscle in the digestive system (→ Fig. 9.21b).
- the enteric division uses a range of neurotransmitters and neuropeptides.

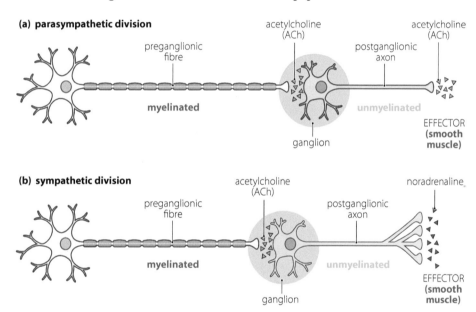

Fig. 9.21 Neurotransmitters in the autonomic nervous system: (**a**) parasympathetic division; (**b**) sympathetic division.

9.9 Pain

Pain is defined as an unpleasant sensory and emotional experience associated with actual or potential disease of the body. It can be experienced as:

- mild, localised discomfort contained within a discrete area
- a specific injury
- diffuse feelings of pain, e.g. fibromyalgia or abdominal pain
- excruciating pain (→ Box 9.34).

Pain activates the sympathetic nervous system, increasing respiration and pulse rates in response, while other signs include grimacing, guarding the area where pain is localised, calling out or moaning to get help.

Box 9.34 Pain assessment scales are used by healthcare practitioners and patients with the aim of assessing different aspects of pain, e.g. disability and mood, and the effect of pain medication (analgesics).

Pain assessment scales are available in different formats so that they can be reliably used with adults or children, those who have disabilities, and people who speak different languages.

Pain can be:
- **physical** when tissues are damaged
- **affective** when it affects the quality of life and interferes with the capacity to sleep, move and maintain everyday activities
- **emotional** when linked with unpleasant feelings; e.g. shame, loneliness, bereavement, divorce, trauma, abuse, bullying or other adverse experiences that can induce highly individual feelings of suffering or torment (→ Box 9.35).

9.9.1 Types of pain

The major types of pain are:
- **nociceptive pain** associated with physical damage to tissues or organs
- **neuropathic pain** associated with dysfunction of sensory nerves.

Distinguishing between these two types of pain is useful because the treatment approaches are different.

Nociceptive pain

Nociceptive pain is associated with physical trauma, e.g. injury, postoperative pain or arthritis. **Nociceptors** (pain receptors) are sensory neurons that detect the damage and transmit impulses to the spinal cord and brain. The pain can be felt as a sharp or dull aching pain, hot or burning, be mild to severe, temporary as occurs with a sprained ankle, or chronic as with arthritis. Nociceptive pain usually responds well to pain medication but usually not to neurostimulation (→ Box 9.36).

Inflammation leads to the release of chemical substances, such as histamine, that stimulate the nerve endings sensitive to pain, sometimes called **pruriceptors**. The pain can be acute and disappear when the inflammation subsides, or chronic as a result of long-term inflammatory conditions such as rheumatoid arthritis.

Neuropathic pain

Neuropathic pain, sometimes called **neuralgia**, can be chronic pain. It includes **phantom limb pain** following amputation and **post-herpetic neuralgia** – pain that occurs at the site of a previous attack of shingles. Direct damage or pressure on the nerve stimulates the pain receptors to send information to the brain, e.g. **sciatica** usually caused by compression or irritation of the sciatic nerve, or **trigeminal neuralgia** – sudden severe facial pain associated with the trigeminal nerve (cranial nerve V). Neuropathic pain can arise in damaged tissue after the initial cause has been resolved. It is often very severe and can be a sharp or shooting pain and does not usually respond as well as nociceptive pain to medication, but can often be managed by neurostimulation (→ Box 9.37). There are also good reports of effectiveness of cognitive behavioural therapy (CBT), relaxation (→ Box 9.36) and mindfulness practice in the modulation (relief) of pain.

9.9.2 Pain pathways

A **pain pathway** is the route taken by nerve impulses when sensory receptors are stimulated and pain is perceived in the brain. The perception of pain involves physiological, psychological and emotional aspects.

Box 9.35 The physiology of pain is a complex problem, not least because of the variety of factors that influence the subjective experience as well as the efficacy of therapeutic interventions and the possibility of recovery. This means that pain is a challenging problem for those who experience it, for society and for healthcare professionals.

Box 9.36 Relaxation techniques, including hypnosis and mindfulness, help to relax tense muscles and promote modulation of pain perception or adjust it to a certain degree.

Box 9.37 TENS (Transcutaneous electrical nerve stimulation) is a form of neurostimulation that uses electrodes placed on the surface of the skin. These impulses reach the brain faster than the pain signals and blocks them, and a tingling sensation is felt instead of pain. This type of pain relief has been successfully used for labour pains.

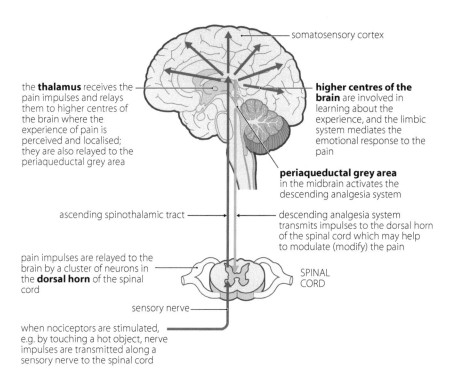

somatosensory cortex

the **thalamus** receives the pain impulses and relays them to higher centres of the brain where the experience of pain is perceived and localised; they are also relayed to the periaqueductal grey area

higher centres of the brain are involved in learning about the experience, and the limbic system mediates the emotional response to the pain

periaqueductal grey area in the midbrain activates the descending analgesia system

ascending spinothalamic tract

descending analgesia system transmits impulses to the dorsal horn of the spinal cord which may help to modulate (modify) the pain

pain impulses are relayed to the brain by a cluster of neurons in the **dorsal horn** of the spinal cord

SPINAL CORD

sensory nerve

when nociceptors are stimulated, e.g. by touching a hot object, nerve impulses are transmitted along a sensory nerve to the spinal cord

Fig. 9.22 Stimulation of nociceptors leads to transmission of information via ascending neural tracts to the brain.

Stages in perception of nociceptive pain

1. **Nociception**. Stimulation of sensory receptors to noxious (harmful) or potentially harmful stimuli initiates a train of impulses (pain signals) to activate the process. The stimulus can be:
   - mechanical stimulus, e.g. squeezing, scratching of skin or a very loud noise
   - thermoreceptors in extreme heat or cold
   - inflammation.
2. **Transmission**. Pain signals are conducted along a sensory nerve to the dorsal horn of the spinal cord where they may:
   - trigger a reflex response to withdraw from the noxious stimulus (→ Fig. 9.16)
   - be transmitted towards the brain via the nerve fibres in the ascending spinothalamic tract. The ascending tracts cross over to the other side of the CNS following a well-defined path to the brainstem, reticular activating system and thalamus in the brain. The pain signals ascend from the thalamus to the somatosensory cortex which enables pain to be localised, and to the limbic system which is responsible for the emotional response to pain.
3. **Modulation**. Transmission of nerve impulses may be blocked by descending modulatory circuits at the spinal or brainstem level so that the pain is not perceived. This top-down, inhibitory pain modulation from the brainstem is thought to be engaged to protect people from pain (→ Box 9.38).

The primary centre for modulation of pain transmission is called the **periaqueductal grey** (PAG) which is located in the midbrain (→ Fig. 9.22). This columnar nucleus (cluster of neurons) receives input from the cortex

Taking it Further
Relief of pain is an important aspect of healthcare practice. You can find out more about pain and analgesia in online Chapter 18.

Box 9.38 Endogenous opioids (often known as **endorphins**) are found at every level within the CNS and are called **neuromodulators** because they diffuse through nervous tissue to bind to opioid receptors. They trigger a cascade of interactions that are important for reducing the sensation of pain.

and activates the powerful, descending, **opioid-mediated analgesic** (pain-inhibiting) effect. The final effector of this system is the projecting neurons which terminate in the dorsal horns of the spinal cord which are responsible for transmission of pain. Their activity is modulated, depending on the context, to

- facilitate nociceptive transmission to the brain, or
- inhibit nociceptive transmission to the brain.

The PAG does more than simply modulate the subjective experience of the painful stimulus. It is now thought to play a role in adjusting the respiratory rate, cardiovascular variables and other autonomic responses to pain.

4. **Perception.** The individual experience of pain depends on previous experience, learned responses, stress and context. The context of pain refers to the individual's condition, e.g. when people are more anxious or very tired, the perception of pain may be heightened (→ Box 9.39).

There are many interconnected brain regions involved in perception of pain including the somatosensory cortex, insula, prefrontal cortex and limbic system and, together, these give rise to the uniquely personal, subjective experience. Interactions between these sites give meaning to painful experiences (→ Table 9.1).

Persistent pain

People who live with persistent (chronic) pain experience negative psychological, emotional and social effects, as well as altered physiological sensitivity, e.g. pain worsens when the person is trying to sleep. Living with chronic pain is not easy because the pain may impact on decision-making and problem-solving skills, it affects quality of life and is also associated with mental health problems such as depression, anxiety and suicide.

9.9.3 Biopsychosocial model of pain

The **biopsychosocial model of pain** states that health and illness are determined by a dynamic interaction between biological (genetic), psychological (thoughts, emotions, behaviours) and spiritual aspects of health and wellbeing. The same principles can be applied to the assessment of pain (→ Table 9.1).

Box 9.39 Neuroimaging studies have shown that perception of noxious stimuli activates several brain regions including limbic centres responsible for emotional processing and mood, and cortical centres responsible for giving meaning to pain.

Taking it Further
You can find out more about diagnostic imaging in online Chapter 17.

Table 9.1 Assessment of pain

	Acute	Chronic
Duration	temporary	persistent
Onset	sudden	more than 6 months
Cause	can be somatic, visceral or referred	may be unknown, e.g. back pain, or phantom limb pain
Physiological response	apparent, e.g. tachycardia, muscle tension	subtle and less obvious
Psychological response	anxiety	depression; reduced self-esteem
Behavioural response	may include crying, avoidance, agitation and grimacing	may include panic, loss of libido, disturbed sleep and relationship difficulties

9.10 Disorders of the nervous system

Consciousness is one of the most remarkable qualities of the human brain that distinguishes us from other species and earlier pre-human ancestors. Not only does the human brain enable people to walk upright, but it enables us to be self-aware, create new knowledge, enjoy the richness of relationships with other people, question the nature of the world around us and invent new technology. However, the downside of having such an amazing level of intellectual curiosity and free will is the overwhelming variety of abnormal states of mind and disorders that can affect people's development and personality.

A neurological disorder is any disorder of the nervous system. It includes structural, biochemical or electrical abnormalities in the brain, spinal cord, nerves or neurons (→ Box 9.40). With some illnesses of the mind there is no obvious physical damage but people may have problems with everyday living. Defining behaviour as abnormal is fraught with difficulties but people who find it difficult to cope with normal demands of everyday living are usually regarded as mentally ill (→ Box 9.41).

It is beyond the scope of this book to explore all of the wide variety of disorders of the nervous system, but the more common ones are:
- mood disorders, e.g. depression, bipolar disorder
- seizure disorders, e.g. epilepsy
- psychotic disorders, e.g. schizophrenia
- acquired brain injury, e.g. accidental trauma, stroke
- degenerative diseases, e.g. Parkinson's disease and Alzheimer's disease
- infections, e.g. meningitis
- developmental disorders, e.g. spina bifida, autism, Asperger's syndrome and foetal alcohol syndrome
- tumours, e.g. brain tumours.

People from different communities and cultures can exhibit signs of nervous system disorders in various ways. In some cultures, uncontrollable crying or headache may be a primary symptom of distress while people of a different cultural background might experience difficulty in breathing (→ Box 9.42).

9.10.1 Headache

Headaches are multifactorial but can often result from irritation of the meninges or blood vessels within the cranium. The inflammation involves the trigeminal nerve, other cranial nerves and brain centres. Nociceptors (pain receptors) are also thought to be stimulated by compression or inflammation of cranial and spinal nerves or spasm of cranial and cervical muscles. Pain may also originate in the sinuses, orbit of the eye, ears or teeth.

When a headache occurs that is similar to those previously experienced, e.g. tension headache, migraine or neck arthritis headache, and is accompanied by no other new symptom, it is not necessarily a sign of a serious health problem (→ Box 9.43).

Box 9.40 Brain imaging techniques developed in late 20th century and studies of molecular mechanisms of structural changes provide the underpinning evidence and data for modern **neurophysiology** – the physiology of the nervous system.

Box 9.41 Mental health problems are common and affect approximately one in every four people at some stage in their life. Mood disorders, substance misuse and other mental health difficulties constitute a major public health issue across the world.

Many people who experience **mental illness** recover fully, or are able to manage and live with their symptoms, especially if they get help in the early stages.

Unfortunately, lack of understanding, negative attitudes (**stigma**) and stereotyped beliefs about people who have a mental health condition are also common. For this reason, those who are affected by mental health problems often report that they experience strong social disadvantage which can lead to discrimination.

Box 9.42 An important aspect of the work of all health professionals is to recognise and understand the origins of disorders of the nervous system which will help them to gain a fuller and more accurate understanding of the impact of health problems on each individual.

Box 9.43 Headache is one of the most common reasons why people consult a health professional. There are about 200 different types of headache but 90% are of the non-dangerous type.

Several mechanisms have been debated including changes in vascular tone within the brain in response to afferent impulses in the trigeminal nerve (→ Fig. 9.14).

Tension headache

Tension headache is defined as a pressing or tightening, mild to moderate pain on both sides of the head that is not accompanied by nausea or vomiting and not aggravated by physical activity. These headaches are very common and can be due to stress, drinking too much alcohol, not getting enough sleep, becoming dehydrated and being unable to relax after work (→ Box 9.44).

Stress and emotional conflict are frequent triggers in predisposed individuals. In some people, a genetic predisposition may lead to sensitisation within pain processing systems in the CNS, allowing a vicious cycle where irregular headaches evolve into chronic syndromes (→ Box 9.45).

Migraine

Migraine is a severe, recurrent and disabling headache, often described as a pounding or throbbing pain on one or both sides of the head. It is regarded as a complex neurovascular disorder that originates in the sensory and nociceptive nerve fibres that supply blood vessels within the head and neck, causing abnormal activity in some parts of the brain. Each attack may be associated with physiological or emotional stressors, and the pain of the headache can be accompanied by sensory or visual disturbance (aura).

Different headaches

In rare cases, headache can be a symptom of a condition such as a stroke, meningitis, or a brain tumour. It is more likely to be serious if a headache is different, occurs suddenly (like a thunderclap), is very severe, doesn't go away and gets worse over time, or is associated with generalised fever, stiff neck, comes with one-sided muscle weakness, vision loss/change/aura or other disturbance, or is a new progressively worsening headache in someone over 50.

9.10.2 Mood disorders

A mood disorder (also known as a mental disorder, mental illness, mental ill health, psychological disorder or psychiatric disorder) is a mental or behavioural pattern that causes either suffering or the inability to function normally in ordinary life (→ Box 9.46).

All children and adults experience behavioural ups and downs with their mood, energy levels and patterns of activity. What sets mood disorders apart is the profound and unusual behavioural shifts, which can be severe. There are several hypotheses related to the major mental health problems including those below.

- The **monoamine hypothesis** proposes that alterations in the levels of neurotransmitters (dopamine; serotonin; GABA) within some key centres in the brain can alter behaviour and perception.
- The **stress–diathesis hypothesis** suggests that some people may be genetically more vulnerable to stress, while others may have had stressful experiences that have an ongoing impact on behaviour and mental wellbeing later in life, e.g. domestic violence, bullying, rape, abuse or neglect in childhood.

Box 9.44 Tension headaches can sometimes be relieved by rest and relaxation, drinking enough fluids or a mild analgesic (pain reliever). If they are severe, migraine-specific medication may be needed.

Box 9.45 Several genes are known to influence the stress response and how resilient people are in the face of troubles.

Box 9.46 Psychopathology is the scientific study of disorders that affect a person's mood, thinking and behaviour, e.g. depression, anxiety disorders, schizophrenia, eating disorders and addictions. Science and physiology can now track emotion and motivation to the limbic system of the brain (→ 9.3.4) based on neuro-imaging techniques. New ways of explaining mood disorders and other forms of mental ill health are based on ideas relating to disturbances in neural networks in the brain that regulate mood and memory.

- Living with a chronic, disabling condition such as arthritis or Parkinson's disease.
- Over-activity in the limbic system responsible for emotions, motivations and behaviours (→Fig. 9.9).
- History of alcohol or sexual abuse, or of illicit drugs.

Clinical depression

Clinical depression is feeling persistently and deeply sad for weeks or months, not just unhappy or fed up for a few days. It can follow on from life-changing events, e.g. bereavement, unemployment, having a baby (→ Box 9.47), or for no apparent reason. The disorder is quite common and affects about one in 10 people at some point in their lives – men, women and children. People with a family history of depression are also more likely to be affected.

Clinical depression is an illness with a variety of symptoms:
- **emotional symptoms** range from lasting feelings of sadness and hopelessness, to losing interest in the things that used to be enjoyed, to frequent weeping. Many people with depression also have symptoms of anxiety
- **physical symptoms** range from feeling constantly exhausted, sleeping badly, having no appetite or sex drive, and complaining of various aches and pains
- **severity of symptoms** can vary from feeling persistently low in spirits (low mood) to feeling that life is no longer worth living and suicidal (→ Box 9.48).

Bipolar affective disorder

Bipolar affective disorder (BPAD) is a lifelong and life-threatening illness that tends to run in families and which usually appears in early adulthood, affecting equal numbers of men and women. It is characterised by alternating periods of highs – episodes of **hypomania**, and lows – severe **depression**. Bipolar disorder affects about 2.5% of the world's population, with several forms of the illness being recognised (→ Box 9.49).

Hypomania followed by severe depressive swings means that people with BD can have difficulties in leading a normal lifestyle, even with the support of family and friends (→ Box 9.50). Like others who have enduring mental health problems, people with bipolar disorder are also at increased risk of developing obesity, type 2 diabetes, cardiovascular disease and metabolic syndrome (→ Box 9.51) (→ 16.9).

Involvement of the limbic cortex

The limbic cortex, particularly the amygdala (→ Fig. 9.9), has been attributed to mood disorders such as bipolar disorder because these structures are responsible for generating the fight, flight or freeze response to threats. This brain region is supplied with neurons from the prefrontal cortex which modulates emotional behaviours into human interactions and communications, so dysregulation of some of these pathways may lead to mood instability. However, the mechanisms of disruption of homeostasis within these mood networks are poorly understood. Many genes have been implicated in the subtle imbalances in neurotransmission and intracellular signal transduction that impact on cognitive and circadian/seasonal rhythmic processes in people with bipolar disorder.

Box 9.47 Post-natal depression is a severe form of depression that follows childbirth. It is far more serious and long-term than the '**baby blues**' (mild depression) that can occur as the mother's hormones settle down.

Box 9.48 Physical activity – whether regular, brisk walking or taking part in energetic sports – may be a simple strategy for management of clinical depression. Activity stimulates the brain to produce endorphins – opioid molecules that act as neuromodulators and natural painkillers, reduce discomfort and alleviate stress. Many people report that they have an improved sense of wellbeing and they can also feel more confident.

Box 9.49 Self-medication with alcohol, smoking and drugs, combined with a sedentary lifestyle, is a regular finding amongst people with bipolar disorder, which increases the risk of developing the other types of mood disorders.

Box 9.50 Hypomania is characterised by euphoria and elation with a feeling that thoughts are racing, an increased energy level and decreased need for sleep, lasting at least 4 days. The disinhibition is accompanied by a significant degree of persistent talkativeness, grandiosity accompanied by productivity and creative ideas, and hypersexuality.

Box 9.51 The development of metabolic syndrome is closely associated with antipsychotic medication prescribed for bipolar disorder, e.g. clozapine.

Taking it Further
You can find out more about drugs that act on neurons and synapses in online Chapter 18.

9.10.3 Anxiety disorders

Everybody can recognise what it is like to feel fearful, tense or worried about the events that are happening in life and, although the experience is unpleasant and exhausting, it is a perfectly normal reaction. The response incorporates both physical and emotional components related to activation of the sympathetic nervous system in response to a threat (→ Box 9.52). For a time, the worry may affect ability to sleep or to concentrate but usually – when the threat has passed or been dealt with – the physiological response will resolve and homeostasis is restored. It can therefore be difficult to determine when anxiety is becoming a problem for a person and is affecting their ability to carry out the activities of everyday living.

Anxiety is a characteristic symptom of several different problems, including:
- disorders of sleep and circadian rhythms
- substance misuse, e.g. smoking, drinking too much alcohol, using illicit drugs
- altered sex drive (libido)
- compromised immune system leading to impaired wound healing and greater susceptibility to some diseases
- depression
- difficulty in holding down a job
- struggling to maintain relationships or make new ones
- some medical disorders, e.g. hyperthyroidism may mimic symptoms of anxiety disorders.

Generalised anxiety disorder

Generalised anxiety disorder (GAD) is characterised by feelings of worry or fear that range from mild to severe. It is a long-term condition and people who are affected struggle to remember when they last felt relaxed. The ability to carry out activities of daily living (ADL) can be adversely affected and the disorder may be sufficiently severe to interfere with normal relationships with family and friends. Other mood disorders may be associated with GAD including panic disorder and PTSD, phobias and obsessive–compulsive disorder (→ Box 9.53).

Panic disorder

Panic disorder is the name given to recurring but unpredictable panic attacks, often for no reason that seems apparent to other people. A **panic attack** occurs when the body experiences a rush of intense psychological and physical symptoms. The attack is characterised by a pounding heart, breathing difficulties and a feeling of dread – sometimes a feeling that you are going to die; a very unpleasant and frightening experience.

Post-traumatic stress disorder

Post-traumatic stress disorder (PTSD) is an anxiety disorder caused by extremely frightening or life-threatening events, e.g. violent personal assaults (sexual assault; mugging; robbery), or by witnessing violent deaths, military combat or other traumatic experience. PTSD can develop immediately or weeks, months or years later, when the traumatic event is relived through nightmares and flashbacks, producing feelings of panic, isolation, irritability and guilt.

Phobia

Phobia is an extreme or irrational fear of a particular object, place or situation, e.g. agoraphobia – fear of open spaces; claustrophobia – fear of enclosed spaces; arachnophobia – fear of spiders.

Box 9.52 Anxiety can be the cause of physical symptoms such as fainting, dizziness, headache, tremor, sweating, poor concentration, diarrhoea, breathlessness and sexual difficulties.

Box 9.53 The amygdala normally processes sensory information and communicates the level of threat to other processing areas of the brain.

It is located deep in the limbic system of the brain (→ Fig. 9.9) and is part of the brain's system to detect threats and respond to danger. It seems to activate the involuntary responses of the sympathetic nervous system, hypothalamus and pituitary gland, as well as being part of the cognitive processes that people may recognise as 'fear'.

Obsessive–compulsive disorder

Obsessive–compulsive disorder (OCD) is an anxiety disorder that is characterised by recurrent, intrusive thoughts or images (obsessions) that repeatedly come to mind. Compulsions are repeated activities that the person feels they have to do to help diminish the feelings of fear and dread.

9.10.4 Epilepsy

Epilepsy is defined as a transient disturbance in the function of the brain involving the repetitive firing of impulses in large groups of neurons. The disturbance generally develops suddenly and then spontaneously ceases. Epileptic activity in the brain can be detected by an **electroencephalogram (EEG)** which can pick up and record brain wave activity (→ 17.3.2).

The physical manifestation of epilepsy includes seizures and a temporary loss of consciousness that occur when sudden surges of electrical activity in the brain spread to regions that control muscle activity (→ Box 9.54). Depending on the area of the brain affected, a seizure can be classified as partial or generalised (→ Table 9.2).

Partial seizures are those where only a small part of the brain is affected and include:
- **simple partial seizures**. The person remains fully conscious and aware of odd feelings, movements or stiffness. These seizures are sometimes known as 'warnings' or 'auras', because they can be a sign that another type of seizure is on its way.
- **complex partial seizures**. The sense of awareness is lost and there will be no memory of the event. It is often **accompanied by unusual movements** such as smacking the lips, rubbing the hands or making noises. (→ Boxes 9.55 and 9.56).

9.10.5 Schizophrenia

Schizophrenia occurs in roughly 1% of the population. It has a major genetic component, and schizophrenic individuals often have a close relative – mother, father, sibling, cousins – with the disease.

Schizophrenia is a psychotic disorder – a chronic disorder of the mind characterised by confused thinking and odd perceptions. People with psychoses lose touch with reality, two of the main symptoms being delusions and hallucinations. The disorder disrupts the way in which neurons communicate with each other at synapses, leading to disorganised behaviour. The illness usually starts in young adulthood, and the right treatment can result in long periods of normal behaviour.

Neurodevelopmental model of schizophrenia

This hypothesis reasons that environmental factors interact with the genetic factors to create the conditions for development of schizophrenia. Early life traumas including prenatal infections, maternal malnutrition and obstetric complications are thought to predispose abnormal development of the synapses in the foetal brain. Since brain development in humans is not complete until adulthood, other environmental factors including child abuse, loss of parents and neglect may contribute to the abnormalities of thinking and behaviour that are characteristic of schizophrenia.

Box 9.54 Terms no longer in common use:
- convulsion (fit) is now referred to as a **seizure**
- petit mal is now called **absence seizure**
- grand mal has been replaced by **tonic–clonic seizure**.

Box 9.55 Treatment for a seizure
When the seizure has stopped, roll the patient onto their side in the recovery position and loosen anything tight around the neck. Do not restrain the patient's movements except to prevent injury. Gently raise the chin to tilt the head back slightly as this will open up the airway and help the patient to breathe (→ Fig. 9.23).

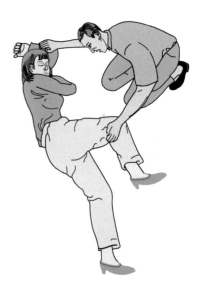

Fig. 9.23 Recovery position – the recommended position for all unconscious people.

Box 9.56 Status epilepticus is an emergency situation when a seizure lasts for more than 30 minutes, or a series of seizures but where the person does not regain consciousness in between.

Table 9.2 Features of different types of generalised seizure which occur when most of the brain is affected

Type of seizure	What happens	Effect
Absence seizures	Loss of awareness for a few seconds; sometimes rapid blinking; interruption to activity	The person may stare vacantly into space and have no memory of the seizure
Myoclonic	Limbs and upper body may twitch or jerk sporadically, often only for a fraction of a second	The person will normally remain conscious during the event
Clonic	Same type of repetitive jerking movements involving both sides of the body and may last for up to 2 minutes	Loss of consciousness may occur
Atonic	Muscles, especially in arms and legs, suddenly relax because they have lost tone	Risk of falling and injury
Tonic	All the muscles of the limbs become stiff	Risk of losing balance and falling
Tonic–clonic	Strong muscle contractions so body becomes stiff then limbs violently twitch	Loss of consciousness; person may cry out, bite their tongue or urinate
Status epilepticus	Seizure persists (lasting 30 minutes or more) because the mechanisms that terminate a seizure fail. Although these are not well defined they may be the result of oxidative stress and mitochondrial failure	A neurological emergency which can lead to neuronal death and is associated with high morbidity (ill health) and mortality (death rate)
Febrile seizure	Most often occurs between the ages of six months and five years when a child has a fever	The child loses consciousness, the arms and legs twitch and the body usually becomes stiff A complex febrile seizure may sometimes indicate more serious disease such as meningitis or encephalitis

Box 9.57 Glasgow Coma Scale (GCS) is a scoring system used to provide an initial assessment of the person's level of consciousness. It is inversely related to intracranial pressure – as pressure rises, the GCS score falls, reflecting deterioration in function of the nervous system (➔ 17.1.10).

Taking it Further
You can find out more about physiological observations and level of consciousness in online Chapter 17.

Box 9.58 Thinking, behaviour and skills are all affected by acquired brain injury but no two people will experience the same difficulties, changes and outcomes.

The consequences and recovery from an acquired brain injury will depend on the structures of the brain which have been affected, so rehabilitation usually requires an individualised, person-centred approach.

9.10.6 Acquired brain injury

Acquired brain injury (ABI) is damage to the brain since birth. The brain and spinal cord are soft delicate tissues that contain very little connective tissue and, therefore, cannot withstand compression. This means that the pressure within the cranium must be homeostatically maintained within normal limits for the brain to function. But, as ABI is likely to be accompanied by inflammation and an increase in intracranial pressure, the activity of important brain structures will be adversely affected. Also, the build-up of pressure on blood vessels restricts the blood flow within that part of the brain and can result in hypoxia (➔ 6.6.10).

The brain can be injured by many situations – traffic accidents, stroke, falls, tumours, toxins, assaults or other trauma to the head. The severity of the injury depends on the part of the brain that is damaged, which can initially be assessed by the Glasgow Coma Scale (➔ Box 9.57). The signs and symptoms of head injury vary widely and can include:
- concussion characterised by headache, confusion and amnesia (memory loss), which can be brief or prolonged
- difficulty in speaking or staying awake
- paralysis and loss of sensation
- loss of hearing
- double vision
- repeated vomiting
- dizziness and difficulties with balance
- blood or clear fluid coming from the ears or nose
- loss of consciousness or coma
- seizures with involuntary movements of muscles and limbs (➔ Box 9.58).

Neuroinflammation and excitotoxicity

In order to function efficiently, cells in the nervous system are very dependent on homeostatic regulation of the level of certain substances within the cytoplasm. Glial cells, such as astrocytes and microglia, play an essential role in clearing away any cell debris or potential toxins.

When the brain is injured or traumatised, hypoxia and inflammation mean that the natural homeostatic processes that clear away debris and toxins including **reactive oxygen species (ROS)** are overwhelmed (→ Box 9.59). This triggers **neuroinflammation** – a special form of inflammation that involves glia (→ 2.5.5) which are activated by the trauma. The response to the trauma can cause neurotransmitters to be released in amounts that poison and damage cells within the nervous system – a process called **excitotoxicity**. Depending on which part of the brain has been damaged, loss of function will follow.

9.10.7 Impaired brain functions after injury

Brain function can be impaired following stroke or brain injury; this can result in executive dysfunction, personality changes, communication problems, emotional changes and physical effects, e.g. hormonal imbalances, coma, reduced awareness, amnesia (→ Box 9.60) and aphasia (→ Box 9.61).

Hemiparesis

Hemiparesis means weakness or paralysis on one side of the body; this most commonly occurs after stroke. When the stroke occurs on the left side of the brain, hemiparesis occurs on the right side of the body; when the stroke occurs on the right side of the brain, the weakness occurs on the left side of the body. The weakness arises on the contralateral (opposite) side because of interruption in the activity of the corticospinal (pyramidal) descending tract that controls body movement (→ Fig. 9.17).

Impaired perception

Although vision and hand coordination may be good, the person may find it difficult to make sense of faces (**prosopagnosia**), pictures, shapes and objects (**agnosia**) or to navigate inside a building. A condition known as **'visual neglect'** may mean that the person may only see one side of objects or plates of food.

Lack of insight

Brain injuries can result in a range of emotional, cognitive, psychological and behavioural changes but the person who has been affected may not be aware of them. The affected person may have uncharacteristic outbursts of inappropriate language and behaviour, e.g. swearing, or make sexual advances due to lack of inhibition, or demonstrate impaired reasoning skills and/or inability to concentrate, which can have a significant impact on decision making (→ Box 9.62).

9.11 Neurodevelopmental disorders

Neurodevelopmental disorders are a group of conditions with their onset during the developmental period – the time from conception to the age of 18 years. Development of the human brain is thought to take place in

Box 9.59 Reactive oxygen species are sometimes referred to as 'free radicals' but, strictly speaking, they are different chemical substances.

Box 9.60 Amnesia is characterised by profound disturbance of memory, including the inability to remember names or recognise faces, and difficulties in learning and remembering what has just been read or said. Many different pathological conditions can lead to memory loss.

Box 9.61 Aphasia is a disturbance in the production and/or expression of language. Different types of aphasia depend on which parts of the brain and which aspects of linguistic processing and/or communicative skills are most compromised. The majority of aphasias are the result of stroke, trauma, cerebral tumours or dementia.

Box 9.62 It can be difficult and distressing for families and loved ones to cope with the changes in the person, and the affected people may find it frustrating when their actions are restricted by those around them. The affected people may also set unrealistic goals for their recovery because of poor understanding of their condition.

stages – from birth to 2 years, 2 to 7 years of age, 7 to 11 years old, and from 11 years upwards, and **development disorders** can become apparent at any stage. The disorders vary from very specific limitations of learning and executive functions of the brain to global development delay. **Global development delay** occurs when a child takes longer to reach the development milestones than other children of the same age, e.g. learning to walk or talk, or interacting with others socially and emotionally. Reduced intellectual ability may also be accompanied by physical or emotional difficulties.

9.11.1 Learning disabilities

Learning disabilities (→ Box 9.63) are defined as neurodevelopmental disorders, as they impact on people's ability to adapt within three domains of everyday function:

- **conceptual domain** – skills in language, reading, writing, maths, reasoning, knowledge and memory
- **social domain** – includes skills in interpersonal communication, empathy and social judgement, including the ability to make friendships
- **practical domain** – skills in self-management, including organisational skills needed for school, household and workplace tasks and responsibilities, personal care, money management.

Down syndrome

The most common learning disability is Down syndrome – a congenital disorder caused by the presence of an extra chromosome 21 (trisomy) in the body's cells that occurs by chance at conception. It affects both mental and physical development and results in intellectual impairment, short stature and broad facial features (→ Box 9.64).

Fragile X syndrome

Fragile X syndrome (FXS) is an inherited condition that can cause a wide range of difficulties with learning, as well as social, language, attentional, emotional, and behavioural problems (→ Box 9.65).

Cerebral palsy

Cerebral palsy (CP) is usually caused by an injury to the brain before, during or after birth. It is a condition that affects muscle control of posture and movement, which can include muscle overactivity and spasticity or weakness and loss of dexterity. This can result in speech and feeding difficulties, balance and coordination problems, hearing and sight problems and learning difficulties. CP is the most common cause of severe physical disability in children, and its incidence is increasing because survival of low birthweight children is improving.

The greatest risk of CP comes with premature deliveries possibly related to:
- cerebral immaturity that results in the presence of underdeveloped white matter in the CNS and fragility of developing blood vessels which leads to ischaemia (poor blood flow)
- infections of the placenta and uterus may initiate premature labour leading to CNS injury and CP because underdeveloped brains are more susceptible to the effects of inflammation
- multiple gestation (twins, triplets, etc.) increases the risk of antenatal complications and CP

Box 9.63 The term 'learning disabilities', formerly known as intellectual disabilities, reflects the change in language that has been happening in the last 20–30 years.

Box 9.64 The likelihood of having a baby born with Down syndrome is higher for older mothers, but the birth rate of Down's babies has fallen in recent decades due to increased numbers of terminations following prenatal diagnosis.

There are over 40,000 people in the UK with the condition. Their average life expectancy is 50–60 years, although a considerable number live into their 60s and beyond.

Box 9.65 Fragile X syndrome is the most common known inherited cause of learning disability and autism. It is the result of silencing of a gene – *FMR1* – on the X chromosome, which is necessary to regulate the synapses which use glutamate as the neurotransmitter. Many of the signs and symptoms of the syndrome arise from changes to synaptic signalling and plasticity (→ 11.1.1), hence the lack of the ability to learn. The syndrome may include autistic features such as social and language deficits, also seizures, hypersensitivity to sensory stimulation, sleep disturbances and macro-orchidism – abnormally large testes.

- problems with the placenta including haemorrhage, pre-eclampsia, placenta praevia, placental abruption or thrombophilias – an abnormal tendency to develop blood clots
- at the time of delivery, complicated labour and asphyxia are commonly associated with CP, but there is no clear association between the quality of midwifery and obstetric care and incidence of CP.

9.11.2 Autistic spectrum disorders

Autistic spectrum disorders (ASD) include autism and Asperger's disorder. ASD is sometimes accompanied by hyperactivity, seizures and sensorimotor abnormalities.

Autism

Autism is a **spectrum condition**, which means that there are varying levels of the disorder. People with autism:
- **may find it difficult to communicate with others**, sometimes not understanding other people's facial expressions, tone of voice or gestures
- **may not show emotions** such as love and affection; sometimes the only emotion is occasional outbursts of frustration or rage
- **might not always understand other people's feelings**, so find it difficult to make friends
- **find it difficult to use imagination**; some people on the autistic spectrum prefer to have a limited range of activities, sometimes carried out rigidly; they may also feel resistance or anxiety to changes in daily routine or unfamiliar surroundings (→ Box 9.66).

Various physiological mechanisms have been proposed to explain the wide phenotypic differences (→ 13.6.1) amongst people who are affected by ASD and their impairments to the CNS. More recent research studies have tended to focus on biochemical differences and nutritional deficiencies that may contribute in the subset of people on the autistic spectrum who are sensitive or intolerant to foods (→ Box 9.67).

Asperger's disorder

Asperger's disorder is considered by some to be a different form of autism and, like autism, Asperger's disorder is a 'hidden' disability because it is not apparent simply by looking at the person. While some individuals with autism have intellectual disabilities, most people with Asperger's disorder possess average or above average intelligence. There may be a limited ability to communicate orally, a lack of common sense and persistence in following particular routines (obsessive behaviour). Although people with this condition are aware of their disability, they often find it very difficult to make friends.

9.11.3 Dyslexia

Dyslexia is a general term for difficulties in learning to read or interpret words, letters and other symbols. It does not, however, affect general intelligence. The disability ranges from mild to severe and is a lifelong condition (→ Box 9.68).

Communication of thoughts involves language skills, and studies consistently show that dyslexia is a deficit of language processing with poor ability in decoding phonemes. Phonemes are linguistic units – the smallest detectable sound in spoken words – which are crucial to developing language and communication skills. Speech requires people to blend

Box 9.66 Some people with autism are very intelligent and may be gifted in certain areas, e.g. music, art or mathematics. But about 50% have learning disabilities – the NHS definition of a learning disability is an IQ below 70.

Box 9.67 Causes of autism are not clear, although suggestions include familial genetic abnormality, complications around the time of birth, exposure to toxins from the environment and early infections, e.g. maternal rubella. There is no evidence to support the hypothesis that autism is linked to childhood vaccinations. Neither is there evidence to suggest that lack of warmth and affection from parents is a contributing factor.

Box 9.68 Neuroimaging studies of dyslexia have implicated variations in parts of the brain's temporal and occipital regions, and genetic research highlights the ways that reading disorders are found in clusters in families, suggesting autosomal dominant transmission (→ 13.6.2).

phonemes into words, but the difficulty associated with dyslexia can arise through problems with recognising the phonemes that form different words, or with blending them. Problems with speed or rapidly naming the words or letters affect fluency (→ Box 9.69).

9.11.4 Attention deficit hyperactivity disorder

Attention deficit hyperactivity disorder (ADHD) is a developmental condition characterised by a group of behavioural symptoms that include:

- short attention span and being easily distracted
- hyperactivity – restlessness, constant fidgeting or over-activity
- impulsiveness and the inability to regulate emotional behaviour.

ADHD can occur in people of any intellectual ability, but is more common in those with learning difficulties; additional problems, such as sleep and anxiety disorders, may also be present.

Symptoms of ADHD tend to be first noticed at an early age, and may become more apparent when a child starts school, with most cases diagnosed between the ages of 6 and 12 years. The symptoms usually improve with age but, in many adults, ADHD will continue to pose difficulties (→ Box 9.70).

9.12 Degenerative diseases of neurons

Degenerative diseases of neurons are caused by the progressive loss of their structure or function, including neuron death which may occur within the CNS or in the periphery.

9.12.1 Multiple sclerosis

Multiple sclerosis (MS) is a progressive autoimmune disease of the central nervous system. Activated immune cells (T cells) infiltrate the blood–brain barrier (→ 9.2.2) of the CNS and attack myelin, causing lesions (damage) and characteristic scarring within the white matter, which affects the ability of the neurons to conduct impulses. The symptoms depend on which parts of the nervous system are affected by **plaques** – deposits of amyloid beta (a protein) in the grey matter of the brain – and may include blurred vision, slurred speech, uncoordinated movements and unsteady walking. Abnormalities in autonomic function are common – this control system acts largely unconsciously and regulates bodily functions and so abnormalities in it can lead to bladder, bowel and sexual problems. The illness is characterised by recurrent relapses followed by remissions, but recovery between episodes is often not complete and illness recurs after short intervals, making a person with MS gradually more disabled (→ Box 9.71).

9.12.2 Parkinson's disease

Parkinson's disease is progressive degeneration of the substantia nigra in the basal ganglia (→ Fig. 9.17) which normally controls movement of voluntary muscles (→ Box 9.72). Stiffness and **tremor** (shaking) of the muscles make movements slow and clumsy (→ Fig. 9.24). Muscles used for speaking are also affected, making speech increasingly slow and delivered in a dull monotone. The symptoms of Parkinson's usually appear after the age of 50, and the disease is often accompanied by chronic depression, anxiety and sleep disturbances.

Many of the neurons within the basal ganglia respond to proprioception input and these may modulate motor output related to specific movements. The slow loss of dopaminergic neurons in the substantia nigra takes place

Box 9.69 Research has found that early educational interventions, ideally before a child reaches seven or eight years of age, are the most effective way of achieving long-term improvements in reading and writing.

Box 9.70 Although the cause of ADHD has not been clarified, several mechanisms have been proposed. The underlying problem may lie within circuitry of the frontal and prefrontal regions and cerebellum, and may be associated with alterations of dopamine and noradrenaline neurotransmitter systems.

Box 9.71 MS affects about twice as many women as men and is usually diagnosed between the ages of 20 and 40 years. It is more common in areas away from the equator, e.g. the UK, Canada or Scandinavia.

Box 9.72 The **substantia nigra** (Latin = black substance) is a column of darkly pigmented neurons in the grey matter within the basal ganglia of the midbrain (→ Fig. 9.17). The function of this region for voluntary movement becomes apparent with the progression of Parkinson's disease. Neurons in the substantia nigra are dopaminergic, i.e. they produce dopamine, the neurotransmitter responsible for regulating movement of the voluntary muscles. Parkinson's disease develops when these neurons die, leading to difficulties with planning and controlling movements.

over many years, and recognisable signs of Parkinson's disease do not usually appear until 70% of them have degenerated. There are several dopaminergic tracts in the brain that connect to the basal ganglia, so disruption explains the effects of the disease (→ Box 9.73).

9.12.3 Motor neurone disease

Motor neurone disease (MND, also known as **amyotrophic lateral sclerosis – ALS**) causes degeneration of the motor neurons and progressive weakness and wasting of the skeletal muscles, which eventually stop working. Muscles used for speech are also affected and it may become increasingly difficult to swallow, but cognitive function (conscious awareness and thinking processes) are not affected. The disease occurs most commonly after the age of 50.

9.12.4 Dementia

Dementia is an umbrella term for a range of degenerative disorders more common in people over the age of 65. It is characterised by death of neurons in the brain, leading to impaired ability to learn and remember, and to behavioural changes. Dementia usually develops gradually with symptoms that include loss of memory, confusion, mood changes and difficulty with day-to-day tasks (→ Box 9.74).

Alzheimer's disease

Alzheimer's disease is named after the doctor who first described it – Alois Alzheimer. During the course of the disease, abnormal proteins build up in the brain to form structures called 'plaques' and 'tangles'. These lead to the loss of connections between neurons, and eventually their death and the loss of brain tissue. One of the first parts of the brain to be destroyed by Alzheimer's disease is the hippocampus – a structure that is key in formation of short-term memories. Thus, people with Alzheimer's disease will become increasingly dependent upon other people.

Vascular dementia

Vascular dementia is the second most common form of dementia. It is caused by problems in the supply of blood to the brain. The way in which vascular dementia affects each person will depend upon which part of the brain is affected by the interruptions in blood supply.

Dementia with Lewy bodies

Dementia with Lewy bodies (DLB) shares characteristics with Parkinson's disease and accounts for about 10% of all cases of dementia. It is caused by a build-up of **Lewy bodies** – tiny deposits of an insoluble protein in nerve cells that are linked to their progressive death and the loss of brain tissue (→ Box 9.75).

9.12.5 Prion diseases

Prions are defective proteins that damage neurons in the brain, leading to dementia, poor coordination and balance, cognitive and visual changes, persistent painful sensory symptoms and other neurological signs that worsen over time. The rare neurodegenerative diseases caused by misfolded proteins include:

- Creutzfeldt–Jakob disease
- Transmissible spongiform encephalopathy (TSE).

Box 9.73 Dopamine replacement therapies offer symptomatic benefits for many people who have Parkinson's disease, although their effects can wear off, and there can be severe side-effects.

Box 9.74 All forms of dementia are the result of death of neurons, often associated with an inflammatory response and the deposition of abnormal forms of the proteins in the brain. There are more than 100 different forms of dementia, the most common being Alzheimer's disease.

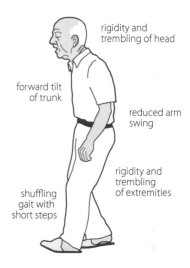

rigidity and trembling of head

forward tilt of trunk

reduced arm swing

rigidity and trembling of extremities

shuffling gait with short steps

Fig. 9.24 Parkinson's gait. People with Parkinsonian gait usually take small, shuffling steps.

Box 9.75 Coping with any form of dementia is distressing to both the person with dementia and to family members and professional carers. The person concerned tends to behave in ways that the carers find more and more upsetting, and does not understand why. Family members who struggle to cope with the continuous and demanding job of caring may become physically and emotionally worn out, and it is important that their own health is safeguarded so that they can continue to care.

9.13 Addiction

Addiction is a compulsion to do something that can interfere with everyday living such as the ability to sustain relationships or to hold down employment. There may also be a physiological component, known as **tolerance**, when the addict needs an increasingly higher dose to gain the same effect, e.g. to a drug such as nicotine, alcohol or cocaine. (*Addictus* is a Latin word meaning 'one who is slave to a master'.)

Addiction is considered to be a disease because the drugs change the structure of the brain and the way in which it functions. Addiction affects some of the motivational pathways and tracts within the brain (→ Box 9.76). The changes can be long-term; the behaviours can be compulsive and self-destructive, with failure to fulfil major role obligations at school, at home or in the workplace. Addiction may not be a specific diagnosis – it may be described as **substance use disorder**, because of a problematic pattern of use of an intoxicating substance.

Common addictions include alcohol, some drugs, shopping, surfing the internet, gambling including slot machines, sexual activity and playing video games. Treatment is aimed at the gradual withdrawal of the cause of the addiction and eventually total abstention.

9.13.1 Drug addiction

Drug addiction is defined as a chronic, relapsing brain disease that is characterised by compulsive drug seeking and use, despite the harmful consequences. Nearly all addictive drugs target the brain's dopaminergic pathways in the parts of the brain that are responsible for motivation, emotion and pleasure. The overstimulation of this system by the substance results in the 'rewarding' feelings of euphoria that teach people to repeat the behaviour to gain the pleasurable, desired effect. Tolerance to a drug requires increasing amounts of the substance to achieve the desired effect.

9.14 Managing disorders of the nervous system

Behavioural and psychological health cannot be separated from overall health and individual physiology. Mental health and physical wellbeing are inextricably linked but are often artificially separated by conceptual and professional boundaries and divisions (→ Box 9.77).

Neurologists are doctors specialising in the diagnosis and treatment of disorders of the brain, spinal cord and nerves, including those of the autonomic nervous and musculoskeletal systems, e.g. strokes, epilepsy, sleep disorders, pain syndromes, multiple sclerosis, Alzheimer's disease and Parkinson's disease.

Neurosurgeons specialise in surgery of the nervous system, especially the brain and spinal cord, e.g. tumours, intracranial bleeding or other trauma.

Mental health nurses are responsible for planning and providing support and medical and nursing care to people in hospital, at home or in other settings who are suffering from mental illness.

Learning disability nurses promote the health, wellbeing and independence of people with a learning disability. They also give help and support to families and carers.

Box 9.76 Addiction is thought to result from activity of the internal reward pathway which originates with the dopaminergic neurons of the median forebrain bundle (→ 9.3.4). When these are activated, they release dopamine, and this neurotransmitter seems to act as a reward and serves as a reinforcer. A **reinforcer** is something that, when presented after a behaviour, causes the probability of that behaviour's occurrence to increase.

GPs (General Practitioners) treat milder forms of depression and anxiety by talking with patients, advising on exercise as the treatment of choice for mild depression, and prescribing medicines such as antidepressants. Those with severe mental illness and neurological disorders are referred to multidisciplinary teams such as stroke nurses, dementia care teams, eating disorder specialists and neurology units.

Geriatricians are doctors who provide specialist expertise that focuses on acute illness and rehabilitation of frail older people. Although the health conditions that affect elderly people can be varied, geriatricians tend to take a holistic view and often coordinate the work of MDTs to provide supportive care of people with movement disorders, including falls, those who have dementia or Alzheimer's disease and those affected by delirium.

Psychiatrists are doctors who specialise in the study and treatment of mental disorders. Being medically trained, they are able to advise on treatments and prescribe medication when necessary. **Psychiatric hospitals** have clinics and beds for inpatients who will be cared for by mental health nurses. When discharged, patients may receive care from a community psychiatric nurse or from multidisciplinary teams in the community.

Clinical psychologists study normal and abnormal behaviour and are trained to assess and treat people who have mental health problems. **Educational psychologists** advise on the management of children and their learning.

Psychotherapists help people to understand their difficulties, weaknesses and anxieties in order to manage them. They generally treat more complex problems that have built up over many years.

Cognitive behavioural therapy (CBT) helps patients to change how they think ('cognition') and what they do ('behaviour'), e.g. sleeping difficulties, relationship problems, depression, anxiety, phobias, eating disorders (→ 19.9.2) and drug and alcohol abuse.

Working with a therapist, the patient looks for explanations for the distressing events in their life. To help this process, the patient may be asked to keep a diary. The diary is then used to identify the pattern of thoughts, emotions, bodily feelings and actions. This makes it easier to see how they are connected and how the patient can best deal with them. The aim of a course of therapy is to enable the patient to develop the skills needed to cope with the negative thoughts and emotions when they occur.

Box 9.77 Myths and misconceptions about serious mental health problems abound, so all healthcare providers have an important role to play in challenging stigma. As with any other illness, when given the right kind of help many people with long-term neurological or mental health disorders do recover and lead healthy, productive and satisfying lives.

It is estimated that about one in four people experience mental illness at some point in their lives. Most mental illness can be treated or controlled either by counselling or medication, but a short stay in a psychiatric hospital may be necessary.

Key points

1. The nervous system is an extensive network of neurons which are specialised to communicate rapidly by means of electrical impulses.
2. The central nervous system (CNS) is made up of the brain and spinal cord and is protected by bony structures and cerebrospinal fluid.
3. Nerves are bundles of nerve fibres that originate from the central nervous system and convey impulses between the sense organs, the CNS and effectors, including muscles and glands.
4. Action potentials (nerve impulses) are brief reversals of the electrical potential, which travel along neurons in one direction and at the same strength.
5. Neurotransmitters are chemical signal molecules that enable communication between neurons at synapses – microscopic gaps between neurons.
6. Movement and locomotion are consciously controlled through the voluntary nervous system while internal organs (viscera) are involuntary, being regulated by the autonomic nervous system.

Test yourself! Go to *www.lanternpublishing.com/AandP* and try the questions to check your understanding.

CHAPTER 10
THE SENSORY SYSTEM

Information about the external environment is obtained by sensory receptors. Collections of these receptors sensitive to light, sound, balance, smell and taste are found in the sense organs – eyes, ears, nose and tongue. Other sensory receptors are specialised to detect touch, temperature, pressure and pain. Proprioception – the sense of the body's position – is sometimes called the body's sixth sense.

10.1 Sensory system

The sensory system is the part of the nervous system responsible for processing sensory information, e.g. vision, hearing, olfaction, gustation and touch. Activation of a sensory system begins with a stimulus, and the response to the stimulus will depend on its:

- **location** – the origin of the stimulus
- **type** (**modality**) – the pattern and rate of impulses fired off in response to the stimulus
- **intensity** – the strength of the stimulus; a minimum intensity (threshold) of a stimulus will be required to produce a response
- **duration** – how long the stimulus lasts.

10.1.1 How sense organs work

All sense organs work in the same way – when the sensory receptors are stimulated, nerve impulses are sent along a sensory pathway to the central nervous system and, depending on which part of the brain they terminate in, they will be perceived as sight, sound, taste, etc. (→ Box 10.1).

Sensory pathways

Each sensory pathway starts in a sense organ when the sensory receptors transduce (convert) the energy of the stimulus into a series of nerve impulses. These travel along nerve fibres to the spinal cord which synapses with **ascending tracts** (bundles of nerve fibres in the spinal cord) before reaching the **thalamus** in the brain (→ Box 10.2). The thalamus acts as a control centre by relaying impulses onwards to the approriate region of the cerebral cortex (→ Fig. 10.1).

Box 10.1 The process of perception begins when an event or object in the external environment stimulates the sense organ(s).

Box 10.2 Sensory information enters the spinal cord on the same side of the body as the stimulus and moves along a sensory pathway in the spinal cord. The ascending tract then crosses over to the contralateral (other) side before reaching the brain. So, if one side of the brain is damaged, e.g. by a stroke, the sensory organs on the other side of the body are affected.

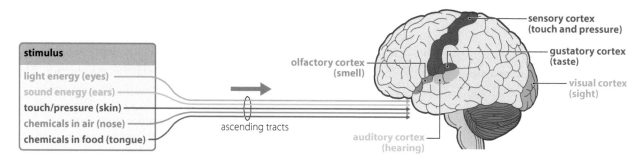

Fig. 10.1 Transduction of a physical stimulus into the experience of a sensation in the cerebral cortex of the brain.

Box 10.3 It is difficult to define a standard value for a sensory threshold because there are so many reasons why it is not consistent, e.g. mental state, age, fatigue and memory.

Box 10.4 The **extraocular muscles** are the six muscles that control movement of the eyeball and one muscle that controls the eyelid. They are all under the control of the **oculomotor nerve** which is very sensitive to changes in intracranial pressure (ICP). When ICP rises, the pupil of the eye becomes less responsive to light – a warning sign of brain injury.

Box 10.5 Saccadic eye movements are tiny, unconscious movements of the eyes as they move rapidly from one point to another when reading, scanning faces or the landscape. They originate in the brainstem and are coordinated with information from the vestibular apparatus (→ 10.4.1) in the ear. These movements of the eyes can be readily observed in a person who is dizzy after spinning round and round or who is suffering from **nystagmus** – the eyes look involuntarily from side to side in a rapid, swinging motion rather than staying fixed on an object or person.

10.1.2 Sensory receptors

Sensory receptors are specialised nerve endings that respond to stimuli by converting them to nerve impulses for transmission to the CNS. Some stimuli are from the internal environment and important for homeostasis, while others are from the external environment and provide a window on the outside world.

Different types of receptor respond to different stimuli:
- **photoreceptors** – **rods** and **cones** – in the eye are sensitive to visible light, which the brain interprets as vision
- **mechanoreceptors** in the **organ of Corti** of the ear are sensitive to vibrations that the brain perceives as sounds
- **hair cells** in the **vestibular apparatus** (semicircular canals) are sensitive to displacements that the brain interprets as the need to readjust balance and posture
- **chemoreceptors** detect blood oxygen and carbon dioxide levels
- **proprioceptors** in the muscles, tendons and joints monitor changes in the position of the body
- **baroreceptors** (stretch receptors) in the blood vessels respond to changes in blood pressure (→ 5.15.3)
- **thermoreceptors** respond to temperature changes in the skin
- **osmoreceptors** respond to changes in fluid balance (water balance)
- **nociceptors** respond to pain (→ 9.9.1).

Sensory adaptation

The minimum amount of a given stimulus that gives rise to a sensation is called the **sensory threshold** (→ Box 10.3). When a stimulus is applied frequently or continuously to sensory receptors, its effect is reduced with time and known as **sensory adaptation**. The degree of adaptation depends on the sensory receptors; for example, touch adapts readily and we soon forget we are wearing a ring, whereas warning sensations such as pain and cold adapt very slowly and incompletely.

10.2 Eyes

The function of the eyes is to receive light rays and convert them into nerve impulses that are sent to the visual cortex of the brain where they are interpreted as 'seeing'. Each eye has the shape of a small ball about 2–2.5 cm in diameter situated in an orbit (socket) in the skull, and is connected to the brain by the **optic nerve** at the back of the eyeball (→ Fig. 10.2).

10.2.1 Eye movements

Movement of the eyeball is carried out by the six **extraocular muscles** attached to it (→ Fig. 10.2); when these are all relaxed, the eyeball faces forward (→ Box 10.4). Contraction of one or more muscles causes the eye to move and receive light from a different direction, and they work together to focus on an object, track the words when reading and follow a moving object (→ Boxes 10.5 and 10.6).

Conjunctiva

The conjunctiva is a thin layer of stratified epithelium (→ 2.5.1) that lines the inside of the eyelids and covers the sclera. It contains goblet cells that secrete a small amount of tear fluid that helps to lubricate the eyeball to enable smooth movement (→ Fig. 10.3).

Lachrymal glands

A lachrymal gland (tear gland) lies deep above the upper, outer corner of each eye and continuously secretes fluid that:
- keeps the surface of the eyeball moist and clear. Every time the eyelids blink, tear fluid is spread over the eyeball with any excess draining away through a duct leading to the back of the nose. When foreign particles irritate the eye, e.g. dust or chemicals, the lachrymal glands secrete extra fluid – **tears** – to wash the irritant away. Emotions such as joy or sadness may also produce tears
- contains lysozyme – an enzyme that destroys bacteria, thus helping to prevent infection.

Box 10.6 Oculomotor dysfunction (OMD) occurs when the saccadic eye movements in one or both eyes do not move smoothly, accurately, and quickly across a line when reading or following a moving object. OMD is often not noticed in young children but becomes problematic when a child is asked to read or copy information. Vision therapy is then required.

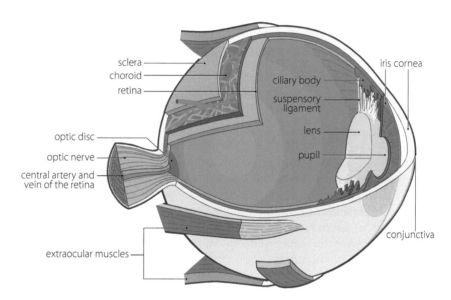

Fig. 10.2 Structure of the eye.

10.2.2 Structure of the eye

Eyeball wall

The eyeball has a three-layered wall (→ Fig. 10.2):
- **sclera** – the 'white of the eye' – is the opaque, fibrous, protective, outer layer; it is continuous with the transparent, bulging **cornea** in the front of the eye (→ Box 10.7)
- **choroid** is the middle layer containing the main arteries and veins of the eye; the black pigment (a form of melanin) in this layer prevents reflection of light within the eyeball. The choroid is continuous with the **ciliary body** to which the **suspensory ligament** is attached
- **retina** – forms a thin lining containing the light-sensitive cells and covers about 65% of the inner surface of the eyeball.

Box 10.7 Slight scratches to the cornea are acutely painful but quickly heal. If the scratch is deep, it should normally be checked by a health professional because a thick scar on the cornea can interfere with vision permanently.

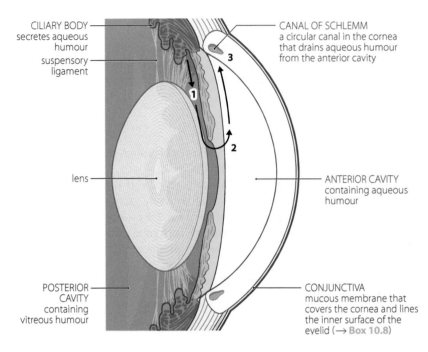

CILIARY BODY
secretes aqueous humour

suspensory ligament

lens

POSTERIOR CAVITY
containing vitreous humour

CANAL OF SCHLEMM
a circular canal in the cornea that drains aqueous humour from the anterior cavity

ANTERIOR CAVITY
containing aqueous humour

CONJUNCTIVA
mucous membrane that covers the cornea and lines the inner surface of the eyelid (→ Box 10.8)

Fig. 10.3 Circulation of aqueous humour in the anterior cavity of the eye, showing the direction of flow of aqueous fluid (1–3).

Box 10.8 Conjunctivitis ('red eye') is infection and inflammation of the conjunctiva caused by bacteria or viruses that can spread rapidly. **Allergic conjunctivitis** is a reaction to pollen or animal hair, dust mites, etc.

Anterior and posterior cavities

Internally the eye is divided into the anterior and posterior cavities. The two cavities are separated by the **lens** which is surrounded and held in position by the suspensory ligament. The **anterior cavity**, located in the space between the cornea and the lens, is filled with transparent watery fluid called **aqueous humour**, secreted by the ciliary body (→ Fig.10.3). The fluid is similar to plasma and flows around the cavity before draining away into the canal of Schlemm that connects with the blood system. As the fluid flows around, it supplies the cornea and lens with nutrients because both these structures lack a blood supply.

Posterior cavity

The **posterior (vitreous) cavity** is the space behind the lens filled with a clear gel called **vitreous humour**. This semi-solid substance helps maintain sufficient pressure to prevent the eyeball from collapsing and to keep the retina in place. Unlike aqueous fluid which is continuously being replaced, vitreous humour remains unchanged (→ Box 10.9).

Box 10.9 'Floaters' are collagen fibres and vitreous matter that shrink with ageing and cast shadows on the retina.

Box 10.10 Crystallins are the family of proteins that enable the lens to refract light while maintaining its transparency.

Lens

The lens of the eye is a nearly transparent, flexible structure suspended behind the iris of the eye (→ Fig. 10.4). The main component in the lens is water (65%); 34% is crystallin (→ Box 10.10), and the 1% of other substances includes lipids and inorganic materials. The function of the lens is to focus light rays onto the retina by the process of refraction (bending). The biconvex shape of the lens is maintained by a protein exoskeleton which, being flexible, means that the lens can change its shape – becoming fatter to focus on objects that are near and thinner to focus on objects that are far away. Organelles such as mitochondria (→ 2.3.1) are absent from the lens since they would alter its refractive properties and reduce transparency.

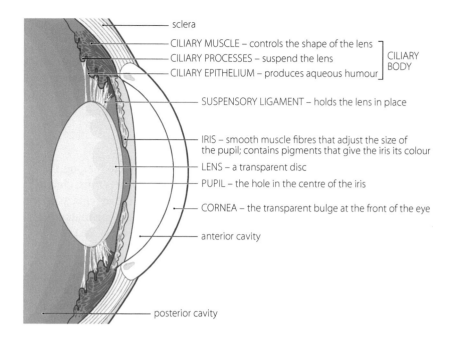

Fig. 10.4 Section through the front of the eye.

10.2.3 Retina

The retina lines the inner surface of the eye and contains three types of photoreceptors – cells sensitive to different qualities of light (→ Fig. 10.5):

- **rods** contain **rhodopsin** (visual purple) and are sensitive to the presence or absence of light but not to colour; they enable us to see in a dim light
- **cones** are sensitive to colour and function best in brighter light. There are three types of cone – one type is sensitive to red wavelengths, another to green wavelengths, and the third type to blue wavelengths. Equal stimulation of all three types of cone gives a sensation of white
- **ganglion cells** contain **melanopsin** and are sensitive to day length (→ Box 10.11). This photosensitive pigment is involved in the regulation of circadian rhythms (→ Box 10.12). Ganglion cells are neurons specialised to receive visual information from the rods and cones, via the bipolar cells, and transmit it to the brain.

Box 10.11 Rhodopsin and melanopsin belong to a group of light-sensitive pigments (**opsins**) that are sensitive to different wavelengths of the visible electromagnetic spectrum.

Box 10.12 Circadian rhythms are physical, mental and behavioural changes that follow a roughly 24-hour cycle, responding primarily to light and darkness in the external environment.

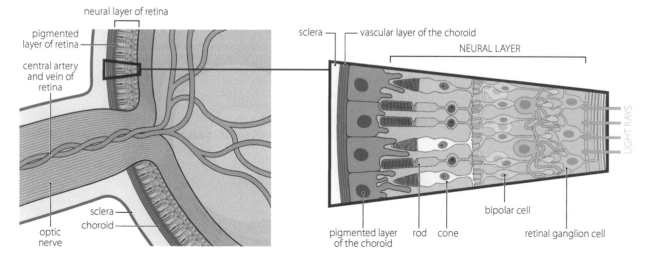

Fig. 10.5 Simplified structure of the retina.

Function

The function of the photoreceptors of the eye is to compress sensory information into a series of nerve impulses that travel via the optic nerve to the **visual cortex of the brain** (→ Fig. 9.7). The densely packed neurons of the visual cortex are arranged in layers, each of which plays a different role in creating perception of the depth, colour and motion of the image.

Distribution of rods and cones

Cones are more numerous in the part of the retina opposite to the pupil called the **macula lutea** (→ Box 10.13). In daylight, an object is most clearly seen when the light rays from it are focused directly onto the macula, with the surrounding objects being indistinct. Moving outwards from the macula, the density of cones decreases and density of rods increases (→ Box 10.14).

10.3 Vision

Vision (**eyesight** or **visual perception**) is the ability to see. In order for vision to occur, light rays must form an image on the retina that stimulates the photoreceptors (rods and cones) to send impulses along the optic nerve (2nd cranial nerve) to the **visual cortex** of the brain, where the image is perceived. The **optic disc** (blind spot) is the point where the nerve fibres from the light-sensitive cells leave the retina to form the optic nerve (→ Fig. 10.2).

Night vision

In a dim light the pupils open wide, allowing light to reach the rods at the sides of the retina. The **rhodopsin** (visual purple) they contain is bleached to visual yellow in bright light and re-forms when the light becomes dim. Consequently, when a person moves from a bright light to a dim light, nothing can be seen at first, but as rhodopsin gradually re-forms it becomes possible to see again – not in colour, but in various shades of grey (→ Box 10.15).

Dazzled by bright light

When going from dim light to a bright light, a person feels dazzled at first. It takes time for the pupils to get smaller, the rhodopsin to bleach, and the eyes to become adapted to bright light and colour.

Colourblindness

Most people can see thousands of different colours, but those who are colourblind do not see colours in the usual way. The condition is often inherited and people who are affected lack one or more of the three different kinds of cone found in the retina. As a result, they may be able to see some colours but not others.

Colourblindness can sometimes make it difficult for children to read and can affect people's career choices, so early assessment can be important for a child's self-esteem.

10.3.1 Pathway of light through the eyes

Light rays pass through the transparent cornea, aqueous humour, lens and vitreous humours to reach the retina where they form an image which is upside down and back to front (→ Fig. 10.6a), which is later corrected by the brain. In order for the light rays to form a clear image on the retina, they undergo four processes.

Box 10.13 The **macula lutea** is the yellow-pigmented area in the central area of the retina which provides sharp, sensitive vision needed for reading and appreciating colour (→ Fig. 10.10). A tiny pit in the macula called the **fovea centralis** contains only cones and provides the clearest acuity (sharpness) of vision (→ Fig. 10.6).

Box 10.14 The retina contains about 7 million cones and about 75–150 million rods.

Box 10.15 Rhodopsin strongly absorbs green-blue light and therefore appears reddish-purple, hence the name 'visual purple'. Vitamin A is one of the required precursors for the formation of rhodopsin, and is found in many foods from both plants and animals.

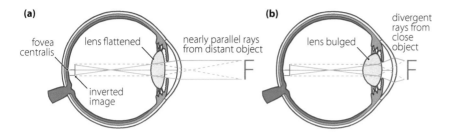

Fig. 10.6 Vision (**a**) Distant vision; (**b**) Near vision.

1. Corneal refraction

Most refraction in the eye takes place as light rays enter the cornea and are refracted (bent) and brought into focus on the retina (→ Fig. 10.6b).

2. Pupil adjustment

The function of the iris is to regulate the amount of light entering the eye through the reflex control of the size of the pupil (→ Fig. 10.7). The pupil contains a sphincter (ring of muscle tissue) around the margin that contracts in bright light, causing the pupil to become smaller. In a dim light the radial muscles in the iris contract and the sphincter relaxes, increasing the size of the pupil and allowing more light to enter the eyeball (→ Box 10.16).

Box 10.16 Mydriasis is dilation of the pupils, a common cause being drugs of abuse, e.g. amphetamines, cocaine, LSD and mescaline. Other drugs, e.g. alcohol and opiates, cause the pupils to constrict (**myosis**).

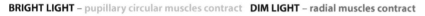

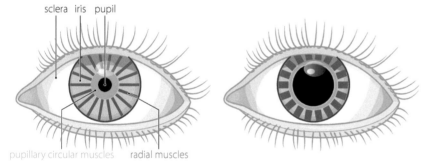

Fig. 10.7 Pupil light reflex.

3. Accommodation (focusing the lens)

Accommodation is the ability of the eye to change its focus from distant to near objects (and vice versa) by action of the ciliary muscles (→ Fig. 10.6). When they contract and relax, the ciliary muscles tighten or loosen the suspensory ligaments, which adjusts the shape of the lens. A convex (outward-curving) lens refracts (bends) light rays more and enables nearer objects to be brought more precisely into focus on the retina (→ Box 10.17).

4. Convergence

Convergence is the simultaneous movement of both eyes to focus on the same object. The nearer the object, the greater the degree of convergence; when looking into the distance, the eyes diverge until parallel. Eye movements are controlled by the extraocular muscles. Convergence is one of several cues that help us to discern depth (→ Box 10.18).

Box 10.17 Accommodation of the eye is a reflex action (→ Fig. 9.6). The **afferent pathway** travels from the retinal cells and optic nerve to the visual cortex. **Interneurons** help to determine whether an image is in focus or blurred and send corrective signals from the visual cortex to initiate and modulate the response. The efferent pathway of the oculomotor nerve (→ Fig. 9.14) arises in the midbrain and supplies parasympathetic (→ Fig. 9.20) fibres to the eye, constricting the pupil and altering the shape of the lens.

Box 10.18 Extreme convergence (cross-eyed viewing) occurs when focusing on the nose.

10.3.2 Binocular vision

When an object is viewed with both eyes, each one receives light from a slightly different angle and sends slightly different information about the image to the visual cortex in the brain. When the images are perceived, the small differences between them produce a three-dimensional effect. This gives an impression of depth and allows more accurate judgement of distance (→ Fig. 10.8). Binocular vision enables people to see where objects are in relation to their own bodies and is particularly important for skills like pouring fluids into containers, throwing and catching, driving a car, crossing a road or reaching out to touch objects.

If the acuity (sharpness) of vision from one of the eyes becomes poor, or the part of the visual cortex that is responsible for comparing the images does not develop properly or becomes damaged, then binocular vision is lost. This is because the brain is unable to work out depth and speed of movement.

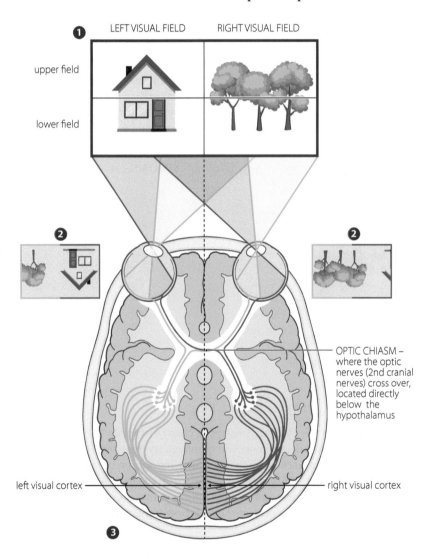

Fig. 10.8 Visual pathway. **Step 1**: Light rays from this view stimulate the eyes to send impulses to the brain. **Step 2**: The image of the external world seen from the right eye becomes inverted. Part of the information about the image comes from the left visual field and part from the right visual field. A corresponding inversion occurs in the left eye. **Step 3**: The two images are corrected in the brain to give a single image with a 3D effect which is the correct way up.

Optic chiasm

The optic chiasm is located in the base of the cerebrum. It is an X-shaped structure formed by the two optic nerves as they partly cross-over on the pathway from the eyeballs to the visual cortex in the brain (→ Fig. 10.8).

At the point of cross-over, nerve fibres from the inner (nasal) side of each retina move across to the other side. This allows visual images from both eyes to reach the visual cortex where they are combined to form a single image. The neurons in the visual cortex are arranged in layers which perceive dark and light areas, movement, and horizontal and vertical planes (→ Box 10.19).

10.3.3 Visual problems

When the eyeball has the normal shape and curvature, light is refracted on the retina; but when the shape is irregular, refractive errors mean that vision is affected and can be the cause of myopia, hypermetropia or astigmatism.

Myopia

Myopia (short-sightedness) occurs when the light rays entering the eye from distant objects are focused in front of the retina rather than on it and cannot be corrected by accommodation. The condition arises when the eyeball is too long from front to back or the cornea has too much curvature. This makes distant objects appear blurred but those close to the eyes can be clearly seen. Myopia is corrected by lenses that refract (bend) the light rays outwards before they reach the eyes, or by laser surgery (→ Box 10.20).

Hypermetropia

Hypermetropia (long-sightedness) occurs when the eye does not focus light on the retina because the eyeball is too short from front to back, or the cornea is too flat. Light rays entering the eye from objects nearby are focused behind the retina rather than on it and appear blurred, whereas distant objects can be seen clearly. The condition is corrected by wearing spectacles with convex lenses that refract the light rays on the retina (→ Box 10.21).

Astigmatism

A normal cornea is round, and evenly curved from side to side and top to bottom. Astigmatism occurs when the cornea is unevenly curved, making objects look crooked and out of shape, and distorting both near and distant and vision.

10.3.4 Visual impairment

Visual impairment is sight loss that cannot be fully corrected by spectacles or contact lenses. **Total blindness**, due to the loss of sight in both eyes, injury to the optic nerves or damage to the visual areas of the brain, is rare. Most visually-impaired people have **low vision**, which has many causes including those mentioned below.

Box 10.19 Neurological test to light When a torch is shone directly into one eye for three seconds, both pupils should constrict briskly to protect the retina from damage to the high intensity of light. Failure to do so can indicate damage of the optic system. Dilation of the pupil on one side only is also abnormal and may be a sign of brain injury or other condition that raises pressure within the cranium.

Box 10.20 Myopia is often inherited but regular eye checks can ensure that corrective lenses are properly fitted. Refractive laser surgery is a more recent option once eyes have stopped growing.

Box 10.21 Presbyopia develops because of gradual changes in the structure of the lens. Eventually the ageing eye is unable to focus on close objects; this often occurs between the ages of 40 and 50. People with presbyopia will tend to squint or hold reading materials at arm's length.

Cataract

A cataract is an opaque (cloudy) lens that usually makes the centre of the eye look milky-white, and vision is blurred or lost completely in the affected eye (→ Fig. 10.9). Surgical removal of the lens restores some sight, and useful vision is obtained by replacing the cataract with an artificial lens. Cataracts are most commonly due to ageing but there are other less common forms (→ Box 10.22). People who have diabetes mellitus are also at higher risk of cataract than those who do not.

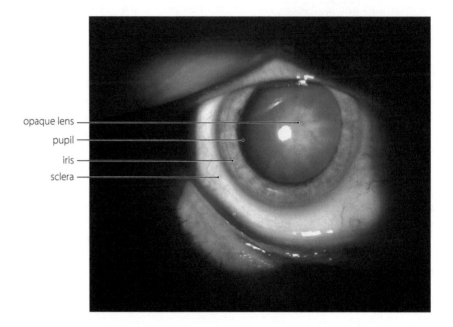

opaque lens
pupil
iris
sclera

Fig. 10.9 Image of a cataract in the lens.

Age-related macular degeneration

Age-related macular degeneration (**AMD**) is a painless eye condition that leads to the gradual loss of central vision due to changes in the macula lutea region of the retina (→ Box 10.13). As central vision becomes increasingly blurred, it leads to difficulties in reading, recognising people's faces and identifying colours. The two types of AMD are:

- **dry (atrophic) AMD** results from reduced blood supply to the macula and is the most common and least serious cause of blindness in the elderly. The loss of vision is gradual and occurs over many years (→ Fig. 10.10)
- **wet AMD** is associated with the growth of new abnormal blood vessels under the retina that leak fluid and blood. One treatment of this condition is injection of growth factor inhibitors into the eyeball.

Retinal detachment

Retinal detachment occurs when the retina at the back of the eye begins to pull away from the blood vessels that supply it with oxygen and nutrients. Without prompt treatment, it will lead to blindness in the affected eye.

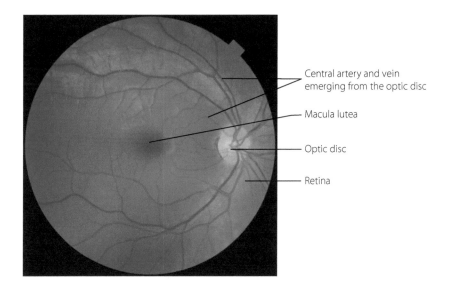

Central artery and vein
emerging from the optic disc

Macula lutea

Optic disc

Retina

Fig. 10.10 Image of a normal retina showing the major blood vessels that radiate from the optic disc.

Glaucoma

Glaucoma is too much fluid within the eyeball usually because aqueous humour is unable to drain away, causing pressure within the eye, pain and blurred vision (→ Fig. 10.3). If increased pressure is diagnosed early, treatment with eye drops, tablets or simple surgery should keep the condition under control. Blindness results if left untreated.

Trachoma

Trachoma is an infectious disease caused by the bacterium *Chlamydia trachomatis*, which causes a roughening of the inner surface of the eyelids. This roughening can lead to pain in the eyes, breakdown of the cornea of the eyes, and eventual blindness. Untreated, repeated trachoma infections can result in a form of permanent blindness (→ Box 10.23).

Strabismus

Strabismus (**squint**) is present when the eyes look in different directions. It originates in the part of the brain where eye movement is coordinated by the extraocular muscles. A squint can be normal in the first few weeks of life, but if it persists or develops later, corrective treatment is necessary to improve the quality of life for people with the condition. This includes exercises for the eye muscles, wearing special glasses or surgery.

10.4 Ears

Only the outer part of the ear is visible. The rest of the ear – the middle and inner parts – are small and delicate and situated within the bones of the skull (→ Fig. 10.11). The two functions of the ear are:

- **hearing**. Sound waves that enter the ears are converted into nerve impulses and transmitted to the brain where they are perceived as sounds. Having two ears helps to determine the direction that the sound waves are coming from, as they will reach one ear before the other ear (→ Box 10.24)
- **balance**. Movements of the head are detected by the inner ear and this information is relayed to the brain.

Box 10.23 Trachoma is responsible for the blindness or visual impairment of about 1.8 million people, and remains a public health problem in 42 countries. Its elimination is an objective of the World Health Organization (WHO).

Box 10.24 When hearing a recording of our own voice we find that it differs from the way we think we sound. This is because when we speak we not only hear the sound through our ears but also the sound which is conducted from the larynx through the skull bones and which resonates in the air-filled sinuses before it reaches the cochlea of the inner ear.

Outer ear

The external part of the ear consists of a flexible flap of tissue called the **pinna** and the **auditory meatus** (→ Box 10.25). The **tympanic membrane** (eardrum) stretches across the inner end of the auditory meatus, separating it from the middle ear. When sound waves travel along the auditory meatus they make the tympanic membrane vibrate.

Cerumen (earwax) is secreted by modified sebaceous glands in the auditory canal. It cleans, lubricates and protects the lining of the ear by trapping dirt and repelling water. Being slightly antiseptic, it also provides some protection against infection.

Pressure on the eardrum. The pharyngotympanic (Eustachian) tube (→ Fig. 10.11) is a narrow canal that connects the middle ear and the pharynx (back of the throat).

The canal is normally closed, but its main function is to balance the pressure differences on either side of the tympanic membrane. Swallowing and yawning cause contraction of muscles connected to the tube, allowing small amounts of air to enter and equilibrate the pressures; this results in a 'popping' sound in the ear.

If the Eustachian tube becomes inflamed or does not open properly, the person may experience distorted hearing, a sense of fullness in the ear or tinnitus (→ Box 10.26).

Box 10.25 Because the auditory canal is curved, the pinna should be gently pulled up and back to straighten the auditory canal when fluid medication is being placed into the ear.

Box 10.26 Tympanic thermometers are now often used by health professionals when taking a patient's temperature. The instructions need to be carefully followed to ensure that the thermometer is correctly placed in the auditory canal to obtain an accurate reading.

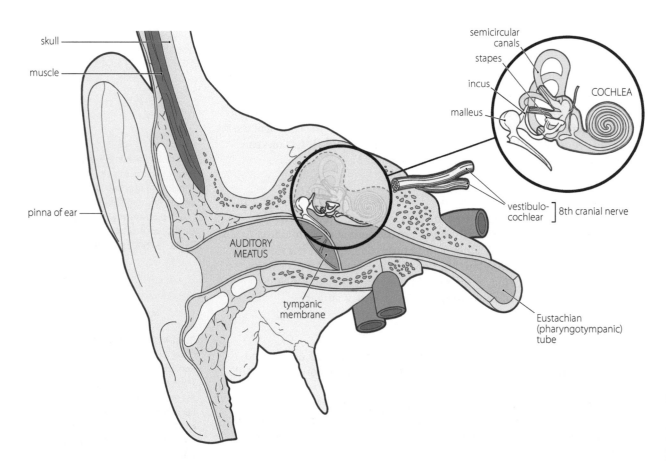

Fig. 10.11 Structure of the ear, with middle and inner ear enlarged.

Middle ear

The middle ear is a small cavity in the skull that contains three tiny bones – **ossicles**. Because of their shape, they are named the **malleus** (hammer), **incus** (anvil) and **stapes** (stirrup), the stapes being connected to the oval window of the cochlea. The ossicles act as a series of levers which move when the tympanic membrane vibrates, thus transmitting sound waves through the middle ear to the cochlea (→ Fig. 10.12).

The **Eustachian tube** (**pharyngotympanic tube**) links the middle ear to the throat (→ Fig. 10.11). This provides a pathway for throat infections such as head colds to reach the middle ear and, especially in children, may lead to middle ear or mastoid infections (→ Box 10.27).

Box 10.27 Otitis media (**glue ear**) is a condition common in childhood in which infection in the middle ear produces thick, sticky fluid which collects and causes temporary deafness. **Mastoiditis** can develop if the infection spreads out of the middle ear and into the mastoid part of the temporal bone (→ Fig. 4.6).

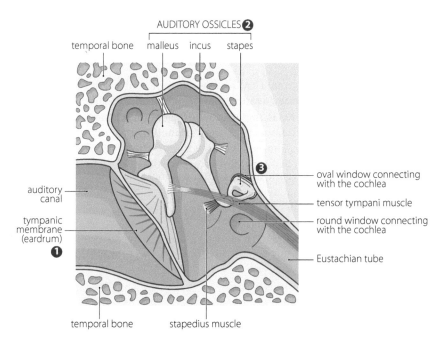

Fig. 10.12 Transmission of vibrations by the ossicles of the middle ear. **Step 1**: When sound waves hit the tympanic membrane they make it vibrate. **Step 2**: The three tiny bones of the middle ear transmit vibrations from the tympanic membrane to the oval window of the cochlea. **Step 3**: As the stapes vibrates, it pushes and pulls on the membrane covering the oval window.

Inner ear

The inner ear, also called the **labyrinth**, consists of fluid-filled tubes embedded in bone. It has two parts – the **cochlea** which is concerned with hearing and three **semicircular canals** which are concerned with balance (→ Fig. 10.13).

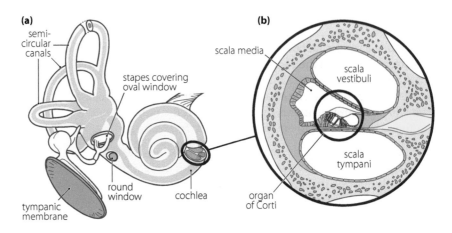

Fig. 10.13 Detailed structure of (**a**) the cochlea; (**b**) a cross-section of the cochlea.

Sound transduction in the cochlea

Vibrations of the membrane covering the oval window cause the fluid in the canals (scala) of the cochlea to move and the basilar membrane to wobble up and down. These movements force the **stereocilia** (auditory receptors) to bend, which initiates nerve impulses to travel along the **vestibulocochlear nerve** (8th cranial nerve) to the auditory cortex of the brain, where they are interpreted as the sounds we hear (→ Fig. 10.14).

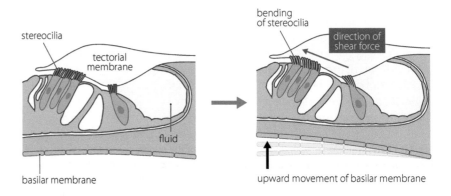

Fig. 10.14 Sound transduction in the organ of Corti (→ Box 10.28).

10.4.1 Balance

The **vestibular apparatus** (labyrinth) of the inner ear contains three **semicircular canals**, plus the **saccule** and **utricle** (→ Fig. 10.15). The semicircular canals are tiny, fluid-filled tubes, each with a small swelling – **ampulla** – at its base that contains sensory cells. When the position of the head moves, the fluid in the semicircular canals stays still, which stimulates the sensory cells to send impulses to the brain informing it of the position of the head. If the person is 'losing their balance', the brain immediately sends motor impulses via the spinal cord to the appropriate muscles so that they can restore the body to its correct position (→ Box 10.29).

The utricle and saccule translate movement of the head into impulses which the brain can interpret, the utricle being more sensitive to horizontal movement and the saccule more sensitive to vertical movement.

Box 10.28 Transduction converts energy from one form to another. This happens when sound vibrations (mechanical energy) are transduced into electrical energy by stereocilia in the inner ear.

Box 10.29 Spinning round and round and then stopping suddenly causes dizziness. This is because the fluid in the semicircular canals continues moving after the body has stopped.

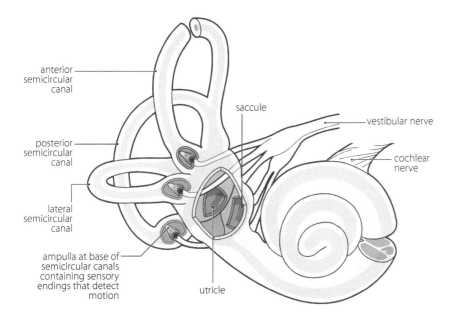

Fig. 10.15 Structure of the vestibular apparatus.

The vestibular apparatus contains small patches of **otolithic membrane** in the ampulla, utricle and saccule. The otolithic membrane contains hair cells which are coupled to a mass of grainy stones made of calcium carbonate embedded in a protein gel (→ Fig. 10.16). When the body changes position and the head moves, the stones start to tumble and bend the hair cells. Movement of the head is transduced (converted) into impulses, which signals its position to the brain. The brain compares input from the utricles and saccules from both ears with input from the visual system to detect whether the head is level or tilted.

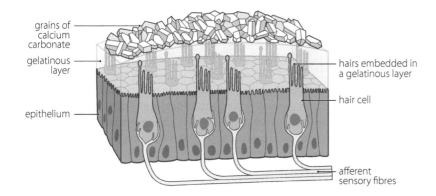

Fig. 10.16 The otolithic membrane of the vestibular apparatus.

Vertigo

Vertigo is the most common type of dizziness and may be associated with nausea, vomiting, sweating or difficulties in walking. Common disorders that result in vertigo are:
- **benign paroxysmal positional vertigo** (BPPV)
- **labyrinthitis** – an inner ear infection
- **vestibulitis** – inflammation of the vestibular nerve of the inner ear.

Box 10.30 Earwax (**cerumen**) is continuously being produced in the ear canal and then gradually pushed out of the ear. If more is produced than drops out, it accumulates and blocks the ear canal, which may impair ability to hear.

10.4.2 Hearing impairment

Hearing impairment (deafness; hearing loss) is partial or complete loss of hearing. It can occur in one or both ears and be:

- **temporary** – due to a build-up of wax (→ Box 10.30) or glue ear (→ Box 10.27)
- **partial** – some sounds are heard but not others, which makes it difficult to understand what other people are saying
- **profound** – no sounds can be heard, even at the highest volume possible; profound deafness is rare.

Some people can be born deaf or become deaf over time because of a genetic abnormality or viral infection of the inner ear or auditory nerve, e.g. mumps, measles or rubella. Generally, hearing impairments are classified as conductive or sensorineural.

Conductive hearing loss occurs when there is a problem in the outer or middle ear – either a barrier that hinders the conduction of sound waves in the auditory canal, e.g. earwax, or the incomplete conduction of vibrations through the ossicles in the middle ear, e.g. glue ear or otosclerosis (→ Box 10.31). Conductive hearing loss is a common factor in deafness that develops later in life, often arising gradually over a period of years following prolonged exposure to environmental noise.

Box 10.31 Otosclerosis is caused by abnormal growth of the ossicles in the middle ear and is a common reason for progressive deafness in young adults.

Sensorineural hearing loss occurs in the inner ear (sensory) or auditory nerve (neural).

- **Sensory hearing loss** is the result of impaired ability of the hair cells within the organ of Corti in the cochlea to generate nerve impulses (action potentials). It is usually permanent because the hair cells have only limited ability to repair themselves.
- **Neural hearing loss** arises if damage occurs to the 8th cranial (vestibulocochlear) nerve, or within the auditory tracts in the brainstem. This kind of hearing loss may be accompanied by loss of acuity (sharpness of hearing), tinnitus or vertigo.

Tinnitus

Tinnitus is the term for hearing sounds made inside the body, not by an outside source. It's often described as "ringing in the ears" although the sounds may be buzzing, humming, hissing, whistling, similar to music or singing, or noises that beat in time with the pulse (pulsatile tinnitus). The sounds can be continuous, or come and go, and may gradually get better. Many cases are associated with hearing loss caused by damage to the inner ear. Severe cases can be very distressing, affect concentration, and cause problems such as insomnia.

10.5 Olfaction and gustation

Olfaction is the sense of smell and **gustation** is the sense of taste. They both depend on **chemoreceptors** – sensory cells that respond to chemical stimuli by initiating nerve impulses in a sensory nerve. Chemoreceptors in the nose respond to chemicals in the air and those in the tongue to chemicals in food, and they work together to detect flavour in foods – a combination of smell and taste (→ Box 10.32).

Box 10.32 Women generally have a more acute sense of smell than men, and it varies across the menstrual cycle. The peaks of sensitivity to smell correspond with peaks in the levels of the hormone oestradiol that occur close to the time of ovulation, and also again in pregnancy.

10.5.1 Nose

The nose extends from the front of the face as far back as the end of the palate and is divided into two nasal passageways lined with mucous membrane. The visible, external part of nose that projects in the front of the face consists mainly of cartilage. The much larger nasal passageways are situated within the skull and their surface area is increased by three ridges of bone (**conchae**) on their lateral walls (→ Fig. 10.17). The two functions of the nose are:

- **olfaction** – sense of smell detected by the olfactory epithelium
- **to warm, moisten and filter the air** on its way to the lungs; this is why the nose has a much larger surface area than is required for olfaction.

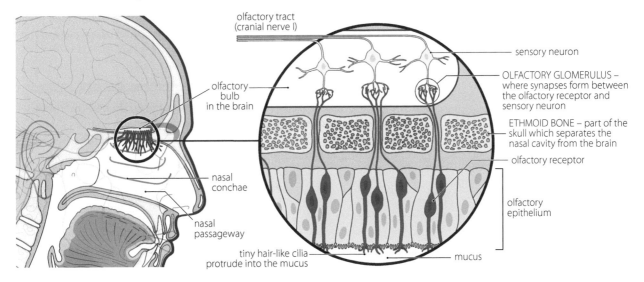

Fig. 10.17 Section through the nasal cavity with details of the olfactory epithelium.

Olfactory epithelium

The **olfactory epithelium** is a small (2.5 cm) patch of highly specialised tissue situated on the roof of each nasal cavity. It is kept moist by a covering of mucus and contains the **olfactory receptors** (chemoreceptors) – neurons specialised for detecting chemical compounds (→ Box 10.33). Each olfactory receptor ends in cilia which project into the mucous layer and can detect an infinite variety of smells that:

- give information about the environment, e.g. the smell of burning or rotten food
- trigger memories and emotions, e.g. perfumes, foods
- enable babies to recognise their mothers; a baby's sense of smell is highly developed at birth and it can differentiate between the odour of its mother and that of other women (→ Box 10.34).

The olfactory epithelium is replaced about every seven weeks, which means it can often be replaced after injury. Permanent damage to the sense of smell is called **anosmia**.

Mechanism for detecting odours

1. Mucus protects the olfactory epithelium and allows odours to dissolve so that they can be detected by the cilia that cover the end surface of the olfactory receptors (→ Box 10.35).
2. The cilia bind to odourant molecules, with each receptor having affinity for a range of hundreds of odourant molecules, depending on their physical and chemical properties.
3. Odourant molecules stimulate the olfactory receptors to transmit impulses via olfactory glomeruli to the olfactory bulb in the limbic system of the brain (→ Fig. 9.9).
4. Synapses form between the branching ends of sensory receptor cells and sensory neurons.
5. The limbic system identifies and determines the odour and it may trigger specific memories or emotional responses.

Box 10.33 The olfactory receptors are extremely sensitive and stimulated by odours in very small concentrations. They adapt easily to odours, which explains why odours that are at first very noticeable are not detected after a short while.

Box 10.34 Odours are characterised by different 'signatures' which activate different patterns of activity in olfactory receptors. The variability of odorant receptors is an important mechanism for activation by chemically diverse odour molecules. Sniffing, for example, can trigger intermittent trains of activity in particular olfactory neurons, identifying memories of particular smells.

Box 10.35 The surface of the cilia is covered with odourant receptors – a very diverse family of G-protein coupled receptors (→ Fig. 11.3) and each responds to multiple chemical stimuli.

Box 10.36 Mouth feel is an expression that is used to describe the texture, sweetness, juiciness and other properties of food that is eaten. All of these properties contribute to the experience of eating and identifying the taste of food.

10.5.2 Gustation

Gustation is the action of tasting substances. Food is tasted when saliva in the mouth moistens food and dissolves some of the chemical substances it contains, which are detected by the hairs of the gustatory receptors in the taste buds. The **flavour of food** is a combination of the smell of the food, detected by the olfactory cells, and the basic tastes of the food detected by the gustatory cells (receptors). Tasting involves perception of the taste of the food, but also depends on texture and 'mouth feel' (→ Box 10.36).

Tongue

The tongue is a solid mass of skeletal muscle covered by mucous membrane. The muscle fibres are arranged in several directions, which enables the tongue to alter its shape and position as it carries out the functions of chewing, tasting, swallowing and speech. The upper surface of the tongue is normally moist, pink and covered with projections of varying size called **papillae** (→ Fig. 10.18a). These are sometimes mistaken for taste buds, but the taste buds are very much smaller and situated in the sides of the papillae at the tip and edges of the tongue and in the roof of the mouth, also in the cheeks, pharynx and upper oesophagus (→ Box 10.37). The basal cells in taste buds are precursor cells that differentiate into mature gustatory cells with an average life span of about 8–12 days.

Taste buds

Taste buds are not just found on the tongue but also in the cheek, epiglottis and upper oesophagus. A taste bud is a tiny sphere containing 50 to 100 **gustatory cells**, each with a gustatory hair that projects through the pore and is sensitive to chemicals in solution (→ Fig. 10.18b). The gustatory hairs, which are able to detect a range of tastes, are stimulated to send information to the gustatory areas of the brain via cranial nerves VII, IX and X (→ Fig. 10.19; Box 10.37).

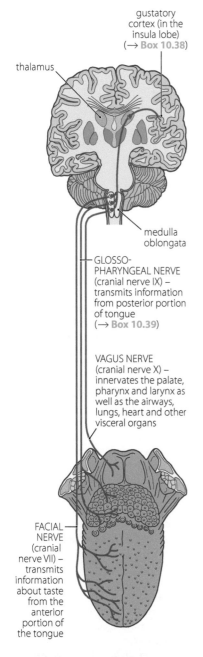

Fig. 10.19 Sensory pathway from the tongue and mouth to the gustatory areas in the insula (→ Fig. 9.7) via the cranial nerves VII, IX and X.

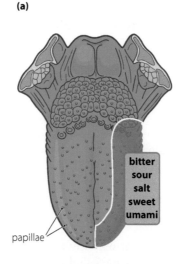

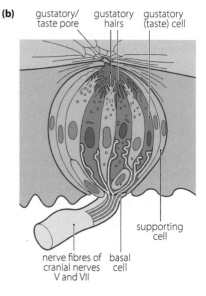

Fig. 10.18 (**a**) Tongue showing papillae – the small, round or cone-shaped protuberances that cover its surface; (**b**) a taste bud.

Taste buds are able to discern five different tastes – sweet, sour, salt, bitter and umami (savoury taste). Pungency (spiciness) that ranges from mild to hot in foods, e.g. ginger and chilli pepper, is not considered a taste in the technical sense.

10.6 Skin

A range of different types of sensory receptors are located in the skin (→ Fig. 10.20).

10.6.1 Sensory pathway from the skin

The sensory pathway consists of sensory receptors that send nerve impulses to the spinal cord where they are transmitted via the ascending spinothalamic tract to the sensory cortex in the brain (→ Fig. 10.21).

Activation of the sensory receptors when stimulated by touch, heat, cold or pain can induce a reflex response such as moving away from a source of heat or pain, rubbing or scratching an itch, all of which will be perceived by the brain (→ Box 10.38).

Box 10.37 Taste sensations are experienced when food is being consumed and taste and smell information activates the gustatory cortex in the brain (→ Fig. 10.1). Efferent pathways that enable digestion to begin are then activated, e.g. saliva flows and peristaltic activity of the gastric wall increases.

Box 10.38 The **pharyngeal (gag) reflex** is triggered when something presses on the soft palate (roof of the mouth). The sensory arm of the reflex involves the glossopharyngeal nerve, while the motor response is activated by the vagus nerve.

The gag reflex enables people to eject food or objects from the mouth before swallowing.

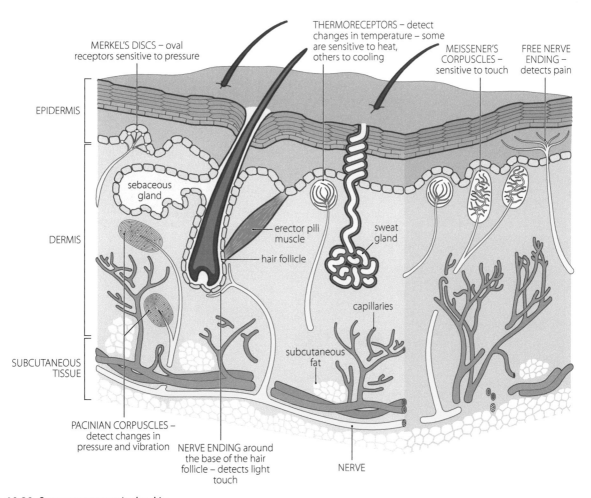

Fig. 10.20 Sensory receptors in the skin.

10.7 Proprioception

Proprioception is the conscious awareness of the position of the parts of the body and the strength required for movement.

Proprioceptors are the receptors (nerve endings) in muscles (muscle spindles), tendons, joints and ligaments that supply information to the cerebellum – the part of the brain that converts the information into awareness of, e.g.:

- the position of the hands when behind the back
- the heaviness of a weight which is being lifted
- righting oneself when stumbling.

10.7.1 Proprioception pathway

The tracts that carry proprioception information from the body extend from the spinal cord to the thalamus and are the same as for touch (→ Fig. 10.21).

❶ First order neurons have their nerve cell bodies in the dorsal root ganglia of the spinal cord.

❷ Second order neurons synapse in the dorsal horn of the medulla in the brain and cross over to the opposite side of the pons before ascending to the thalamus.

❸ Third order neurons from the thalamus carry nerve impulses to the sensory cortex.

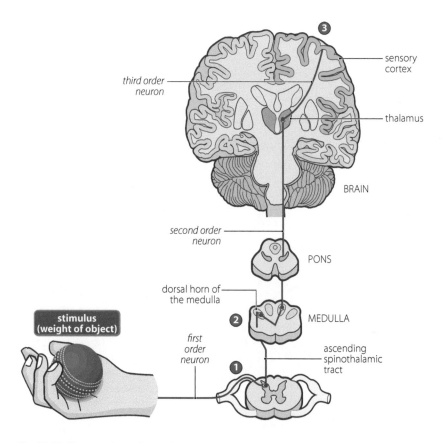

Fig. 10.21 The proprioception pathway.

Key points

1. The function of the sensory system is to gather information about the external and internal environment and to communicate it to the central nervous system where it is perceived.

2. Sensory pathways begin in sense organs which are specialised structures whose function is to transduce (convert) energy from the stimulus into action potentials.

3. The retina of the eye converts light energy into impulses that travel along visual pathways (2nd cranial nerve) to the brain.

4. Sound waves are converted into electrical impulses by the cochlea and they travel in the auditory tracts (8th cranial nerve) to the brain.

5. Olfaction (smell) and gustation (taste) depend on chemoreceptors that work together for the detection of the flavour of foods.

6. The sense called proprioception depends on communication between joints, muscles, tendons and the brain and enables people to maintain posture and balance as well as being consciously aware of the position of the body and limbs.

Test yourself! Go to *www.lanternpublishing.com/AandP* and try the questions to check your understanding.

CHAPTER 11
THE ENDOCRINE SYSTEM

The endocrine system is a collection of glands that secrete hormones – a hormone being a chemical released in one part of the body that affects cells in other parts of the body. The endocrine system works with the nervous system to maintain homeostasis, with the hypothalamus being the major link between them (→ Box 11.1).

11.1 Endocrine glands

A **gland** is an organ or a group of cells that are specialised for synthesising and secreting a substance. There are two different types:
- **exocrine glands** discharge their secretions through a duct into the external environment, e.g. saliva, sweat and tears
- **endocrine glands** secrete **hormones** (chemical signals) directly into the bloodstream and for this reason, they are often called ductless glands (→ Fig. 11.1) (→ Box 11.2).

Box 11.1 Endocrinology is the study of hormones and the clinical practice related to hormones. It draws on many subject disciplines including molecular and cellular biology, genetics, physiology and immunology. The field encompasses a very wide range of endocrine disorders – from diabetes and thyroid disease through infertility and adrenal insufficiency to osteoporosis and growth.

Box 11.2 The so-called 'glands' in the neck are not glands at all but lymph nodes that form part of the immune system (→ 5.17.3).

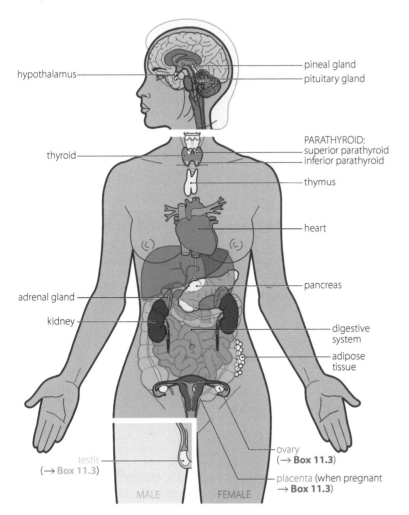

hypothalamus

pineal gland
pituitary gland

thyroid

PARATHYROID:
superior parathyroid
inferior parathyroid

thymus

heart

adrenal gland

kidney

pancreas

digestive system

adipose tissue

testis
(→ **Box 11.3**)

ovary
(→ **Box 11.3**)

placenta (when pregnant → **Box 11.3**)

MALE   FEMALE

Fig. 11.1 Endocrine glands, organs and tissues.

Box 11.3 The ovaries, testes and placenta function both as endocrine glands and reproductive organs and are discussed in Chapter 12. Key hormones from the ovary are oestrogens and progesterone, and those from the testes are androgens, and the placenta is a source of relaxin, oestrogen and progesterone.

11.1.1 Chemical signalling

The vast number of different activities that take place in cells are coordinated by a complex communication system that involves the use of different types of chemical signals. A chemical signal molecule, sometimes referred to as the **first messenger** (→11.2.1), is a substance that is released into body fluids which brings about a cellular response (→ Box 11.4). There are several types of chemical signalling, a key difference between them being the distance that the signalling molecule travels to reach its target.

Autocrine signalling (self-signalling) occurs when a cell secretes a signalling molecule that may bind to receptors on the same cell, e.g. interleukin.

Synaptic signalling occurs at synapses when neurons (nerve cells) secrete chemical signals – **neurotransmitters** – which diffuse across the synaptic gap to adjacent neurons (→ Fig. 9.13), e.g. acetylcholine and noradrenaline (→ Fig. 11.2a).

Paracrine signalling is a form of cell–cell communication in which a cell produces signals that induce a quick response in nearby cells. The signalling molecules are secreted by cells into interstitial fluid and regulate the activity of neighbouring target cells before being rapidly broken down, e.g. histamine and prostaglandins (→ Fig. 11.2b).

Endocrine signalling is carried out by hormones released into the bloodstream which bind with hormone receptors on the target cells. Compared to local signalling, endocrine (also called hormonal) signalling is sometimes relatively slow as it relies on diffusion and blood flow, e.g. hormones that affect metabolism such as insulin, testosterone and progesterone (→ Fig. 11.2c).

Neurocrine signalling occurs when neurons release chemical signals into the bloodstream that affect distant cells, e.g. the hormones adrenaline and oxytocin.

Box 11.4 Cells are continually sending out and receiving signalling molecules to maintain homeostasis in response to a changing external environment, e.g. hormones and neurotransmitters. Individual cells possess highly specific receptors for the signal molecules on their membranes (→ Fig. 11.3) so that, for example, insulin binds to insulin receptors and dopamine activates dopamine receptors.

Having these receptors embedded within the plasma membrane means that signalling molecules can usually bring about their effect from outside the cell in a process called signal transduction (→ Box 11.7).

Taking it Further
A wide range of medicines and other substances pharmacologically alter the function of receptors, e.g. beta blockers inhibit the action of the hormone adrenaline at beta-adrenergic receptors. Find out more about the action of drugs in online Chapter 18.

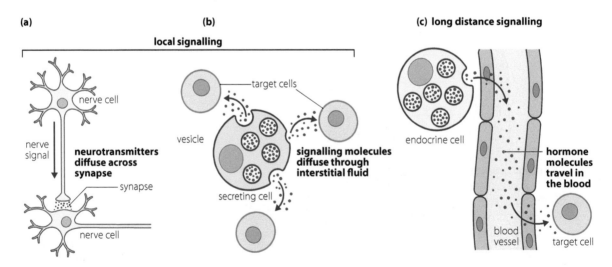

Fig. 11.2 Differences between (**a**) synaptic, (**b**) paracrine and (**c**) endocrine signalling.

11.2 Hormones

Box 11.5 Hormones are very powerful and control much of our general health. If one hormone malfunctions, it can snowball into a physiological or psychological disorder.

A hormone is a chemical signal produced and secreted by an endocrine gland in one part of the body and transported in the bloodstream to affect tissues or organs in another part (→ Box 11.5). Hormone signalling involves the following steps:

- hormone molecules are produced and stored in vesicles within endocrine cells. They are secreted from the cell by the process of exocytosis (→ Fig. 2.4), a little at a time as needed, not continuously
- although travelling to all part of the body, each hormone only affects certain cells, called **target cells** – those with the right hormone receptors (→ Box 11.6)
- when a hormone molecule binds to a target cell receptor, it triggers a reaction. Generally, hormones trigger a reaction in two different ways: on the surface of the plasma membrane (→ Fig. 11.3), or with receptors for lipid soluble hormones which are located in the cytoplasm (→ Fig. 11.4).

11.2.1 Signal transduction by protein receptors

Protein hormones range in size from a few amino acids (peptides) to macromolecules of over 200 amino acids, e.g. insulin. They do not enter cells but transfer their effect by signal transduction (→ Box 11.7), a process that unlocks a series of molecular switches:

1. A hormone (**first messenger**) binds to a protein receptor on the plasma membrane of the target cell in a lock-and-key manner, and changes the receptor's shape
2. The change enables a G-protein in the cytoplasm to couple with the protein receptor (→ Box 11.8)
3. The G-protein immediately exchanges GDP and GTP which initiates a cascade in the cytoplasm
4. The binding of GTP stimulates the production of a **second messenger** – an intracellular signalling molecule that makes the hormone effective inside the cell by causing biochemical reactions, e.g. enzyme production or cell division
5. The second messenger, often cyclic AMP (cAMP), triggers enzyme action (→ Fig. 11.3).

Box 11.6 A hormone receptor is a protein and, like all proteins, is a string of amino acids which is folded, coiled and cross-linked in a way that is specific to each variety of protein (simplified receptors are shown in Fig. 11.3). There are from 2000 to 100,000 hormone receptors on the surface of a cell and their structure and action vary so that target cells are able to recognise and respond to a specific hormone.

Box 11.7 Signal transduction is a cascade of chemical reactions in a cell that occurs when a hormone binds to a receptor on the plasma membrane and eventually produces a response within the cell.

Box 11.8 G-proteins (guanine nucleotide-binding proteins) are substances involved in transmitting signals from a variety of stimuli outside a cell to its interior. Humans have more than 1000 different types of G-protein that couple with protein receptors.

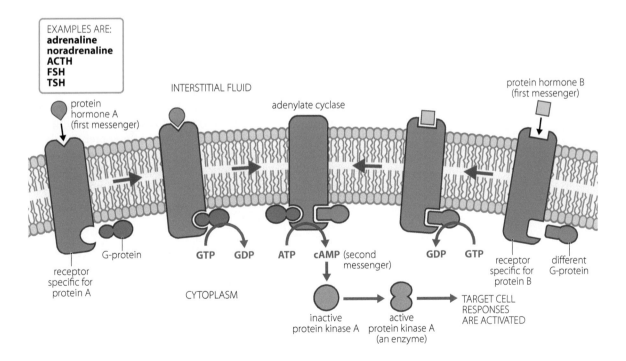

Fig. 11.3 Hormone action in a target cell.

11.2.2 Action by steroid hormones

Unlike protein hormones, steroid hormones act inside the cell, with receptors being found in the cytoplasm or nucleus (→ Fig. 11.4). Steroid hormones are derived from cholesterol and include:

- **corticosteroids** mainly secreted by the adrenal cortex, which are involved in a wide range of physiological processes including the stress response, immune response, and regulation of inflammation
- **sex hormones** made in the gonads or placenta; these hormones build proteins, e.g.:
  - testosterone builds muscle tissue
  - oestrogen builds the endometrium (lining of the uterus)
- **vitamin D** in various forms.

The mechanism by which steroid hormones act on target cells differs from that of protein hormones. Since they are soluble in the plasma membrane and can diffuse across it, their receptors are usually found within the cytoplasm or nucleus (→ Box 11.9).

Steroid hormone action

① The hormone diffuses through the plasma and nuclear membranes into the nucleus (→ Fig. 11.4).
② The hormone then binds to a receptor in the nucleus to form a complex.

Box 11.9 Steroid hormones are lipid molecules based on cholesterol, e.g. oestrogen, progesterone and cortisol, and they enter the cell by means of passive diffusion (→ 2.2.2), binding to receptors in the nucleus. They have their effect on a cell by controlling gene expression – the process by which information from a gene is used in the synthesis of a protein. Steroid hormones therefore influence many aspects of physiology.

Taking it Further
You can find out more about drugs that bind to nuclear receptors, including steroid anti-inflammatory agents and contraceptive hormones, in online Chapter 18.

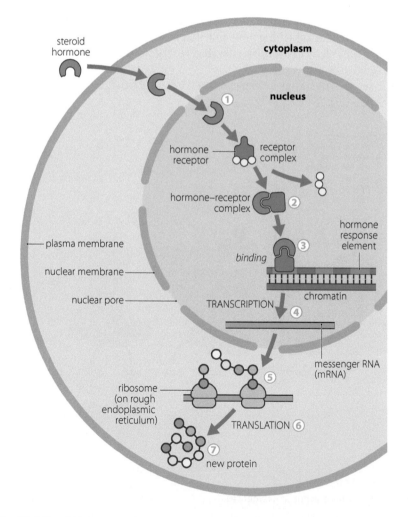

Fig. 11.4 Steroid hormone action.

③ The complex binds to chromatin (contains DNA which carries genetic information).
④ Transcription takes place – this is the first step of gene expression in which a particular segment of DNA is copied into messenger RNA, which now contains a code for making a protein.
⑤ Messenger RNA moves into the cytoplasm and becomes attached to ribosomes.
⑥ Translation of the gene takes place as ribosomes use the code to synthesise a new protein.
⑦ A new protein is made, which is the cell's response to the steroid hormone.

11.3 Hypothalamus and pituitary gland

The hypothalamus is located on the undersurface of the brain. It lies just below the thalamus and above the pituitary gland, to which it is attached by a stalk (→ Fig. 11.5). The hypothalamus is sometimes called 'the master of the endocrine system' because this tiny, complex gland produces its own hormones (neurohormones), controls the release of hormones from the pituitary gland, and plays a vital role in maintaining **homeostasis**.

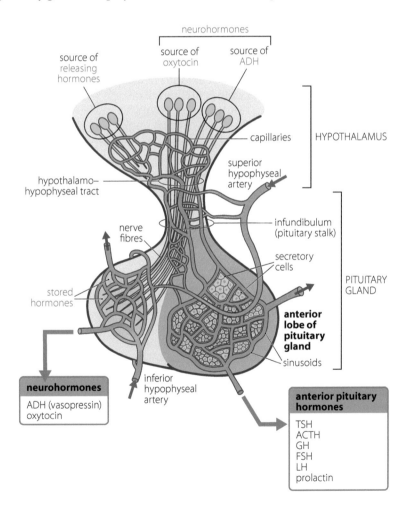

Fig. 11.5 Hypothalamus and pituitary gland.

Being part of the limbic system (→ Fig. 9.9), the hypothalamus receives information from nearly all parts of the nervous system and is also sensitive to the composition of the blood that flows through it. It gathers and integrates information about the external environment and uses it to adjust conditions in the internal environment, which keeps the body in homeostasis, e.g.:

- a stable body temperature
- fluid and electrolyte balance, including thirst
- circadian rhythms (sleep–wake cycles)
- stress response (→ Box 11.10)
- hunger and satiety (feeling of fullness)
- menstrual cycle.

11.3.1 Hypothalamic hormones

Hormones produced by the hypothalamus come from two sets of nerve cells that communicate in different ways with the pituitary gland. One set secretes releasing hormones, the other set secretes neurohormones (→ Box 11.11).

Releasing hormones

Releasing hormones, produced by the hypothalamus, control the production of anterior pituitary hormones, by either stimulating or inhibiting their release. These hormones are secreted directly into the bloodstream and reach the **anterior lobe** of the pituitary gland via a network of blood vessels that run down through the pituitary stalk. The releasing hormones are:

- **thyrotropin-releasing hormone** (TRH) stimulates the release of thyroid-stimulating hormone (TSH) and prolactin (PRL)
- **gonadotrophin-releasing hormone** (GnRH) is the key hormone for adult sexual physiology. It stimulates the onset of puberty and sexual development in both males and females
- **corticotrophin-releasing hormone** (CRH) stimulates the release of adrenocorticotrophic hormone (ACTH) and other melanocortins
- **growth hormone-releasing hormone** (GHRH; somatotrophin) stimulates the secretion of growth hormone (GH)
- **dopamine** inhibits the release of prolactin from the pituitary gland.

Neurohormones

Neurohormones pass along nerve fibres in the pituitary stalk to the **posterior lobe** of the pituitary gland where they are stored until required and then released into the bloodstream (→ Box 11.12). The two neurohormones produced in the hypothalamus are:

- **antidiuretic hormone** (ADH). This hormone is primarily known as ADH because of its action on the kidneys (→ 8.2.4). It is sometimes called **vasopressin** when secreted in high concentrations to stimulate contraction of smooth muscle in the walls of arterioles, e.g. in response to haemorrhage or dehydration
- **oxytocin** stimulates the uterus to contract at the end of pregnancy. It is also essential for the milk ejection reflex which releases the flow of milk in the breasts of nursing mothers (→ 12.8.4).

11.3.2 Pituitary gland

The pituitary gland is a small pea-sized structure at the base of the brain just below the hypothalamus, to which it is attached by a stalk containing nerve fibres. It consists of two distinct parts – the posterior pituitary and anterior pituitary (→ Fig. 11.6) (→ Box 11.13).

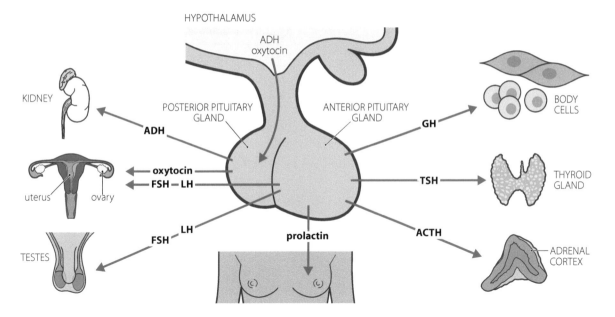

Fig. 11.6 Hormones from the pituitary gland and their targets.

Posterior pituitary

The posterior pituitary (neurohypophysis) stores and releases the neurohormones produced by the hypothalamus.

Anterior pituitary

Most hormones from the anterior pituitary (adenohypophysis) are activated or inhibited by releasing hormones from the hypothalamus (→ Box 11.14).

- **Growth hormone** (GH; somatotrophin) stimulates growth of bones and muscles. It also stimulates the liver to produce **somatomedins** – proteins that promote cell growth and division in response to stimulation by growth hormone.
- **TSH** (thyroid-stimulating hormone) controls the secretion of thyroxine and plays a key role in the regulation of metabolic rate.
- **ACTH** (adrenocorticotrophic hormone) controls the secretion of hormones from the adrenal cortex and plays a key role in regulation of the stress response.
- **FSH** (follicle-stimulating hormone) controls the production of eggs in ovaries and sperm in the testes.
- **LH** (luteinising hormone) controls the secretion of sex hormones.
- **Prolactin** stimulates breast development and milk production in women. It is also responsible for changes in the maternal brain that are thought to help prepare for the demands of becoming a new parent.

Box 11.14 The hypothalamic–pituitary–adrenal axis describes the complex inter-relationships between these endocrine glands. Production of each hypothalamic releasing hormone and its secretion into the bloodstream influences the release of the appropriate anterior pituitary hormone into the circulation.

11.4 Thyroid gland

The thyroid gland is a butterfly-shaped gland situated at the base of the neck and in front of the trachea (→ Fig. 11.7). It produces:

- **thyroid hormone** containing iodine which is essential for determining the basal rate of metabolism and normal growth and development. There are two forms:
  - **T4 (thyroxine)** – the main hormone from the gland. It is a prohormone that is converted to T3 as it passes through the liver and kidneys
  - **T3 (triiodothyronine)** is the active form of the hormone which increases oxygen consumption and determines how cells use energy (→ Box 11.15).

Box 11.15 Homeostasis of thyroxine is an example of negative feedback. Thyroxine levels in the blood are continually monitored by the hypothalamus and pituitary. These glands, in their turn, adjust the output of TRH and TSH so that thyroxine levels in blood remain within the normal range.

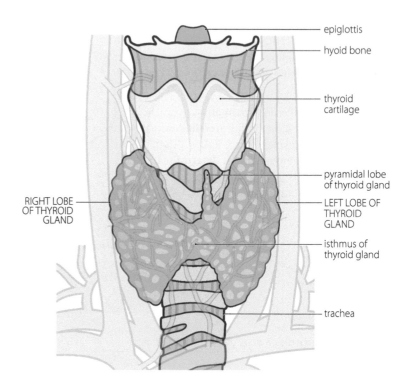

epiglottis

hyoid bone

thyroid cartilage

pyramidal lobe of thyroid gland

RIGHT LOBE OF THYROID GLAND

LEFT LOBE OF THYROID GLAND

isthmus of thyroid gland

trachea

Fig. 11.7 Anterior view of the thyroid gland.

Box 11.16 Graves' disease is the most common cause of hyperthyroidism. It is an autoimmune disorder in which the body makes antibodies that act like TSH (a pituitary-stimulating hormone), causing the thyroid to make more thyroid hormone than the body needs. Graves' disease occurs more often in women than in men and tends to run in families, which suggests a genetic link.

Box 11.17 Hashimoto's disease is the most common cause of an underactive thyroid. It develops when the immune system attacks the thyroid gland and damages it.

Box 11.18 The neonatal blood spot test (heel prick test) is carried out to check for rare but serious health conditions including congenital hypothyroidism.

- **calcitonin (CT)** which lowers the level of calcium and phosphate in the blood when it has risen above its set point. Calcitonin opposes the effects of parathyroid hormone (PTH), which acts to increase the blood calcium level (→ Box 11.19).

11.4.1 Hyperthyroidism

Hyperthyroidism (overactive thyroid) means that too much thyroid hormone is produced, increasing the body's metabolic rate more quickly than normal, which results in symptoms that include hyperactivity, tachycardia (fast heart rate), nervousness, irritability, tremor of the hands, increased appetite and loss of weight (→ Box 11.16).

11.4.2 Hypothyroidism

Hypothyroidism (underactive thyroid) is a relatively common endocrine disorder (→ Box 11.17). It develops when the thyroid gland is not producing enough T4 or T3.

In adults the symptoms of hypothyroidism are often subtle and not very specific, including fatigue, cold intolerance, forgetfulness, constipation, hoarseness and weight gain.

If the condition is present at birth and left untreated, an underactive thyroid results in severe hypothyroidism (a condition previously known as cretinism), leaving a child undersized and with learning disabilities (→ Box 11.18).

11.4.3 Goitre

Goitre is a benign enlargement of the thyroid gland seen as a swelling in front of the neck as the gland enlarges in an attempt to normalise thyroid hormone levels. Worldwide, the most common reason is iodine deficiency, but there are a range of other causes.

11.5 Parathyroid glands

The parathyroid glands are four tiny glands about the size of a grain of rice embedded in the back of the thyroid gland in the neck (→ Fig. 11.8). They secrete **parathyroid hormone** (PTH) which acts with vitamin D to regulate calcium and phosphorus levels in the blood and bone (→ Box 11.19).

Box 11.19 PTH indirectly stimulates **osteoclasts** to break down bone tissue and the calcium it contains is then released into the blood. **Osteoblasts** use calcium from the body to build new bone tissue. Together, these cells facilitate bone remodelling and bone growth (→ 4.1.4).

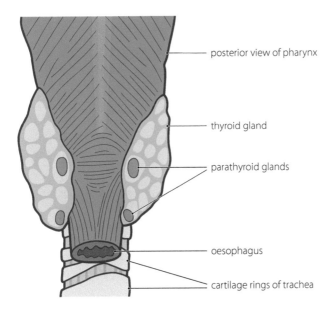

Fig. 11.8 The four parathyroid glands embedded in the thyroid gland.

11.6 Pancreas

The pancreas is part of both the digestive and endocrine systems. It functions as a digestive gland by secreting pancreatic enzymes and as an endocrine gland by secreting hormones.

11.6.1 Islets of Langerhans

The pancreas contains millions of microscopic structures called islets of Langerhans which are scattered within the gland tissue that produces pancreatic juice (→ Box 11.20). The islets contain several types of cell, including three that secrete hormones (→ Fig. 11.9):
- **Alpha cells** secrete **glucagon** which raises the level of glucose in the blood, thus protecting the body from hypoglycaemia (→ 16.2.1). It does this by stimulating the liver and skeletal muscles to break down glycogen to release glucose into the bloodstream
- **Beta cells** secrete **insulin** that lowers blood glucose levels by stimulating cells and tissues to remove glucose from the blood when it is abundant, by converting it into glycogen
- **Delta cells** make **somatostatin**, a hormone secreted in the pancreas and pituitary gland which inhibits the release of gastric juice (→ Box 11.21).

Box 11.20 An **acinus** is a group of epithelial cells, called acinar cells, arranged around a lumen which connects to the pancreatic duct. The acinar cells make alkaline pancreatic juice containing enzymes which are important for digestion in the duodenum.

Acinar cells are exocrine cells because the pancreatic juice that they secrete is carried away in ducts to the duodenum (→ Fig. 7.4).

Box 11.21 Somatostatin also stimulates the ducts in the mammary gland to contract for milk ejection and the reproductive tract muscles to contract at orgasm.

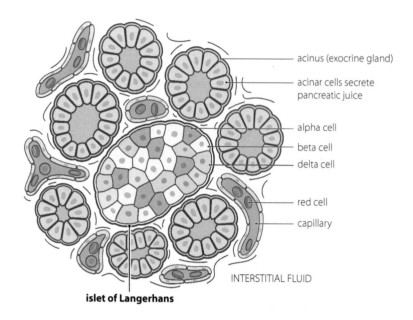

acinus (exocrine gland)

acinar cells secrete
pancreatic juice

alpha cell

beta cell

delta cell

red cell

capillary

INTERSTITIAL FLUID

islet of Langerhans

Fig. 11.9 Pancreatic tissue showing an islet of Langerhans.

11.7 Adrenal glands

The adrenal glands are small organs that sit on top of the kidneys (→ Fig. 11.1).
There are two separate parts to each adrenal gland: the outer part – the
cortex – which surrounds the central part – the **medulla** (→ Fig. 11.10).
Hormones from the cortex are steroid compounds derived from cholesterol.
The medulla is neuroendocrine tissue which secretes adrenaline into the
bloodstream in response to activation of the sympathetic nervous system.

11.7.1 Adrenal medulla

The adrenal medulla secretes **adrenaline** into the bloodstream with a little
noradrenaline (→ Box 11.22) when a person is frightened, alarmed or excited.
These hormones prepare the body for action ('fight, flight or freeze') by:
- increasing the rate and force of heartbeat
- increasing the rate of breathing
- converting glycogen to glucose
- diverting blood from the skin and gut to the skeletal muscles; this may
  manifest as, e.g. turning 'pale with fear' or a 'sinking feeling in the
  stomach'
- altering bladder and/or bowel control; vomiting
- dilating the pupils.

Box 11.22 Noradrenaline is
primarily a neurotransmitter within
the sympathetic nervous system
that plays an important part in the
physiological changes that take
place when people experience a
stressful event (→ 9.8.2).

11.7.2 Adrenal cortex

The adrenal cortex secretes a number of hormones called **corticosteroids**
(→ Box 11.23). Corticosteroids include:
- **cortisol**, which helps to control the use of glucose and also has anti-
  inflammatory effects. Secretion of cortisol follows a circadian rhythm,
  with high levels early in the morning and low levels at time of sleep.
- **aldosterone**, which helps to control blood pressure by regulating the salt
  and water in the body by promoting sodium and water retention in the
  distal tubule of the nephrons in the kidneys (→ 8.2.2).

Box 11.23 When corticosteroids
are used as medicine they are
usually referred to as 'steroids'. They
are prescribed to reduce swelling,
redness, itching, and allergic
reactions, and are often used as part
of the treatment for diseases such
as severe allergies, skin problems,
asthma, or arthritis.

11.7.3 Stress response

Stress is the adverse reaction to perceived pressure when that pressure exceeds the individual's ability to cope. The hypothalamus in the brain is in charge of the stress response and, when triggered, it sends signals to two other structures: the pituitary gland and the adrenal medulla. The adrenal glands respond to either short-term or long-term stressors by releasing different hormones that act differently on the body (→ Fig. 11.10).

Short-term response

The short-term response involves the adrenal medulla. When a person is anxious or frightened, nerve impulses from the hypothalamus are routed through the sympathetic nervous system and to the adrenal medulla. They stimulate the secretion of **adrenaline** which prepares the body for 'fight, flight or freeze' (→ Box 11.24).

Long-term response

If the threat continues, the long-term response involves the adrenal cortex. **Corticotrophin-releasing hormone** (CRH) from the hypothalamus travels in the bloodstream to the anterior pituitary and stimulates the release of **adrenocorticotrophic hormone** (ACTH). This hormone, in turn, stimulates the adrenal cortex to secrete **aldosterone** and **cortisol**. These hormones enable the body to adapt to the ongoing challenge associated with the stressor.

Box 11.24 The stress response is important for survival as it is an immediate physiological reaction in response to a perceived harmful event. It is also called the fight-or-flight response, alarm response, hyperarousal, or the acute stress response.

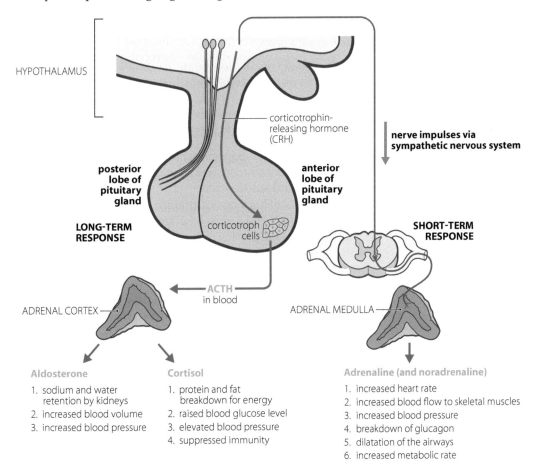

Fig. 11.10 The hypothalamic–pituitary–adrenal axis plays an essential role in regulation of both the short-term and long-term response to stressors.

11.8 Pineal gland

The pineal gland (pineal body) is a pea-sized mass of nervous tissue located deep in the centre of the brain which produces the hormone melatonin (→ Fig. 11.1). **Melatonin** is important in controlling the circadian rhythms and reproductive hormones of the 'body clock'. This hormone is produced in darkness but not in bright light, and it encourages sleep by activating certain types of receptors in the brain.

11.8.1 Sleep homeostasis

Sleep performs an essential homeostatic function that maintains equilibrium. When deprived of sleep, people feel tired, may become more irritable, and often make mistakes. Sleepiness therefore serves a similar physiological function to thirst or hunger as a physiological drive.

The hypothalamus is responsible for the timing of sleep–wake cycles through an internal 'clock' that is normally synchronised with the light–dark cycle over a 24-hour period. This circadian (daily) rhythm, sometimes called **Process C**, also regulates core body temperature, hormone secretion and brain level of alertness as well as sleepiness (→ Box 11.25).

A further process – sometimes called **sleep–wake homeostasis** or **Process S**, is responsible for the drive to sleep, which gets stronger the longer a person has been awake. The internal process increases as the day progresses, and is essentially reminding the body and brain that it needs to sleep; the longer the time spent awake, the greater the sleep pressure and the more likely a person is to fall asleep.

Eventually, usually late in the evening, levels of melatonin begin to rise and the person feels drowsy. When sleep takes place, the sleep pressure dissipates.

11.9 Endocrine function of the kidney

In addition to the endocrine organs mentioned in this chapter, many other organs have endocrine functions including the kidney, which is part of both the urinary and endocrine systems. It functions as an endocrine gland by secreting a variety of hormones including:

- **erythropoietin** (EPO) – released in response to hypoxia (low levels of oxygen) in blood passing through the kidneys. It then stimulates erythropoiesis (production of red blood cells) in the bone marrow (→ Boxes 11.26 and 11.27)
- **renin** – secreted whenever blood flow to the kidney is reduced; it stimulates the production of the hormone **angiotensin**
- **vitamin D** – activated by the kidneys to take part in calcium homeostasis (→ 11.10.1).

11.10 Other hormones

Although most hormones are produced in endocrine glands, a small number are made in other tissues and organs, e.g. vitamin D, prostaglandins, leptins and ghrelin.

Box 11.25 Night shift working and jet lag mean being awake at times when the circadian pacemaker is at its lowest, leading to lack of synchrony between the sleep–wake cycle, light levels and activity of the hypothalamus. In the longer term, these changes are associated with poor sleep quality, impaired cognitive performance, mood disorders and metabolic disturbances.

Box 11.26 People with kidney failure who are undergoing dialysis therapy need regular injections of EPO to avoid the development of anaemia.

Box 11.27 People who go to a high altitude respond to the lower oxygen availability by increasing production of EPO. Knowledge of this hormone is being applied to treat anaemia in people who have kidney disease, AIDS, myeloma, or are receiving chemotherapy.

11.10.1 Vitamin D

Vitamin D plays an essential role in calcium homeostasis – a complex system maintained by two hormones, **parathyroid hormone** (**PTH**) and **calcitonin** (**CT**) from the thyroid gland.

Vitamin D is also called **vitamin D$_3$** or **calcitriol**. It is sometimes known as the 'sunshine hormone' because its precursor – **pre-D$_3$** – can be made in the skin by the action of the sun's rays, then converted into active vitamin D by the liver and kidneys (→ Fig. 11.11).

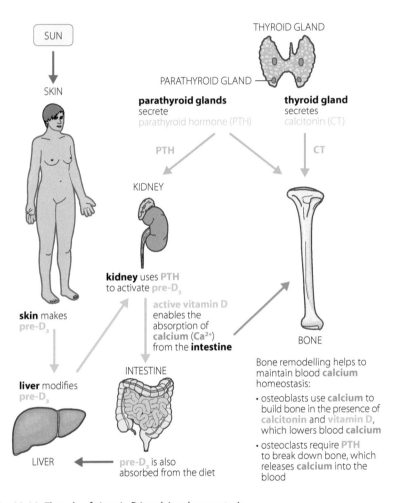

SUN

SKIN

THYROID GLAND

PARATHYROID GLAND

parathyroid glands secrete parathyroid hormone (PTH)

thyroid gland secretes calcitonin (CT)

PTH

CT

KIDNEY

kidney uses PTH to activate pre-D$_3$

skin makes pre-D$_3$

active vitamin D enables the absorption of **calcium (Ca²⁺)** from the **intestine**

BONE

liver modifies pre-D$_3$

INTESTINE

LIVER

pre-D$_3$ is also absorbed from the diet

Bone remodelling helps to maintain blood **calcium** homeostasis:

• osteoblasts use **calcium** to build bone in the presence of calcitonin and vitamin D, which lowers blood **calcium**

• osteoclasts require PTH to break down bone, which releases **calcium** into the blood

Fig. 11.11 The role of vitamin D in calcium homeostasis.

Calcium homeostasis

Calcium homeostasis (calcium metabolism) refers to the movement and regulation of calcium ions into and out of the body fluids in the gastro-intestinal tract, blood, bone and kidneys. As part of this process, blood acts as a source of calcium and bone as a storage centre.

The concentration of calcium ions in blood plasma is kept within very narrow limits by negative feedback (→ Fig. 11.12).

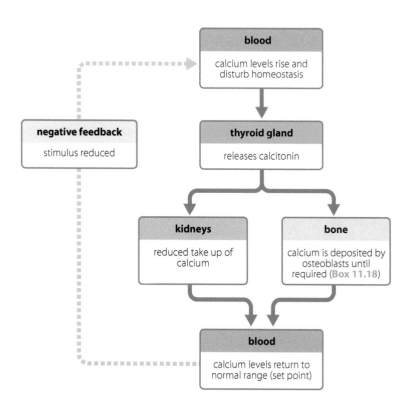

Fig. 11.12 Homeostasis of blood calcium.

11.10.2 Prostaglandins

The prostaglandins (PG) are a group of substances synthesised from fatty acids in the walls of blood vessels in nearly all the tissues of the body. They are powerful, locally acting vasodilators which inhibit the aggregation of blood platelets and prevent clot formation. They are usually short-lived substances as they are rapidly broken down close to where they are produced.

Prostaglandins are formed by the action of enzymes called cyclo-oxygenases which help the inflammatory response. Anti-inflammatory drugs including aspirin and ibuprofen inhibit the enzymes, thus reducing levels of prostaglandin, relieving inflammation and preventing unwanted clotting.

11.10.3 Ghrelin and leptin

Ghrelin and leptin are two hormones involved in the control of appetite and body mass. Both are under the influence of the hypothalamus in the brain but they have opposite effects as ghrelin increases appetite and leptin suppresses it (→ Fig. 19.13).

Ghrelin

Ghrelin is secreted by the lining of the stomach. It is a fast-acting hormone and its levels tend to increase dramatically when people feel hungry and before eating a meal. Many factors – age, gender, BMI, growth hormone, insulin and glucose levels – can influence ghrelin secretion. Higher levels of ghrelin may be secreted when people are stressed, which may go part of the way to explaining why some people may overeat or comfort eat when they are feeling stressed (→ Box 11.28).

Taking it Further
There is more information about non-steroidal anti-inflammatory drugs in online Chapter 18.

Box 11.28 Plasma levels of ghrelin decrease when gastric volume is reduced by **bariatric surgery** (e.g. gastric sleeve procedure) and this may help to explain why this procedure reduces weight.

Leptin

Leptin is an appetite suppressant as it reduces desire and motivation to eat (*leptos* (Gk) = thin). This hormone is derived from adipocytes (fat cells) and, because it comes from fat cells and inhibits hunger, it is sometimes known as the 'satiety hormone' or 'fat controller'. The amount of leptin circulating in the body is directly related to the mass of adipocytes:
- the more fat a person has in their body, the more leptin will normally be circulating in blood
- the less body fat the person has, the less leptin will normally be circulating so when a person is losing weight, leptin levels tend to be falling.

Effects of leptin on appetite

- The desire to eat depends on many other factors including when the person last ate a meal and on sleeping patterns.
- Some obese people may have built up resistance to the effects of leptin so they may keep eating despite adequate, or excess, nutrition.
- When people are losing weight, leptin stimulates appetite instead of suppressing it – because the body thinks it is being starved (➜ Box 11.29).

Surviving starvation

Deficiency of leptin is thought to signal to the brain that energy reserves are under threat from starvation. This then triggers adaptations that promote efficient use of available energy in the regulation of metabolism by:
- lowering the level of thyroxine
- lowering the level of activity of the sympathetic nervous system
- reducing fertility.

11.10.4 Incretins

Incretins are hormones derived from the wall of the small intestine and which are released (within minutes) in response to the ingestion of food. Two incretin hormones circulate in blood and stimulate the release of insulin from beta cells in the pancreatic islets of Langerhans (➜ 11.6.1), which lower plasma glucose levels (➜ Box 11.30).

Different incretins have effects on other organs, including delayed gastric emptying and suppression of appetite.

Box 11.29 Understanding the mechanisms that regulate appetite for food is an important area of research because it can have the potential to improve the understanding of obesity, which is becoming prevalent across the globe.

Box 11.30 The 'incretin effect' accounts for at least 50% of the secretion of insulin, but type 2 diabetes is a disorder that is characterised by insulin resistance and a reduced 'incretin effect'. In recent years, new drugs have been developed which contain enzyme inhibitors that block the breakdown of incretins.

Key points

1. A number of glands which are able to secrete chemical signal molecules, called hormones, into the bloodstream make up the endocrine system.
2. Homeostasis is maintained through the action of hormones on their target organs.
3. Hormones bind to receptor molecules whose structure varies so that target cells are able to recognise and respond in specific ways.
4. The hypothalamus plays a key role in maintaining homeostasis because it regulates the release of hormones from the pituitary gland and influences the output of autonomic centres in the brainstem.
5. Other endocrine glands in the human body include the pancreas, the kidneys, the pineal gland and adipocytes.

Test yourself! Go to *www.lanternpublishing.com/AandP* and try the questions to check your understanding.

CHAPTER 12

THE REPRODUCTIVE SYSTEMS

The male and female reproductive systems ensure survival of the human race. Their development and functioning are under hormonal control and are affected by the emotions, physical disorders and sexually transmitted infections.

12.1 Sex determination

A baby's gender is determined at **conception** when the egg is **fertilised** by a sperm. If the sperm contains an X chromosome the resulting embryo will be a genetic female (XX); if the sperm contains a Y chromosome it will be a genetic male (XY). The Y chromosome is essential for the development of the male reproductive organs because of the presence of the sex-determining gene known as the **sex-determining region Y (SRY)** (→ Box 12.1).

In both sexes the essential organs of reproduction are the **gonads** – the organs that produce **gametes** – sperm or eggs. The gonads in the male are the testes (sing. testis); the gonads in the female are the ovaries. In the earliest stages of development, the embryos of both sexes contain two embryonic tubes called the Wolffian duct and the Müllerian duct.

If the embryo is a male the SRY region of the Y chromosome promotes the development of the testes which helps to stimulate the Wolffian duct to develop the male genitalia. Sertoli cells in the testes secrete anti-Müllerian hormone (AMH) that degrades the Müllerian duct (→ Fig. 12.1).

If the embryo is female the gonads develop into ovaries that secrete oestrogen. The Müllerian duct develops into the female sex organs, and the Wolffian duct degrades, its remnants forming the female clitoris.

Box 12.1 Variation in sexual determination is a complex process. Although not fully understood, factors include chromosomes, genes, hormones and environmental factors.

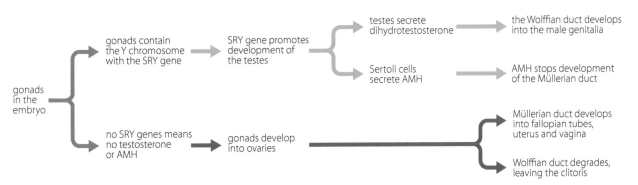

Fig. 12.1 Effect of the SRY gene of the Y chromosome in sex determination.

12.1.1 Sex hormones

Sex hormones influence the growth, development and function of the reproductive organs and the development of secondary sex characteristics. They are **androgens** – the male sex hormones, and **oestrogens** – the female sex hormones. Males normally have a small amount of oestrogens and progesterone, and females normally have a small amount of androgens. These sex hormones are responsible for the changes that occur at **puberty** – the stage during which the reproductive organs mature and become capable of reproduction (→ Box 12.2).

Androgens

Testosterone is the most important male sex hormone and its presence increases protein production and the formation of muscle tissue. Testosterone is also responsible for the development and maintenance of the male reproductive system and secondary sexual characteristics:

- the body becomes more muscular and taller
- hair grows on the face and body
- the sex organs grow and function to produce sperm
- the voice deepens
- changes in behaviour and attitudes occur.

Oestrogens

Oestrogens are the primary female sex hormones, responsible for development and regulation of the female reproductive system and secondary sex characteristics:

- development of breasts
- further development of the uterus and vagina
- broadening of the pelvis
- growth of pubic and axillary hair
- increase in adipose (fat) tissue
- the menstrual cycle (for a possible pregnancy)
- changes in behaviour and attitudes.

Progesterone

Progesterone belongs to a group of steroid hormones, called **progestogens** and is secreted by the corpus luteum of the ovary after ovulation. It prepares the uterus for a possible pregnancy. If the egg is not fertilised, the corpus luteum degenerates and the production of progesterone falls (→ Fig. 12.12). If a pregnancy occurs, progesterone continues to be produced in the placenta (→ Box 12.3).

Human chorionic gonadotrophin

Human chorionic gonadotrophin (hCG) is produced after a fertilised egg has begun to implant in the lining of the uterus. It comes from the trophoblast which develops into the placenta and its level continues to rise for about 3 months before declining (→ Fig. 12.13). hCG is the basis of a pregnancy test as it can first be detected by a blood test about 11 days after conception and by a urine test 12–14 days after conception (→ Box 12.4).

Box 12.2 Sex hormones are **steroids** – a large group of chemical substances with a specific carbon structure. All steroids are based on the cholesterol molecule, but differ in their chemical structure. The three major groups of steroids in the human body are:
- sex hormones
- glucocorticoids
- mineralocorticoids.

Box 12.3 The **placenta** is a temporary organ that develops in the uterus to join the foetus to the mother. It is also an endocrine gland that secretes several hormones including progesterone, oestrogen and gonadotrophin (hCG).

Box 12.4 hCG can be used therapeutically to treat infertility in women, increase sperm count in men, and for young boys when their testicles have not dropped down into the scrotum.

12.2 Male reproductive system

The male reproductive system is situated in the lower part of the abdominopelvic cavity. Its function is to make **testosterone** (male hormone) and **sperm** (male gametes), and deliver the sperm into the female for fertilisation (→ Fig. 12.2).

Box 12.5 Circumcision is the removal of the **prepuce** (foreskin) by surgery, and is carried out by some religious groups. Its removal can reduce the spread of HIV, the cause of AIDS.

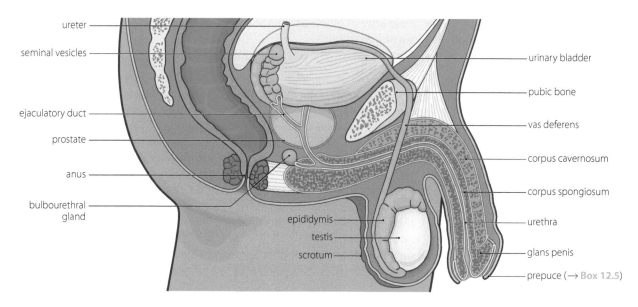

Fig. 12.2 Male reproductive system (sagittal view).

12.2.1 Testes

The testes (**testicles**) are two small ovoid structures about 5 cm in length, with the left testicle generally located about 1 cm lower than the right. They are suspended in the scrotal sac by the **spermatic cords** that run from the abdominal cavity to the testicles in the scrotum (→ Box 12.6). Nerves and the **vas deferens** connect with the testicles by passing through the spermatic cord (→ Fig. 12.3). A fibrous **capsule** surrounds each testis and sends out partitions to divide the interior into 200 or more lobules. Each lobule contains:

- tiny coiled **seminiferous tubules** in which sperm are produced by the process of spermatogenesis (→ Fig. 12.3)
- **Leydig cells** that lie in the interstitial spaces between the tubules and are specialised to secrete testosterone in response to stimulation by the luteinising hormone from the anterior pituitary gland.

Box 12.6 During foetal life, or shortly after birth, a boy's testes descend out of the abdomen into the scrotal sac. The cause of undescended testicles (**cryptorchidism**) is not fully understood but may be the result of hormonal problems.

Epididymis

The **epididymis** is a tightly coiled tube in a fibrous casing that lies along the top and behind the testis and connects the testis to the vas deferens. Sperm from the testis take several days to move passively along the epididymis which is about 7 metres long, during which time they become mature and capable of fertilisation. Sperm are then stored in the tail (lower) region of the epididymis until ejaculation.

Vas deferens

The **vas deferens** is the duct (channel) that connects the epididymis to the urethra by passing through the spermatic cord and into the abdomen. It goes over the top of the bladder before joining with the seminal vesicle to form the ejaculatory duct which opens into the urethra – the tube that carries both urine and sperm. The vas deferens has thick muscular walls that help in propelling sperm through the ducts during ejaculation (→ Box 12.7).

12.3 Spermatogenesis

The testes are located in the scrotum as spermatogenesis requires a testicular temperature that is 4–5˚C lower than core body temperature. Heat is lost:

- from arterial blood arriving at the testes as it passes to the copious surrounding veins
- through the large surface area and thin skin of the scrotum, and the lack of sub-cutaneous fat.

Spermatogenesis is the development of mature spermatozoa (sperm) from **spermatogonia** – stem cells that begin to multiply after puberty, and go through several stages. The entire process takes 70–80 days (→ Box 12.8).

1. **Spermatogonia** line the walls of the seminiferous tubules and act as stem cells by dividing continuously by **mitosis** to produce spermatocytes (→ 13.4.2).
2. **Spermatocytes** divide by **meiosis** (→ 13.4.3) to produce **spermatids**. Sertoli cells are the elongated cells in the seminiferous tubules to which the spermatids become attached and from which they apparently derive nourishment.
3. **Spermatids** are transformed into mature **spermatozoa** which can move independently by using their long tail to swim (→ Fig. 12.4).

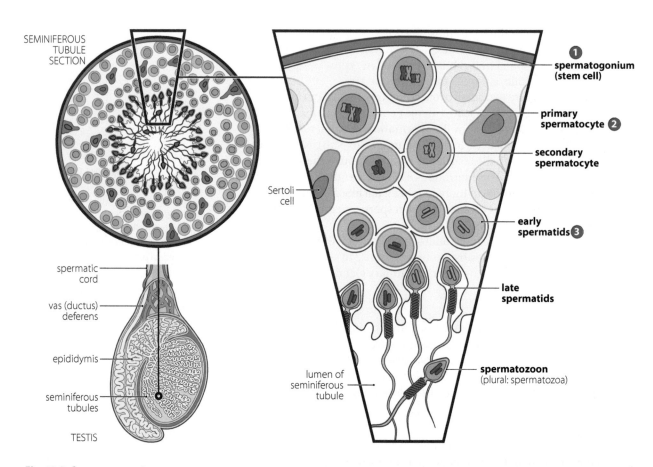

Fig. 12.3 Spermatogenesis.

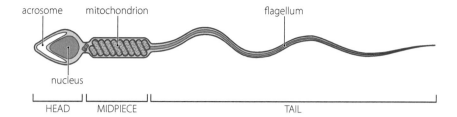

acrosome   mitochondrion   flagellum

nucleus

| HEAD | MIDPIECE | TAIL |

Fig. 12.4 Spermatozoon.

12.3.1 Hormonal control of spermatogenesis

Spermatogenesis is highly sensitive to fluctuations in the environment, particularly temperature and hormones.

- **Gonadotrophin-releasing hormone** (GnRH) secreted by the hypothalamus stimulates the release of FSH and LH from the pituitary gland (→ Fig. 12.5).
- **Follicle-stimulating hormone** (FSH) causes the Sertoli cells of the testes (which help nurse developing sperm cells) to begin the process of spermatogenesis.
- **Luteinising hormone** (LH) acts on the Leydig cells in the interstitial spaces between the tubules in the testes and stimulates them to secrete testosterone, which diffuses into the seminiferous tubules and regulates spermatogenesis. The interstitial spaces also contain capillaries through which blood circulates.
- Rising testosterone levels and high sperm production are the stimulus for Sertoli cells to produce **inhibin** – a hormone that reduces secretion of GnRH, FSH and LH from the pituitary gland by negative feedback (→ Box 12.9).

Box 12.9 Sertoli cells form a blood–testis barrier that protects the developing sperm from contact with blood which could trigger an autoimmune response. The Sertoli cells control the environment in which the sperm cells develop because they provide a selectively permeable barrier that prevents the passage of damaging or toxic substances from blood into the seminiferous tubules.

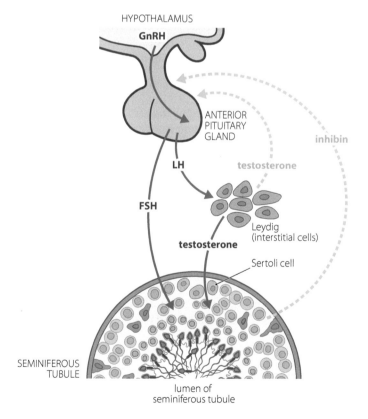

Fig. 12.5 Hormonal control of spermatogenesis – a negative feedback system from the gonads to the pituitary gland.

Sperm count

Sperm are produced in the testes and a system of ducts transport them to the exterior, so problems with any part of this process can affect sperm production. **Semen analysis** (**seminogram**) investigates some characteristics of a man's semen including a sperm count. A sperm count is considered to be low (**oligospermia**) if it contains fewer than 15 million sperm per millilitre and could cause inability to conceive a child. Complete absence of sperm from semen is called **azoospermia**. A wide range of different causes can result in a sperm count that is lower than usual, including infection, **varicocele** (swelling of veins that drain the testes), hormone disturbances, cystic fibrosis, overheating of the testes, tobacco smoking, excess weight and some medications (→ 12.9).

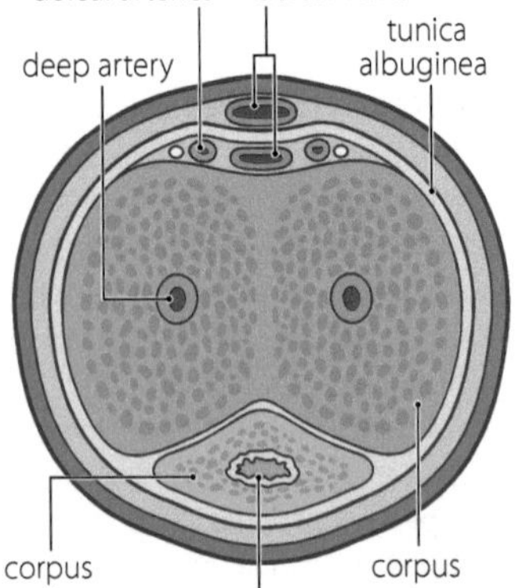

12.3.2 Penis

The **penis** is the male organ containing the urethra, through which both urine and semen are discharged (→ Fig. 12.6). It has a long shaft with a bulbous tip (the **glans**) and is able to become erect during sexual arousal. Erection occurs when the **corpus spongiosum** and **corpus cavernosum** (spongy erectile tissue) become filled with blood, which enlarges the penis and makes it firm (→ Box 12.10). The glans is covered by the **prepuce** (foreskin) – a fold of skin that retracts as the penis becomes erect.

12.3.3 Coitus

Coitus (sexual intercourse) occurs when the erect penis enters the vagina and peristalsis pumps sperm from the epididymides through the vas deferens and urethra into the vagina as orgasm occurs. On the way the sperm are mixed with seminal fluid to make a thick, sticky fluid – **semen** – which is ejaculated from the penis into the vagina. **Orgasm** in men is the climax of sexual excitement accompanied by the ejaculation of semen, each ejaculate containing as many as 300–500 million sperm.

Seminal fluid

Seminal fluid (semen) is fluid secreted by the seminal vesicles, prostate gland and bulbo-urethral glands, and may not contain sperm.

Seminal vesicles

The seminal vesicles are a pair of glands that produce fluid rich in fructose which serves as an energy source for sperm motility after ejaculation.

Prostate gland

The **prostate gland** is a small gland that lies just below the bladder. It is about the size of a large walnut and shaped like a doughnut with the urethra passing through its centre. It secretes a slightly alkaline, milky-white fluid which forms the main constituent of semen. The alkalinity of semen helps neutralise the acidity of the vaginal tract and prolong the lifespan of sperm.

Bulbo-urethral glands

Bulbo-urethral glands (Cowper's glands) are a pair of small glands about the size of a pea that open into the urethra at the base of the penis. During sexual arousal each gland secretes a clear, salty, viscous fluid known as pre-ejaculate. This fluid helps to neutralise traces of acidic urine in the urethra and to lubricate the urethra for sperm to pass through.

Fig. 12.6 Transverse section of the penis.

dorsal arteries
dorsal veins
deep artery
tunica albuginea
corpus spongiosum
corpus cavernosum
urethra

Box 12.10 Erectile dysfunction (ED) is the inability to get or keep an erection firm enough to have sexual intercourse. The cause can be
• **medical**, usually the result of an underlying medical condition affecting the blood vessels or nerves supplying the penis
• **physical**, e.g. prescription drugs, recreational drugs, alcohol, and smoking
• **psychological**, e.g. anxiety or depression.

Many men experience ED at some time in their life and a wide range of treatments are available.

12.4 Female reproductive system

The female reproductive system is situated in the lower part of the pelvic cavity and its functions are to produce the female **hormones** (oestrogen and progesterone), produce **eggs** (female gametes), enable internal fertilisation, nurture a developing baby and give birth (→ Fig. 12.7).

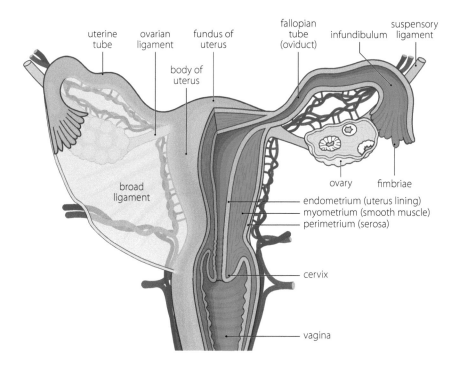

Fig. 12.7 Female internal genitalia.

12.4.1 External female genitalia

The external female genitalia – **vulva** (→ Fig. 12.8) – includes the:

- **labia majora** ('large lips') – two folds of skin that form the lateral boundaries of the vulva
- **labia minora** ('small lips') – two small folds of skin either side of the vaginal opening; situated between the labia majora
- **vaginal orifice** (opening)
- **hymen** – the membrane that covers the opening of the vagina at birth and usually perforates spontaneously before puberty. If the opening is small, it may tear and bleed slightly at the first occasion of intercourse
- **perineum** – the area of thick skin between the vagina and the anus, which may tear during childbirth
- **clitoris** – a small organ composed of erectile tissue located just behind the junction of the labia minora; it is the female counterpart of the penis
- **Bartholin's glands** – two glands that secrete fluid during coitus. If infection blocks an orifice, the gland expands as it fills with fluid and a cyst develops
- **mons pubis** – a pad of fat lying over the pubic symphysis (→ Fig. 4.15).

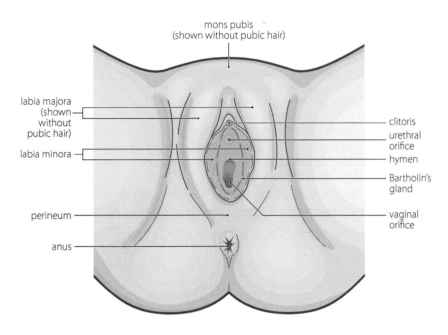

Fig. 12.8 Vulva – the external female genitalia.

uterine artery

radial artery

spiral artery

ENDOMETRIUM

MYOMETRIUM

PERIMETRIUM

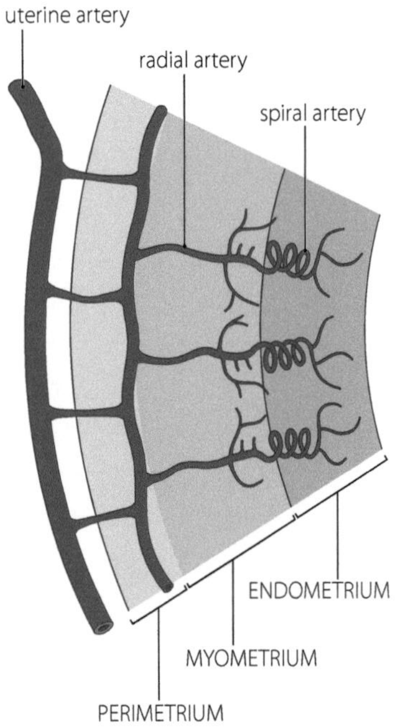

Fig. 12.9 Section through the uterus wall.

12.4.2 **Uterus**

The uterus (womb) is an upside down pear-shaped organ about 7.5 cm in length with a thick wall of smooth muscle that grows and enlarges in pregnancy to keep pace with the developing baby. The small central cavity is lined with a special mucous membrane called **endometrium** which is shed during the menstrual cycle (→ Fig. 12.7).

Uterus wall

The uterus wall is composed of three layers (→ Fig. 12.9):
- **perimetrium** – a layer of serosa that surrounds the uterus and is continuous with the broad ligament
- **myometrium** – a thick layer of smooth muscle; female orgasm is accompanied by rhythmic contraction of the myometrium and pelvic muscles
- **endometrium** – the mucosal lining that thickens during the menstrual cycle in preparation for the possible implantation of an ovum.

Spiral arteries are the small arteries that develop to supply blood to the endometrium during the luteal phase of the menstrual cycle (→ Fig. 12.12). It the event of a pregnancy, the spiral arteries supply nutrients to the placenta and foetus (→ Fig. 12.9).

Cervix

The cervix (neck of the uterus) projects into the vagina (→ Fig. 12.10). It is lined with mucous membrane, and the **cervical mucus** (**CM**) it produces undergoes changes in consistency under the influence of oestrogen. At the time of ovulation, it becomes slippery and with a pH that favours sperm survival and their penetration into the uterus. The **endocervix** opens slightly during menstruation to permit passage of the menstrual flow and is capable of softening, shortening and wide dilation during childbirth. The **ectocervix** is capable of wide dilation during childbirth (→ Box 12.11).

Box 12.11. Cervical screening test (smear test) is a method of detecting abnormal cells on the cervix. About 1 in 20 women show some abnormal changes which may need to be removed in case they became cancerous. About 3000 cases of cervical cancer are diagnosed each year in the UK, mainly affecting sexually active women between the ages of 30 and 45.

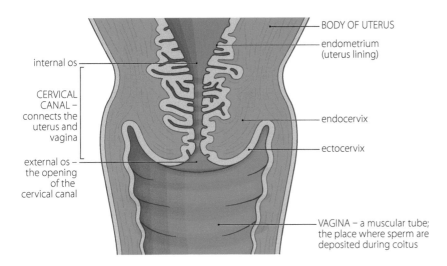

internal os

CERVICAL
CANAL –
connects the
uterus and
vagina

external os –
the opening
of the
cervical canal

BODY OF UTERUS

endometrium
(uterus lining)

endocervix

ectocervix

VAGINA – a muscular tube;
the place where sperm are
deposited during coitus

Fig. 12.10 The cervix (anterior view).

12.4.3 Ovaries

The two ovaries are the shape and size of large almonds; they are situated on either side of the uterus and held in place by ovarian ligaments (→ Fig. 12.7). Their two functions are:

- development and maturation of **ova** (eggs) and their discharge into the pelvic cavity
- secretion of the female hormones – mainly oestrogen and progesterone.

Fallopian tubes

The **fallopian tubes** (oviducts; uterine tubes) are a pair of ducts about 10 cm long that connect the ovaries to the uterus (→ Fig. 12.7). The end close to the ovary is funnel-shaped with fringe-like projections – **fimbriae** – surrounding the opening. Movements of the fimbriae at ovulation assist in gathering the ovum into the fallopian tube where it is moved along to the uterus by cilia of the mucosa lining the tube.

12.4.4 Oogenesis

Oogenesis is the development of an ovum. At birth a female has about 1 million immature ova in the ovaries and no more are produced. Fewer than 500 of these eggs will complete their development at the usual rate of one egg during each menstrual cycle, from puberty to the menopause – a span of 30–40 years. The rest of the eggs gradually disappear from birth onwards.

Each ovary is enclosed in a layer of germinal epithelium and below this are thousands of microscopic structures known as **primary follicles** containing a female sex cell – an **ovum** – which, after puberty, are in various stages of development (→ Box 12.12).

Box 12.12 The **ovum** is the biggest cell in the human body, being about the size of a grain of sand.

Ovarian cycle

The ovarian cycle (→ Fig. 12.11) consists of:

- the **follicular phase**. On the first day of the cycle several primary follicles, each with an enclosed ovum, begin to grow and develop under the influence of FSH, and start to produce oestrogens (→ Fig. 12.12). Usually only one follicle matures into a fluid-filled **Graafian follicle** and moves to the surface of the ovary.

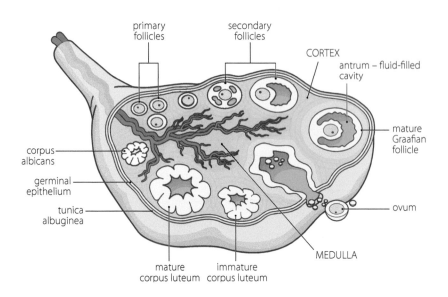

primary follicles
secondary follicles
CORTEX
antrum – fluid-filled cavity
mature Graafian follicle
ovum
MEDULLA
immature corpus luteum
mature corpus luteum
tunica albuginea
germinal epithelium
corpus albicans

Fig. 12.11 Stages of the ovarian cycle.

Box 12.13 Sperm can survive for 5–7 days in the female reproductive tract, but the ovum can only survive for 12–24 hours. If sperm are present in the fallopian tube during this 'window' then the egg can be **fertilised**.

- **ovulation**. A surge of LH triggers the rupture of the follicle and the mature ovum is released into the fallopian tube (→ Box 12.13).
- the **luteal phase**. The cells of the remaining follicle enlarge, become filled with a golden-coloured lipid substance to form the **corpus luteum**. This grows for 7–8 days, secreting oestrogen and progesterone. If fertilisation has not taken place, the size of the corpus luteum and the amount of progesterone it secretes gradually diminish, leaving a white scar – the **corpus albicans**.

Ovarian reserve

The ovarian reserve is an estimate of the number of eggs that could be fertilised during a woman's reproductive life. Since an egg is released during each menstrual cycle, the ovarian reserve declines with age.

12.5 Menstrual cycle

The menstrual cycle is a regular series of changes that take place in the female reproductive system to prepare for fertilisation and pregnancy. It is a complex cycle that includes the ovarian cycle, uterine cycle and hypothalamic–pituitary cycle, which are inter-related and interdependent (→ Fig. 12.12).

The menstrual cycle takes, on average, 28 days to complete (normal range 21–45 days). During this time the **uterine cycle** goes through several stages:
- **menstrual phase** – the endometrium comes away from the wall, bit by bit, and is removed in a flow of blood – menstruation (a period)
- **follicular phase** – FSH and LH stimulate the ovarian cells to secrete oestrogen which stimulates the endometrium to form a new lining. At the same time, an ovum completes its development in the ovary
- **ovulation** – the ovum is released after a surge of luteinising hormone (LH). Although the preovulatory phase of the cycle is highly variable, the postovulatory (luteal) phase is constant in all women, taking 10–12 days to complete. Therefore ovulation usually happens 10–12 days before onset of menstruation
- **luteal phase** – the endometrium grows in thickness under the influence of progesterone from the corpus luteum of the ovary. If the ovum has been

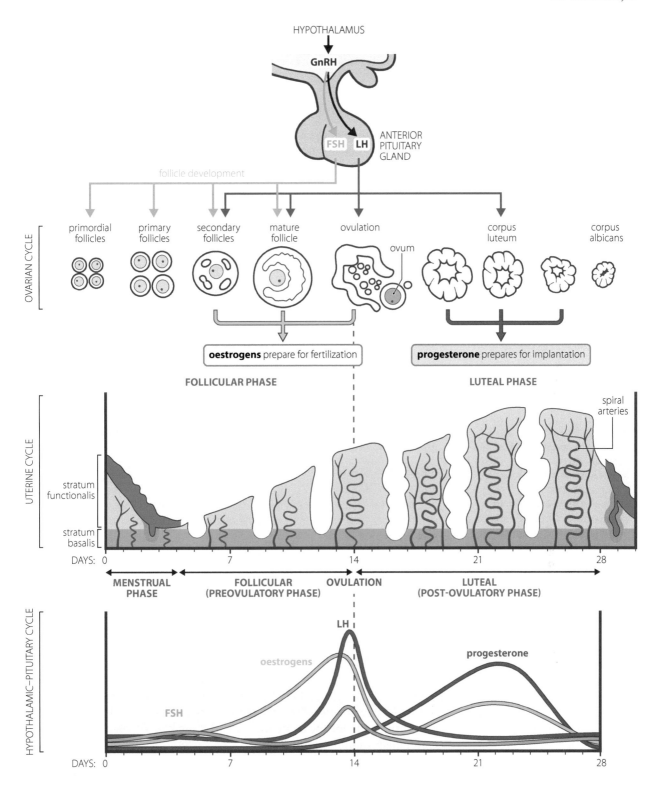

Fig. 12.12 Hormonal control of an **average** (28-day) menstrual cycle. Ovulation does not necessarily take place on day 14 in shorter or longer cycles.
GnRH – gonadotrophin-releasing hormone secreted by the hypothalamus stimulates the anterior pituitary gland to secrete FSH and LH; **FSH** – follicle-stimulating hormone stimulates a follicle to develop and the ovum it contains to mature; **LH** – luteinising hormone causes ovulation and the development of the corpus luteum; **oestrogens** – prepare the lining of the uterus for implantation; **progesterone** – prepares the endometrium to receive a fertilised ovum.

fertilised, it will embed in the endometrium and pregnancy will begin. If the egg is not fertilised, the corpus luteum dies back, progesterone levels fall and the lining of the endometrium is shed during menstruation (→ Box 12.14).

12.5.1 Menarche

Menarche is the name for the first menstrual period. It signals the onset of oestrogen-induced growth of the endometrium and the beginning of **fertility**. The first cycles are often anovulatory, although it is possible for a girl to become pregnant before her first menstrual period. The age of menarche is inherited but affected by nutritional factors as it requires the proportion of body fat to reach about 17% of body mass.

Girls begin to menstruate – have periods – sometime between the ages of 10 and 17 years. Periods are likely to be irregular and scanty at first and it is not uncommon for the interval between the first and second period to be up to a year, but gradually they become more regular.

After puberty cycles usually become more regular with menstruation lasting from 3–7 days, with 21–35 days between one period and the next. The average total blood loss during a period is 30 cm^3 but it can be as much as 180 cm^3.

Menorrhagia is excessive menstrual bleeding and needs medical advice. A hormone imbalance between oestrogen and progesterone can lead to excess development of the endometrial layer which in turn leads to excessive bleeding. Other causes of heavy or prolonged bleeding include anovulatory cycles, conditions including polycystic ovary syndrome (PCOS), thyroid disease, obesity, fibroids and some medications.

Absence of periods. Periods stop during pregnancy and for several months afterwards. They may also stop for a while during illness, poor nutrition or emotional stress. **Amenorrhoea** is the absence of periods in women of child-bearing age and needs medical advice if more than two periods are missed (→ Box 12.15).

Premature ovarian failure

Premature ovarian failure (POF) occurs in women whose ovaries stop working before they reach the age of natural menopause, usually taken as before the age of 40. There may be few or no ovarian follicles following chemotherapy, radiation therapy or as a result of inherited disorder; or there may be intact follicles but autoimmune processes may have affected FSH receptor function.

Physiologically POF is therefore different from a natural menopause because it is the result of dysfunction of the ovaries or early surgical removal of the ovaries leading to infertility. High levels of FSH accompanied by low levels of oestrogens define the condition, which women often experience as an emotionally traumatic diagnosis.

Some cases of POF are attributed to Turner syndrome and fragile X syndrome but in many women no cause can be detected.

12.5.2 Menopause

The menopause (**climacteric**) is a physiological process that is marked by one year having passed since the cessation of menstrual periods. It is a universal and irreversible part of the ageing process.

During a woman's reproductive life, the number and quality of follicles within the ovary declines. At first, menstrual cycles may become irregular and shorter, but pregnancy can still occur because the transition to menopause takes some years; the median age for reaching menopause is 52 years (→ Box 12.16).

Increasing levels of FSH and LH from the pituitary gland are characteristic of the **perimenopausal** period, but the ovaries become increasingly insensitive to the effects of these hormones, so oestrogen production falls dramatically and the ovaries gradually diminish in size. Because no ovulation occurs, levels of progesterone fall too.

The **temperature regulation** centre within the hypothalamus becomes increasingly sensitive to relatively smaller changes in temperature than before the menopause, leading to the experience of unpredictable hot 'flushes' (flashes). Other neurovascular changes include palpitations, light-headedness, dizziness or vertigo (→ Box 12.17).

After the menopause

The structure of **breast tissue** changes after the menopause because ductal and lobular tissue is replaced with soft adipose tissue. In some women, the **pelvic floor** and ligaments soften and become more lax, increasing the risk of prolapse of the pelvic organs into the vagina.

Without oestrogen and progesterone, the **endometrium** begins to atrophy (waste away) and the vascular supply to the epithelial lining of the **genital tract** changes. In some women, these changes can lead to increased infection and feelings of dryness and irritation but in others, e.g. those who have experienced endometriosis or painful periods, menopause may provide relief. Oestrogen has a cardioprotective action which is lost after the menopause, so women's risk of **heart disease** rises to match that of men.

The risk of **osteoporosis** increases after menopause because loss of oestrogen sensitises bone to respond more strongly to the action of parathyroid hormone (→ 11.5). As a result bone remodelling alters, with osteoclast activity becoming more dominant, which leads to loss of calcium from bone and a reduction in density.

Hormone replacement therapy

Women who experience severe symptoms may be offered hormone replacement therapy (HRT), the hormones used being oestrogen and progesterone. Besides reducing the perceived unpleasant effects of the menopause, HRT reduces the loss of calcium from bones and thus leads to a reduction in osteoporosis (weak bones) and the likelihood of fractures.

12.6 Conception

Conception (**fertilisation**) is the fusion of a male and a female gamete. It takes place after an **ovum** has been released from one of the ovaries and is moving slowly along the fallopian tube, where it can survive for 12–24 hours. If coitus has occurred around ovulation, the **sperm** will be active and moving around by the lashing movements of the tail, making their way through the cervix and uterus and into the fallopian tube containing the ovum. Although a number of sperm surround the ovum, only one will penetrate it, which triggers rapid changes in the membrane of the ovum and prevents other sperm from entering (→ Box 12.18). When a sperm fertilises the ovum, its tail drops off and the head (sperm nucleus) moves towards the nucleus of the ovum and the two fuse together. Sperm can survive for five days, so coitus does not need to coincide with ovulation. The fertilised ovum (**zygote**) now

Box 12.16 Across the world, women's subjective perception of **menopausal changes** – as a medical event, as an expected life transition or as a distressing experience – is very variable. Several theories have been proposed to account for the evolutionary role of menopause but no single mechanism is agreed.

Box 12.17 Perimenopausal women often experience a range of effects that are caused by the falling and low levels of oestrogens, including irregular periods, mood swings, headaches, insomnia, vaginal dryness or itching, and weight gain or bloating.

Box 12.18 Multiple pregnancies are caused either by the division of one fertilised egg into two or the release of two or more eggs at the same time which are all fertilised. **Identical twins** come from the same fertilised egg, have the same genes, same gender and are very similar in appearance. **Non-identical (fraternal) twins** may be of the same or different gender and are no more alike than other brothers or sisters in the family. **Conjoined twins** (formerly known as Siamese twins) are identical twins that failed to separate into two individuals.

starts to divide by mitosis (→ 13.4.2) first into two cells then into four, and
so on as it continues its way along the fallopian tube (→ Box 12.19). By the
time the zygote reaches the uterus about 7 days after ovulation, it is a hollow
ball of cells called a **blastocyst** and embeds itself into the lining of the uterus
wall – a process called **implantation**.

The blastocyst contains the stem cells that develop into the **embryo**
(→ Fig. 12.13). The blastocyst wall – **trophoblast** – gives rise to the placenta,
umbilical cord and **amnion**. The amnion is the membrane that forms a bag
containing **amniotic fluid** in which the baby develops.

Human chorionic gonadotrophin (hCG) is produced by the trophoblast
after the blastocyst has begun to implant in the uterus wall. The role of hCG
is to sustain the corpus luteum if pregnancy occurs, and the level of hCG
continues to rise for about 3 months before declining. hCG is the basis of a
pregnancy test as it can first be detected by a blood test about 11 days after
conception, and by a urine test 12–14 days after conception (→ Box 12.4).

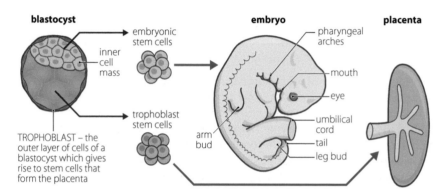

Fig. 12.13 Development of blastocyst to embryo and placenta during the first month after
fertilisation.

12.6.1 Embryology

One month after conception an embryo is curved into a C-shape
(→ Fig. 12.13). It is possible to identify head and tail ends, pharyngeal arches
as deep folds in the neck area, developing eyes, ears and limb buds. The
primitive heart is bulging from the upper body and blood starts to circulate on
day 20 (→ Box 12.20). The umbilical cord and primitive placental structures
for exchange of materials between mother and embryo are forming.

At 2 months, the embryo has grown to look more human-like (→ Fig. 12.14).
The main structures of the body are more or less in place and the heart is
beating (→ Box 12.21). Growth of the head exceeds that of all other regions
because the brain is developing quickly. Nerves are present, muscle mass is
increasing and muscles are being innervated. Eyes and ears are developing,
the buccal cavity is forming, the oesophagus and trachea are differentiating,
while the digestive system is becoming established. The external genitalia
are developing but it is still too early to tell the gender. The end of week 8
marks the beginning of the foetal period.

At 3 months, development of nerves and muscles enables the foetus to
frown, clench the fist, turn the head and kick. Body growth has been so
rapid that the crown–rump length has doubled. The spleen starts making
red blood cells, involuntary muscle is developing in the visceral organs and
the process of ossification of the skull and long bones is initiated. The lower
limbs are not so well developed as the upper limbs.

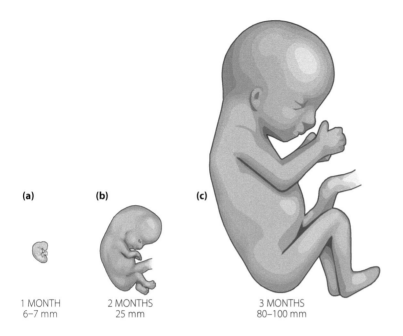

Taking it Further
You can find out more about ultrasound scanning of the developing foetus in online Chapter 17.

(a)   **(b)**   **(c)**

1 MONTH   2 MONTHS   3 MONTHS
6–7 mm   25 mm   80–100 mm

Fig. 12.14 Actual size: (**a**) embryo at 1 month, (**b**) embryo at 2 months, (**c**) foetus at three months.

At 5 months, the mother can feel movements made by the foetus. Very fine hairs (lanugo) now cover its skin and the sex organs have developed sufficiently for an ultrasound scan to reveal its gender.

At 7 months, development is almost complete and the foetus will spend the next two months in the uterus growing larger and stronger. Fat becomes stored under the skin, making a full-term baby look plump.

12.6.2 Placenta

The embryo obtains nourishment from a **yolk sac** until the placenta has had time to develop and function as the organ that feeds the foetus and removes its waste. The placenta starts to develop as soon as the egg is embedded in the uterus wall and becomes a thick, disc-like structure firmly attached to the uterus wall. It continues to grow to keep pace with the developing foetus and weighs about 500 g at term. The umbilical cord grows to be about 50 cm long and 2 cm wide.

Exchange through the placenta

Blood from the growing foetus flows continuously to and from the placenta through the **umbilical cord**. In the placenta, the blood from the foetus comes very close to the mother's blood, but they do not mix (➔ Fig. 12.15). They are, however, close enough for substances to be exchanged.
- Nutrients and oxygen pass from mother to foetus.
- Carbon dioxide and other waste substances pass from the foetus to the mother for excretion.
- Antibodies from the mother pass to the foetus and help to protect it from infectious disease because the foetus has little immunity.

Other substances in the mother's blood can also cross the placenta and affect the foetus:
- **cigarette smoke**. Carbon monoxide, nicotine and other chemicals cross the placenta and can affect the foetus (➔ Box 12.22)

Box 12.22 Women who are heavy smokers are more likely to have a miscarriage, a smaller weaker baby or one that is stillborn.

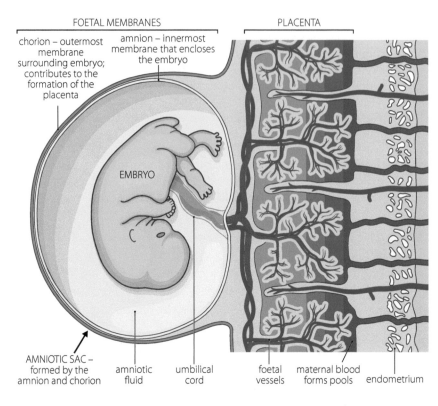

FOETAL MEMBRANES

chorion – outermost membrane surrounding embryo; contributes to the formation of the placenta

amnion – innermost membrane that encloses the embryo

PLACENTA

EMBRYO

AMNIOTIC SAC – formed by the amnion and chorion

amniotic fluid

umbilical cord

foetal vessels

maternal blood forms pools

endometrium

Fig. 12.15 Embryo and placenta at 2 months.

Box 12.23 Foetal alcohol syndrome (FAS) is a pattern of mental and physical defects associated with high levels of alcohol consumption during pregnancy, the main effect being permanent damage to the baby's brain.

Box 12.24 While in the uterus, the mother breathes for the baby, but this ceases at birth. Entry into the air stimulates the baby to take its **first breath** within a few seconds of delivery. The foetal circulation also has to adapt quickly to air breathing by closing the foramen ovale – 'the hole in the heart'.

Box 12.25 Foetal haemoglobin is used to transport oxygen during the last seven months of development in the uterus. It has a greater affinity for oxygen than adult haemoglobin, giving the developing foetus better access to oxygen from the mother's bloodstream. Foetal haemoglobin is replaced by adult haemoglobin postnatally within about six months.

- **medicines**. It is advisable that no medicines are taken in early pregnancy unless vital for the health of the mother, as some may harm the embryo and growing foetus. Women who are planning a pregnancy can work with their doctors and other health professionals to determine if alternative forms of treatment are possible
- **alcohol**. Pregnant women are advised to avoid drinking alcohol. The foetal liver is not fully developed and cannot metabolise alcohol quickly enough to prevent a high blood alcohol concentration that can affect the growth and development of the foetus (→ Box 12.23)
- **vertically transmitted infections**. These are caused by pathogens that are passed from mother to embryo or foetus before or during childbirth. The **TORCH** complex describes some of them:

  T = toxoplasmosis – found in infected meat, infected cat faeces, and unpasteurised goat's milk

  O = other infections, e.g. chlamydia, chickenpox, HIV, syphilis

  R = rubella – also known as German measles

  C = cytomegalovirus – can cause chickenpox

  H = herpes virus that causes cold sores

- **hepatitis B** can also be vertically transmitted but it is a large virus particle which does not cross the placenta. Instead, it is transmitted when the maternal–foetal barrier is broken, e.g. by amniocentesis or bleeding at delivery.

12.6.3 **Foetal circulation**

Foetal circulation differs from a baby's circulation in that:
- **foetal circulation** contains shunts that direct blood flow away from the lungs and liver, as they are still developing and not yet functioning (→ Box 12.24)
- **foetal blood** contains a special form of haemoglobin which has a very high affinity for oxygen (→ Box 12.25).

Foetal shunts

A **shunt** diverts blood from one place to another. The foetal circulation contains three shunts, two that bypass the lungs, shunting blood to the placenta, and one that bypasses the liver, as it flows back towards the heart (→ Fig. 12.16).

❶ **Foramen ovale** – a small opening in the septum between the atria (upper chambers) of the foetal heart. This opening between the right atrium and the left atrium makes it possible for most of the foetal blood to pass directly into the aorta. The umbilical arteries branch off from the descending aorta and carry deoxygenated blood to the placenta to collect oxygen and excrete waste.

❷ **Ductus arteriosus** – a second shunt that allows foetal blood to bypass the lungs by diverting most of the blood from the right ventricle into the descending aorta. The umbilical arteries then carry blood to the placenta.

❸ **Ductus venosus** – a slender vessel that connects the hepatic portal vein to the umbilical vein and carries oxygenated blood directly to the inferior vena cava. This enables some of the umbilical blood to bypass the foetal liver and travel directly to the heart.

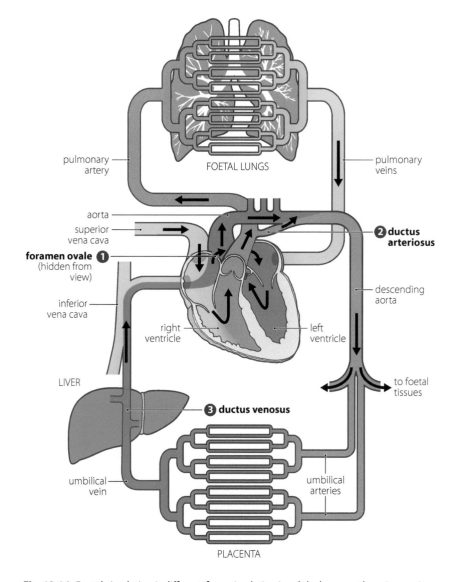

Fig. 12.16 Foetal circulation is different from circulation in adults because the primary site for exchange of gases, nutrients and waste is the placenta which lies outside the body cavity.

12.6.4 Towards the end of pregnancy

The mother's uterus is in a relatively quiescent and tranquil state throughout pregnancy but in the final weeks a series of changes in the cervix and uterus culminate in delivery of the newborn (→ Box 12.26). Towards the end of pregnancy:

- progesterone levels tend to reach a plateau around seven months, while oestrogens continue to rise. As a result, the smooth muscle of the uterus becomes increasingly more sensitive to oestrogenic stimuli and progesterone no longer inhibits contraction
- the mother will notice sporadic tightening of the uterus known as **Braxton Hicks contractions** or 'prodromal labour'
- foetal cortisol levels rise during the final weeks and this boosts placental oestrogen production and prepares the foetus for delivery
- gradually, the uterus becomes more sensitive to the pituitary hormone oxytocin because more oxytocin receptors are being expressed on the myometrial cell membranes
- the foetal head begins to press on the softening cervix, which stimulates labour contractions (→ Box 12.27). This pressure further stimulates oxytocin secretion from the pituitary through a positive feedback mechanism (→ Fig. 12.17; Fig. 1.11 example 1).

The sum of all of these changes in the uterus initiate the regular contractions that are called 'true labour'.

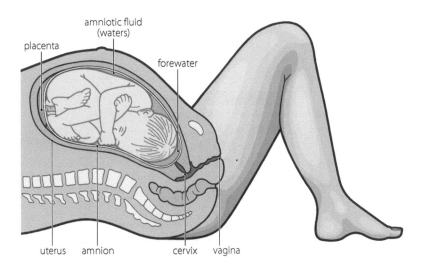

Fig. 12.17 Foetus ready to be born.

Box 12.26 Paracrine (→ Fig. 11.2) and endocrine signalling from both mother and foetus initiate the process of labour but their relative contributions remain to be clarified.

12.7 Parturition

Parturition (labour followed by delivery) is the action of giving birth. Pregnancy lasts approximately 270 days (38.5 weeks from the date of fertilisation, which is assumed to have occurred about 2 weeks after the mother's last period). The estimated date of delivery (EDD) – the date on which the baby is most likely to be born – is therefore calculated by adding 40 weeks to the first day of the mother's last menstrual period. Towards the end of the pregnancy, the baby moves into the correct position to be born, with its head presenting downwards (→ Box 12.27). The process of giving birth is referred to as **labour** and has three stages.

Box 12.27 In fewer than 5% of all births, the foetus is orientated with its buttocks first, known as a **breech presentation:**
- **frank breech** when the legs are pointing upwards
- **complete breech** when legs are crossed and folded downwards.

Many breech births are managed with caesarean section.

Stage 1 Dilation of the cervix and opening of the birth canal

One or more signs indicate that dilation (opening) of the cervix has started:
- **a 'show'.** This is a small discharge of blood and mucus that formed the plug, which comes away from the cervix as it softens
- **release of the forewater** of the amniotic fluid. The amnion may rupture and release this fluid, or will do so later on
- **contractions occur.** These contractions of the uterus wall (uterine muscle) start slowly and irregularly (→ Box 12.28).

As the first stage of labour proceeds, the contractions become stronger, more frequent and more painful as the uterine muscle gradually dilates the cervix. Each contraction reduces the flow of oxygenated blood to the uterus so it is important for the uterus to relax between contractions to allow time for recovery (→ Box 12.29). The contractions of the uterine muscle gradually draw the cervix back and around the presenting part, which is usually the baby's head.

Contractions increase in intensity because of a positive feedback control mechanism (→ Fig. 12.18):
❶ Pressure from the foetal head (or presenting part) on the cervix stimulates sensory endings in the cervix
❷ Nerve impulses are sent along sensory nerves to the hypothalamus and pituitary gland, which respond by secreting increasing amounts of oxytocin
❸ Oxytocin makes the uterus contract, dilating the cervix
❹ Contractions are pressing the baby's head more deeply into the birth canal, which increases feedback to the hypothalamus and pituitary; this results in greater secretion of oxytocin.

During labour the the cervix becomes softer and becomes thinner (effaced) (→ Fig. 12.19). The length of labour varies widely and is generally longer in 1st stage mothers and faster in those who have previously delivered a baby. Labour comes to an end when the cervix is dilated to 10 cm in diameter and the uterus, cervix and vagina now form a continuous **birth canal**.

Stage 2: Full dilation of the cervix and expulsion of the newborn

The second stage takes about 2 hours to complete and begins when the baby's head enters the birth canal (→ Box 12.30). The uterus wall is contracting strongly and, as it does so, it pushes the head first through the birth canal, with the **occiput** (back of the foetal head) usually the presenting part. The moment when the head emerges from the birth canal is called **crowning** (→ Fig. 12.20).

Stage 3 Delivery

The midwife eases the shoulders through the birth canal (→ Fig. 12.21) and the baby slides out into the world. At this point the baby starts to breathe independently (→ Boxes 12.31 and 12.32). Once the baby is delivered, the spiral arteries of the endometrium constrict and stop blood flow to the endometrium. The uterus continues to contract under the influence of oxytocin, and becomes smaller. The placenta starts to separate from the myometrium and pushing, gravity and nipple stimulation from breast-feeding helps it to detach. Once it has stopped pulsating, the umbilical cord is often clamped (→ Fig. 12.22). When separation is complete, the mother pushes the placenta out through the vagina.

Box 12.28 Contractions can cause pain in labour and can be relieved by:
- **relaxation and breathing exercises** that can work well during the early stages
- **Entonox** – a gas mixture of oxygen and nitrous oxide that is inhaled when contractions are strong
- **epidural** injection removes much sensation in the lower body
- **pethidine** to help relax the muscles
- **water bath** – the warm water helps the mother to relax
- **TENS** (transcutaneous electrical nerve stimulation) machine for pain relief during the early stages.

Box 12.29 When there is no relaxation between contractions, **foetal distress** may become apparent as an increased foetal heart rate with its increased risk of hypoxia. This situation can be a cause of emergency delivery with forceps, ventouse or caesarean section.

Box 12.30 The nature of contractions changes during the **2nd stage** of labour because it is the active 'pushing stage' which begins once the cervix has dilated to 10 cm in diameter. The mother's breathing patterns change, with an overwhelming urge to push as the baby moves from the uterus to the outside world.

Box 12.31 The midwife may clear mucus from the nose and mouth and the baby may start to breathe, and even cry when delivered.

Box 12.32 Once the baby is breathing, the umbilical cord is often clamped in two places to prevent blood loss from the baby, and the cord between the clamps is cut to separate the baby from the mother (→ Fig. 12.22). Delayed clamping of the umbilical cord for at least 1 minute is recommended for all newborns not requiring resuscitation.

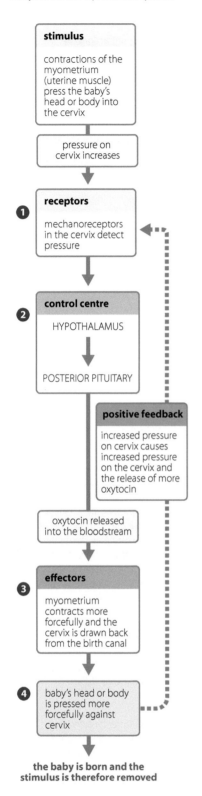

stimulus

contractions of the myometrium (uterine muscle) press the baby's head or body into the cervix

↓

pressure on cervix increases

↓

receptors

❶ mechanoreceptors in the cervix detect pressure

↓

control centre

❷ HYPOTHALAMUS

↓

POSTERIOR PITUITARY

positive feedback

increased pressure on cervix causes increased pressure on the cervix and the release of more oxytocin

↓

oxytocin released into the bloodstream

↓

effectors

❸ myometrium contracts more forcefully and the cervix is drawn back from the birth canal

↓

❹ baby's head or body is pressed more forcefully against cervix

↓

the baby is born and the stimulus is therefore removed

Fig. 12.18 Positive feedback of the regulation of labour.

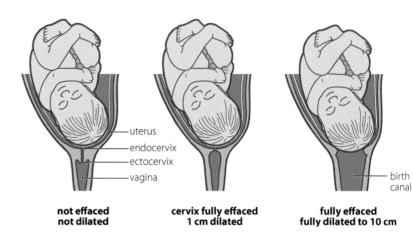

uterus
endocervix
ectocervix
vagina

birth canal

not effaced not dilated   **cervix fully effaced 1 cm dilated**   **fully effaced fully dilated to 10 cm**

Fig. 12.19 Dilation of the cervix and formation of the birth canal in stage 1.

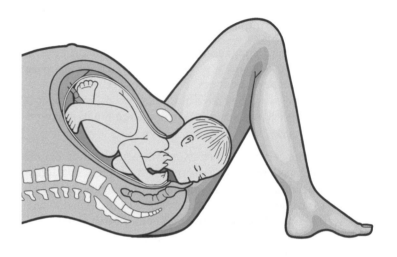

Fig. 12.20 Crowning of the baby's head in stage 2.

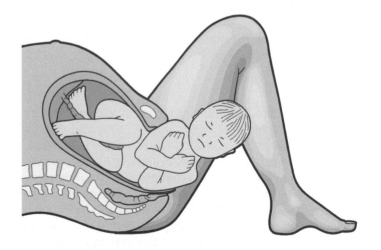

Fig. 12.21 Delivery of the baby's shoulders and body.

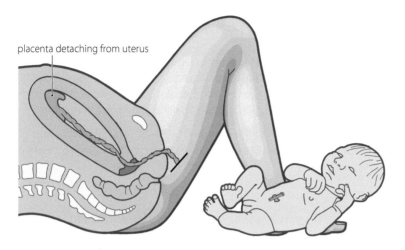

placenta detaching from uterus

Fig. 12.22 The umbilical cord has been cut by a midwife in stage 3.

12.7.1 Other methods of delivery

Induction

The process of labour is started artificially because the birth is very overdue or the health of the mother or baby is at risk, e.g. if the pregnancy goes 10–12 days beyond term the placenta may no longer be working optimally. It may be possible to induce the birth by breaking the forewaters; the mother may also be given the hormone **oxytocin** to stimulate the uterus to start contracting.

Forceps or ventouse (vacuum) delivery

Sometimes the safest method of delivery of a baby is by means of assisted vaginal birth (**operative vaginal delivery**) using obstetric forceps which curve around the baby's head or ventouse (vacuum extraction using a suction cup on the baby's head). This type of delivery may happen if the mother needs help with the birth when the baby is moving slowly through the birth canal, or there are concerns about the baby's health.

Caesarean section

A caesarean section (C-section) is the delivery of a baby through a surgical incision in the mother's abdomen and uterus rather than through the birth canal.
- **Elective** (planned) **C-section** takes place to prevent critical problems that might otherwise arise as a result of placental disorders, e.g. **placenta praevia** (placenta is near or covers the cervical opening), **placental abruption** (placenta detaches prematurely from the uterus), breech presentation or **cord prolapse** (→ Box 12.33).
- **Emergency C-section** may be performed if the baby or the mother become distressed.

Box 12.33 Cord prolapse occurs when the umbilical cord drops (prolapses) through the open cervix into the vagina ahead of the baby. The cord can then become trapped against the baby's body during delivery, which can reduce the amount of blood flowing through the cord. This situation is rare, but may require immediate C-section delivery because of reduced oxygen supply to the foetus.

12.7.2 Neonatal period

The **neonatal period** is the time between birth and 28 days of age, and includes the transition from foetal to adult circulation and breathing.

During foetal life the lungs are filled with fluid, which contributes to increased pulmonary resistance and reduced blood flow to the lungs. Foetal lungs begin to produce surfactant (→ 6.3.1) so that, by 35 weeks of gestation, they are ready to breathe air after delivery. During labour, fluid in the lung moves into the spaces around the alveoli and is reabsorbed so that the lungs are ready to fill with air.

After delivery, exposure of foetal lungs to oxygen reduces pulmonary resistance and increases blood flow to the lungs. Changes outside the uterus – touch, cooler temperature and changes in blood gases – stimulate the respiratory centres in the medulla to trigger diaphragm contraction and breathing.

Shortly after birth, closure of the ductus arteriosus, foramen ovale and ductus venosus begins and the transition to independent life is complete.

12.7.3 APGAR score

This assessment is generally done at one minute after birth and again at five minutes. It may be repeated later if the score is low. It is used to assess the physiological status of the newborn and the need for any intervention to establish breathing by observing five vital signs (→ Table 12.1):

- **A**ppearance – the colour of the baby's skin
- **P**ulse – the rate of heartbeat
- **G**rimace (distressed facial expression) assessed by a reflex response to a stimulus such as being touched; the response might be a grimace, cry or cough
- **A**ctivity – muscle tone and the amount of movement
- **R**espiration – the ability to breathe after delivery.

Taking it Further
You can find out more about newborn blood spot screening and other physiological observations in online Chapter 17.

Table 12.1 APGAR score

APGAR score	0	1	2
Appearance	blue, pale	body pink, toes/fingers blue	completely pink
Pulse	absent	slow – below 100 per min	fast – above 100 per min
Grimace*	no response	grimace	cry/cough
Activity	limp	some movement	active movement
Respiration	absent	slow, irregular	good, crying

A high score of 8, 9 or 10 indicates a healthy baby.
A score of 5–7 indicates that the baby may need some help with the transition to postnatal life.
A low score of under 5 warns that immediate medical care is needed, but may not necessarily predict long-term health issues.
* Reflex irritability.

12.7.4 Neonatal examination

A physical examination of the newborn is carried out within three days of birth and again at 6–8 weeks. It includes checks for:

- eye conditions such as congenital cataracts, **congenital** meaning present at birth
- congenital heart disease
- developmental dysplasia of the hip (→ Box 12.34)
- undescended testicles.

Box 12.34 Developmental **dysplasia of the hip** was formerly referred to as congenital dislocation of the hip. The head of the femur is not stable within the acetabulum (socket), which may loosen the ligaments of the hip joint. Treatment is needed to prevent a permanent limp.

Newborn blood spot screening (heel prick test)

Ideally, this test takes place at five days old (→ 17.5.4). The baby's heel is pricked to obtain a few drops of blood which is analysed to check for a number of conditions including:

- **sickle cell anaemia** (→ 5.9.1)
- **cystic fibrosis** (→ 13.8.2)
- **phenylketonuria** (PKU) due to lack of the enzyme that deals with phenylalanine – an amino acid present in milk and other foods; absence of the enzyme can cause learning disability
- **congenital hypothyroidism** caused when the thyroid gland fails to produce thyroid hormone needed for normal growth and development (→ 11.4.2) (→ 17.5.4)

12.7.5 Post-partum period

The **post-partum** (**post-natal**) period begins immediately after the birth and extends for about six weeks, when the mother's body, including hormone levels and uterus size, returns to a non-pregnant state.

During this time, the uterus shrinks rapidly in size although it never quite returns to the pre-pregnant state. The myometrium contracts strongly, forming a 'living ligature' that reduces blood flow from the site where the placenta was attached in the uterus. The uterus will continue to contract as long as it does not contain any clots. Alternating contractions and relaxations of the uterus at this time may cause cramping which is known as **afterpains**.

After a vaginal delivery, most women experience some swelling of the vulva and perineum and, possibly, vulval varicose veins or haemorrhoids, which can initially cause pain but usually resolve as the perineum (area between anus and vulva) begins to heal. Women can usually begin to resume activities of daily living as long as they are not in discomfort, bearing in mind the often unexpected level of fatigue associated with caring for a newborn baby.

Women who have had a caesarean delivery will experience pain and discomfort from the abdominal incision and may need to wait a little longer to resume some everyday activities, in order to avoid surgical complications.

In all women, the endometrial lining is gradually restored, although the site of placental attachment takes longer. The mixture of blood, mucus and uterine tissue – called the **lochia** – continues for 4–6 weeks after the birth, changing from the initial red colour to a much smaller volume that is yellowish. This process leaves the endometrial layer smooth, spongy and without scar tissue.

Ovarian function after the birth of the baby is highly variable, being greatly influenced by breastfeeding the infant. The average time for resumption of ovulation is about 6 weeks in non-breastfeeding mothers. Breastfeeding delays the return of ovarian cycles and menstruation (**lactational amenorrhoea**) but the timing of the delay depends on the frequency of breastfeeds, giving of supplemental feeds and the duration of the lactation.

It typically takes 6 months, but occasionally longer, after the birth for the menstrual cycle to restart, although it may be possible to become pregnant before periods return. It is also possible, but less likely, to become pregnant while still breastfeeding.

Pregnancy greatly stretches the skeletal muscles of the abdomen and after the birth they feel very loose and floppy. The muscles of the pelvic floor are also stretched and weakened during delivery. All these muscles gradually regain tone and special post-natal exercises will help them to regain their former shape.

12.8 Lactation

Lactation is defined as the secretion of milk by the mammary glands (breasts) to provide nutrition and immunity for the baby. The period of time during which a mother feeds her baby is known as breastfeeding or nursing.

12.8.1 Breasts

Early in pregnancy, under the influence of oestrogen, progesterone and prolactin, the breasts enlarge as the glandular tissue develops in readiness for milk production, and the pigmented area around the nipple – the **areola** – changes from pink to brown (→ Box 12.35).

Each breast contains the 15–20 milk-producing glands called **lobules**, surrounded by fatty tissue and ligaments (→ Box 12.36). The lobules contain **alveoli** (hollow cavities) lined with milk-secreting columnar epithelium. A system of mammary ducts convey milk to the nipple to be stored in ampullae (→ Fig. 12.23).

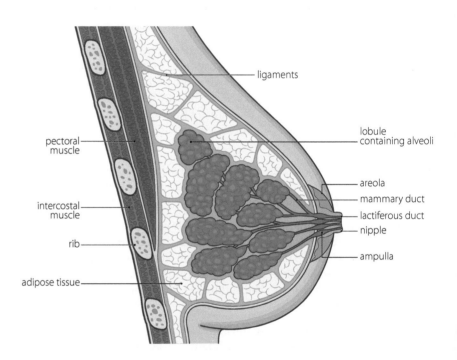

Box 12.35 Montgomery tubercles in the areola are adapted sebaceous glands that have been described as looking rather like goose-bumps. They produce an oily fluid that lubricates the nipple.

Box 12.36 The size and shape of the breasts before pregnancy depends on the amount of fat tissue present and not on the number of milk-producing glands. So breast size is not an important factor in breast-feeding.

Fig. 12.23 Section through a lactating breast.

Box 12.37 Anti-infective agents in breast milk protect against infection by bacteria, viruses and other microorganisms. They include a variety of bioactive substances, e.g. macrophages, immunoglobulins, cytokines, antimicrobial agents and growth factors, all of which help to safeguard the baby's survival.

12.8.2 Colostrum

Towards the end of pregnancy, the breasts start to secrete a yellow, thick and sticky fluid called **colostrum**. This is a concentrated mixture of proteins, vitamins, growth factors and antibodies that helps the newborn baby adapt to life outside the uterus in the first few days of life (→ Box 12.37). Colostrum, although small in volume, helps the newborn to pass **meconium** (the first faeces which are black and sticky) and provides protection through the transition from a sterile, intrauterine environment to life in the outside world.

12.8.3 Transitional milk

A few days after the birth, colostrum is replaced by **transitional milk**, which is a more dilute fluid containing water and thousands of distinct, physiologically active substances that protect the newborn baby against inflammation and infection. It is uniquely suited to the baby both in terms of nutritional content and growth factors and its composition changes as the baby grows. **Growth factors** in breastmilk have wide-ranging effects including protection for the lining of the infant intestine and development of the enteric nervous system, stimulation of red blood cell production and metabolic regulation.

By 4–6 weeks postpartum, human milk is considered to be fully mature although small changes occur in its composition during the remainder of the lactation. Some of the nutrients in breastmilk originate from the alveoli of the breast, some from the mother's diet and some from maternal stores, e.g. adipose tissue.

12.8.4 Milk ejection reflex

The hormone oxytocin is secreted by the hypothalamus and stored in the posterior pituitary. The rooting reflex (search reflex) in newborn babies leads them to the breast, which stimulates tiny nerve endings in the nipple. This signals the release of **oxytocin** into the bloodstream, where it stimulates the muscles surrounding the breast to squeeze out the milk.

12.8.5 Hormonal control of lactation

Prolactin, the hormone that is essential for milk production, is produced during preganancy, but the high levels of oestrogen and progesterone produced at the time inhibit prolactin receptors and milk production. After the delivery, these hormones fall away allowing prolactin to signal to the breasts to make milk. During the first few months of the post-partum period, circulating levels of prolactin gradually fall, but it continues to be produced in pulses every time the baby suckles at the breast, stimulating more milk production in response to the demand (→ Fig. 12.24).

The areolar region of the breast contains densely packed sensory endings – **mechanoreceptors** – and suckling by the baby stimulates them to send signals (nerve impulses) to the hypothalamus, which triggers the release of **oxytocin** from the posterior pituitary gland. In turn, this hormone makes the **myoepithelial** cells that line the lactiferous ducts contract, thus increasing pressure and squeezing milk through the duct system and out through the nipple into the baby's mouth – a **let-down**. There may be a number of let-downs during a breastfeed although mothers are not always aware of them.

Breastfeeding mothers may describe the sensation of the let-down reflex and milk moving down the ducts as tingling or discomfort. The reflex often takes 1–2 weeks to settle down and, after a first baby, it becomes a conditioned (learned) reflex. Stress and anxiety, or trauma to the nipple, e.g. cracks, can disturb or inhibit the reflex (→ Box 12.38).

Typically a newborn baby feeds very frequently, maybe 15–16 times in 24 hours, and this drives the production of more milk. The early milk during each breastfeed (**foremilk**) is a lower fat mixture, but the milk gradually changes as the breast becomes less full, with the later portion (**hindmilk**) being higher in fat and energy.

Box 12.38 Dysphoric milk ejection reflex (D-MER) is an abnormality of the milk ejection reflex that produces a state of unease just prior to milk ejection that can continue for several minutes and may also produce a hollow or churning feeling in the pit of the stomach.

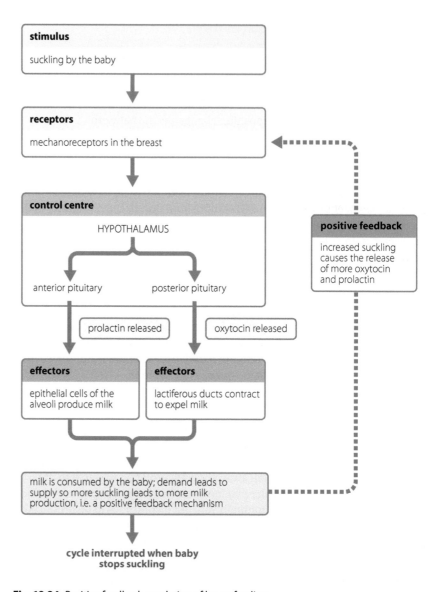

Fig. 12.24 Positive feedback regulation of breastfeeding.

12.9 Infertility

Infertility is the inability of a sexually active couple to achieve pregnancy in one year (→ Box 12.39).

12.9.1 Male infertility

There are many causes of male infertility, including the following:

- a **low sperm count**, or no sperm at all; fewer than 15 million sperm per ml of ejaculated semen would be considered to be a low value (→ Box 12.40).
- **shape and size of the sperm**: fertile sperm have a uniform shape and size and are highly motile. Although only one sperm fertilises an ovum, millions of sperm are necessary for fertilisation to occur.
- **unexplained causes**, possibly involving a variety of congenital or acquired factors, including urogenital abnormalities, varicocele, testicular failure, endocrine disturbances, immunological problems, cancer or exposure to agents that are toxic to spermatogenesis.

Box 12.39 Couples under the age of 40 years who are having regular unprotected sex every 2–3 days have an 80–85% chance of conceiving within a year. Of the remaining couples, about half will conceive in the second year.

Box 12.40 Semen analysis is when a sample of a man's semen is investigated in a laboratory to check the quality and quantity of the sperm it contains.

A normal sperm count ranges from 15 million to more than 200 million sperm per millilitre (ml) of semen.

12.9.2 Female infertility

Female infertility is the inability to conceive and bear children and there are many causes, mainly those mentioned below.

- **Failure to ovulate** – the ovaries do not release eggs or do so only occasionally, due to conditions such as **polycystic ovary syndrome** (PCOS). PCOS is characterised by high levels of androgens and insulin resistance, which make it difficult for the ovaries to produce an egg (→ Box 12.41).
- **Pelvic inflammatory disease** (PID) – an infection of the upper female genital tract that damages and scars the uterine tubes, making it virtually impossible for an egg to travel down into the uterus. Microorganisms can enter through the vagina and cervical canal which is slightly open during menstruation. After gaining entry, they migrate and multiply to involve other structures including uterus, fallopian tubes, ovaries and pelvic ligaments. PID is often caused by a sexually transmitted infection.
- **Endometriosis** – a condition in which tissue similar to that in the endometrium (uterus lining) grows in the ovaries, fallopian tubes, uterus wall or other places within the pelvis. This disturbs maturation of the egg, ovulation or implantation (→ Box 12.42).
- **Fibroids (uterine leiomyomas)** are non-cancerous growths that develop in and around the uterus. They are the most common form of female reproductive tumour but rates of growth are very variable. They are often asymptomatic, but can cause **menorrhagia** (excessive menstrual bleeding), anaemia, constipation and abdominal distension. Impact on pregnancy is rare except if the fibroids interfere with implantation, but they may increase in size during pregnancy due to oestrogen stimulation.
- **Cervical mucus** which is too thick and sticky – rather than thin, clear and stretchy – around the time of ovulation can prevent sperm swimming through into the uterus.
- **Overactive or underactive thyroid gland**. Thyroid disorders are relatively common in women and may be a cause of infertility, although the mechanism is poorly understood.
- **Premature ovarian failure** – the ovaries stop working.
- **Some medicines and drugs** are known to affect fertility.

12.10 Contraception

Contraception is the deliberate prevention of pregnancy. There are many forms of both temporary and permanent contraception available, their aim being to help avoid unwanted pregnancies. Which of them is the most suitable depends on personal preference, religious beliefs, age and whether a short-term or long-term method is required. The various methods of contraception work by preventing ovulation, fertilisation or implantation (→ Box 12.43).

12.10.1 Prevention of ovulation

Ovulation is prevented by the use of **synthetic hormones** – progestogen and oestrogen. The hormones mimic those produced physiologically during the menstrual cycle. They send a strong negative feedback signal to the hypothalamus which suppresses the secretion of gonadotrophin-releasing hormone (GnRH) (→ Fig. 12.12). Hence the anterior pituitary gonadotrophins, FSH and LH are inhibited which means that ovarian follicles do not develop or mature in the follicular phase of the cycle, and the LH surge does not occur so ovulation is prevented (→ Box 12.44).

Besides preventing ovulation, the synthetic hormones also thicken cervical mucus which bars sperm from entering the uterus, and they thin the uterus

Box 12.41 Treatment is aimed at managing the symptoms of PCOS as there is currently no cure.

Box 12.42 Although many theories have been proposed to explain endometriosis, the cause is largely unknown. Bleeding into the various structures can cause a great deal of pelvic pain. Endometriosis can contribute to formation of pelvic adhesions which distort pelvic anatomy. This can then lead to painful urination, pain on defecation and impaired egg release and transport.

Box 12.43 Contraception and Sexual Health (CASH) is an area of specialist healthcare practice in which clinicians and nurses have further training and accreditation that enables them to safely help meet reproductive and sexual health needs. They provide contraceptive advice and support related to STIs, and help people avoid unwanted pregnancy, a service formerly known as family planning.

Box 12.44 Lactational amenorrhoea method (LAM) is a short-term family planning method based on sustained, intensive breastfeeding which maintains a low level of progesterone that inhibits ovulation. It is about 98% effective in women for 6 months after their baby is born as long as they are fully breastfeeding and ovulation and menstruation have not yet returned.

lining so a fertilised egg could not implant itself there. However, they do not prevent transmission of sexually transmitted disease so a barrier method should also be used.

Hormone contraceptives

Taking it Further
For more information on hormonal therapy see online Chapter 18.

All hormone contraceptives contain progestogen and many also contain oestrogen. Contraception can be in the following forms:

- **pill** – the minipill contains progestogen; the combined pill contains both progestogen and oestrogen
- **implant** – a small flexible tube inserted under the skin of the upper arm which slowly releases progestogen over the course of around 3 years
- **patch** – a small, sticky patch applied to the skin that slowly releases both hormones into the bloodstream; the patch is changed every week for 3 weeks, followed by a week without a patch
- **injection** – this contains progestogen and protects from pregnancy for 8–13 weeks, depending on the brand.

12.10.2 Prevention of fertilisation

1 **Permanent methods** render the person infertile for the rest of their life:
   - **vasectomy** (male sterilisation) – a surgical procedure that disrupts the transport of sperm so that semen is produced without any sperm
   - **female sterilisation** – sperm are prevented from reaching eggs in the fallopian tubes (oviducts) because the tubes are surgically ligated (tied).
2 **Barrier methods** stop the sperm and egg from meeting, so there is no fertilisation. These methods are relatively cheap, easily available and have an additional benefit of protection against infection by sexually transmitted disease including HIV. The barrier can be a:
   - **male condom** – covers the erect penis which prevents sperm from being deposited in the vagina at orgasm
   - **female condom** – a lubricated polyurethane pouch which is placed inside the vagina
   - **cap** which covers the cervix or a **diaphragm** which fits into the vagina. Both cover the cervix and block entry of sperm into the cervical canal and the uterus. They need to be used with a spermicide which kills the sperm. They do not provide protection against sexually transmitted infections (STIs) and women require training to use them effectively.

12.10.3 Prevention of implantation

An **intrauterine device** (IUD; coil) is a T-shaped device inserted into the uterus for long-term protection. The presence of the IUD – a foreign object – prevents implantation of the blastocyst. Although its mode of action is incompletely understood, the IUD may bring about an inflammatory response.

12.10.4 Natural family planning

Natural family planning (NFP) is a range of methods based on awareness of the physiological signs and changes associated with fertility and infertility that couples need to be taught. NFP can be a very effective method if genital contact and intercourse are avoided during fertile times of the woman's cycle.

12.10.5 Emergency contraception

When coitus has taken place without contraception or if the contraceptive method has failed, pregnancy can be prevented by the **emergency contraceptive pill** (morning after pill) or the insertion of an IUD (intrauterine device).

12.11 Sexually transmitted infections

Sexually transmitted infections (STIs) (→ Table 12.2) are usually, but not always, spread from one person to another by genital contact and oral, anal and vaginal intercourse (→ Box 12.45).

Symptoms that may indicate infection of the sex organs are:
- unusual discharge from the penis or vagina
- blisters, rash, itching, burning or tingling around the genitals or anus
- pain or a burning feeling when urinating
- heavier periods or bleeding between periods, or pain during sex in women.

Absence of symptoms does not mean absence of infection because:
- an infection takes time to develop
- some people are asymptomatic so the infection could remain undiagnosed, e.g. about 50% of women do not have symptoms of chlamydia infection and most men with herpes do not have sores.

Antibiotic medication. Syphilis, chlamydia and gonorrhoea are bacterial infections which have usually been managed using antibiotics. These infections are becoming more difficult to treat as a result of overuse and misuse of antibiotics, and the older and cheaper antibiotics have often lost their efficacy.

Box 12.45 There are dozens of **STIs** that can spread from one person to another through intimate sexual contact. Infection from these diseases can be avoided by:
- abstention from sexual contact
- safer sex – when condoms are used
- having a partner who is free from sexually transmitted disease.

Genitourinary medicine (GUM) clinics, also known as Sexual Health Clinics, give advice on sexually transmitted infections. Many STIs are easily treated with medications such as antibiotics or antifungal creams.

Taking it Further
You can find out more about the mode of action of antibiotic drugs in online Chapter 18.

Table 12.2 Common sexually transmitted infections

Chlamydia	The most common STI in the UK. It is easily passed on during sex and as most people don't experience any symptoms and are unaware they're infected. When symptoms of chlamydia appear they can cause pain or a burning sensation when urinating and: • **in women**, a vaginal discharge, pain in the lower abdomen and bleeding during or after sex, or between periods, or heavier periods • **in men**, a white, cloudy or watery discharge from the tip of the penis and pain or tenderness in the testicles. It is also possible to have a chlamydia infection in the rectum, throat or eyes.
Candidiasis	An infection caused by a species of yeast (*Candida albicans*) that commonly occurs on the skin. It is usually harmless but can cause an infection – **thrush** – in the mouth, vagina or penis. **Invasive candidiasis** is a serious infection that develops when the fungus enters the bloodstream and spreads systemically to infect other parts of the body, e.g. heart, brain, eyes, bones.
Gonorrhoea	Caused by bacteria that can only live in the warm, moist area of the genital regions; it is easily spread by casual sex. It can also infect the throat.
Genital herpes	Caused by *Herpes simplex* – a different strain of the same virus that produces cold sores around the mouth. Most people do not know they are infected, partly because the herpes virus can lie dormant for some years. When symptoms occur, there can be small blisters that open to form ulcers which cause pain and may be accompanied by flu-like symptoms. Rarely, newborn babies become infected when the virus is present in the birth canal at the time of delivery, which results in serious illness for the baby.
Genital warts	Caused by the **human papillomavirus** (**HPV**) and easily passed on through unprotected vaginal, anal and oral sex whether or not there are visible warts (painless bumps or fibrous growths).
Trichomoniasis (TV)	A tiny parasite that infects the vagina in women and the urethra in both men and women.
Syphilis	A bacterial infection that is spread only by sexual intercourse. It is less common than some STIs but it is on the rise in the UK. Screening is offered to women during pregnancy because there is a risk of miscarriage, stillbirth or congenital syphilis (the baby is born with the disease).
HIV (human immunodeficiency virus)	Most commonly passed on through unprotected sex but can also be transmitted by contact with infected blood. The HIV virus attacks and weakens the immune system, making it less able to fight infections and disease. There's no cure for HIV, but there are treatments that allow most people to live a long and otherwise healthy life.

12.12 Diseases of the male reproductive organs

12.12.1 Prostate gland

Benign prostatic hyperplasia (**BPH**), often known as **enlarged prostate**, is a common condition associated with ageing, and it is estimated that 60% of men over 60 years of age have some degree of prostate enlargement (→ Box 12.46). Because the prostate gland surrounds the outlet from the bladder, an enlarged prostate puts pressure on both the bladder and the urethra. This affects urination, causing:
- a frequent urge to urinate
- getting up during the night to urinate
- difficulty urinating and dribbling urine.

Prostatitis

Prostatitis refers to inflammation or infection of the prostate gland. Symptoms include pelvic pain, pain when urinating and pain when ejaculating semen (→ Box 12.47).

12.12.2 Penile disorders

Disorders of the penis include:
- **balanitis** – inflammation (redness, irritation and soreness) of the glans (head of the penis). It can be caused by a build-up of **smegma** – the natural lubricant from the glans – to become a smelly breeding ground for infections, which can be prevented by regular washing
- **irritation** to the skin caused by soap, medication or condoms
- **priapism** – an abnormally prolonged (more than 4 hours) painful erection of the penis that is unrelated to sexual stimulation. It is an emergency because the prolonged erection can result in ischaemia (poor perfusion) of the erectile tissue of the corpora cavernosa, and is associated with a high risk of subsequent impotence if it does not resolve. Priapism can occur at any stage of the lifespan, with sickle cell anaemia being one of the most common causes. Secondary causes include neurological problems (stroke, spinal injury) and haematological problems such as leukaemia, or renal failure
- **urethritis** – inflammation of the urethra. Symptoms include a white or cloudy discharge from the tip of a sore penis, a burning or painful sensation when urinating and the frequent need to urinate. Urethritis is normally caused by an STI (→ 12.11), but if the cause is unknown it is called **non-specific urethritis** (NSU).

12.12.3 Testicle disorders

There are many other causes besides cancer for unusual lumps or swellings in the testicles, four main types being:
- **varicocele**, a swelling caused by dilated (enlarged) veins within the scrotum
- **hydrocele**, a swelling caused by fluid around the testicle
- **epididymal cyst**, a lump caused by a collection of fluid in the epididymis; if it contains sperm, it is known as a **spermatocele**
- **testicular torsion**, a sudden painful type of swelling that occurs when a spermatic cord becomes twisted, interrupting the blood supply to the testicles; immediate surgery is needed to save the testis (→ Box 12.48).

Box 12.46 The prostate doubles in size when young men go through puberty. A second growth phase begins after 25 years of age, so by the time men reach 60, more than half have **BPH**. Family history, hormonal changes, obesity and a sedentary lifestyle are common risk factors.

Box 12.47 Prostatitis is poorly understood but is thought to be the result of disturbed homeostasis of cell proliferation and apoptosis (cell death) which results in overgrowth of mucosal glands within the prostate. However, there is little correlation between the degree of enlargement and the symptoms of obstruction of urine flow; some men have no symptoms despite having a greatly larger prostate; others have severe problems with little sign of enlargement.

The discovery that the proliferation depends on a form of testosterone that is formed within the gland (dihydrotestosterone; DHT) has led to some of the drug therapies that are used to manage the condition.

Box 12.48 Men are recommended to examine their testicles once a month after a warm bath or shower when the scrotal skin is relaxed. If any lumps or swellings are found, they should be checked by a doctor as soon as possible. It is unusual to develop symptoms in both testicles at the same time, so testicles can be compared as to whether they feel normal.

Key points

1. The chromosomes in a fertilised egg determine a baby's biological gender.
2. Sex hormones – androgens, oestrogens and progesterone – are responsible for physical changes at puberty, which initiate the normal function of the adult reproductive tracts.
3. Under the influence of testosterone, the male reproductive system makes sperm which are ejaculated through the penis and are capable of fertilising an ovum (egg).
4. Female reproductive life is characterised by cyclic changes in oestrogen and progesterone which alter the structure of the uterine lining, regulate the release of eggs from the ovary and regulate menstruation.
5. Human pregnancy lasts on average 40 weeks, during which time the growing foetus is sustained by gaseous and nutrient exchange via the placenta.
6. Foetal circulation changes to adult circulation when the baby is delivered at the end of labour (parturition).

Test yourself! Go to *www.lanternpublishing.com/AandP* and try the questions to check your understanding.

CHAPTER 13
THE HUMAN GENOME

The human genome is the body's complete set of genetic instructions in the nucleus of the cell. Each gene is a code for making a protein which has a part to play in the structure (anatomy) and functioning (physiology) of the body. Genetics is the science of inheritance and the mechanism by which characteristics (traits) are transmitted from one generation to the next.

13.1 The human genome

The human **genome** is the body's complete set of genetic instructions (genes) found in the form of **chromatin** – the material of which chromosomes are made. All human cells are derived from the fertilised egg, so every cell has identical copies of the same genes, but different cells express the genes needed for that particular type of cell, e.g. genes being expressed in a cardiac muscle cell are different from those being expressed by a liver cell or an epithelial cell.

13.1.1 Genes code for proteins

The genetic instructions to make proteins are coded in **DNA** (**deoxyribonucleic acid**) – long, thin macromolecules that make up the chromatin. A **gene** is a segment of chromatin that contains the code for a particular protein. To make a protein, the gene's DNA is first copied into a strand of mRNA (ribonucleic acid), and the mRNA is the template for producing the protein (→ Fig. 13.1). There are about 20 000 genes in the human nucleus, each being expressed when that protein is required.

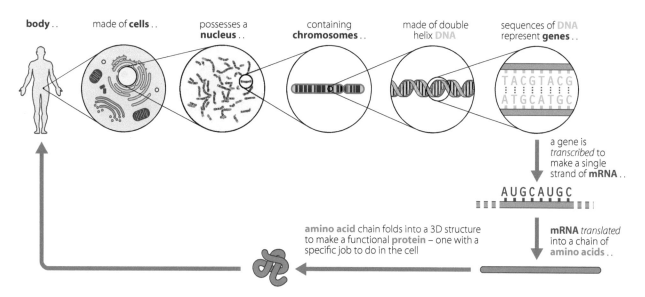

Fig. 13.1 Summary of how a gene is a blueprint for a functional protein.

13.2 Structure of DNA

DNA is a molecule composed of nucleotides arranged in two chains of nucleotides that coil around each other to form a **double helix** (→ Fig. 13.2a). DNA molecules condense (coil up tightly) and become visible as chromosomes during cell division (→ Fig. 13.8).

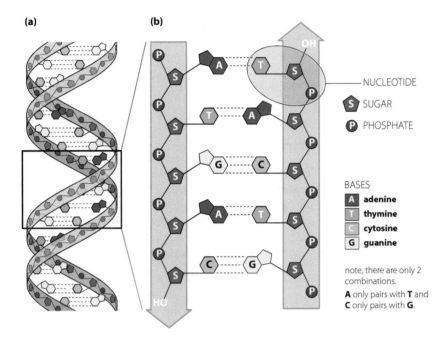

Fig. 13.2 Part of a DNA molecule (chromosome): (**a**) the double helix, (**b**) 5 base pairs.

13.2.1 Nucleotides

A nucleotide consists of three parts:
- sugar molecule
- phosphate group
- a base (→ Fig. 13.3).

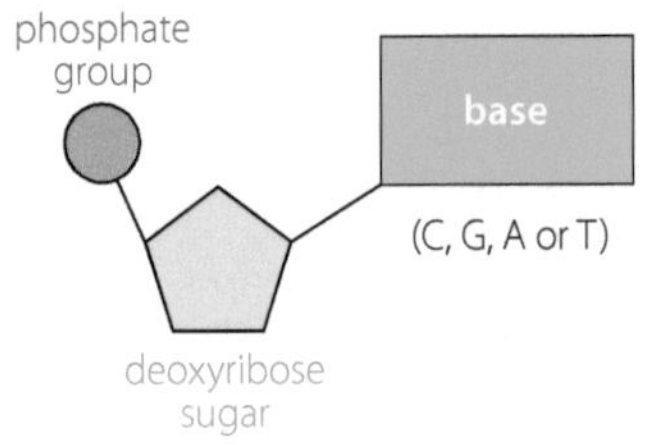

Arrangement of the nucleotides

The nucleotides are arranged in the chromosome so that:
- the sides of the double helix are formed from alternate phosphate and sugar molecules
- the rungs of the double helix are formed from **base pairs**. Although only these two types of base pair exist within DNA, variation in their number and their order in the sequence provides the genetic code (→ Box 13.1).

Base pairs

There are four different bases within DNA – **adenine (A)**, **thymine (T)**, **cytosine (C)** and **guanine (G)**. These DNA bases pair up with each other to form **base pairs**:
- C pairs with G
- A pairs with T (→ Fig. 13.2b).

Fig. 13.3 Nucleotide.

phosphate group
base
(C, G, A or T)
deoxyribose sugar

Box 13.1 DNA is almost the same for each individual, but 1–2% is unique, with every person having a distinct **genetic profile** – a genetic fingerprint – which can be used for detecting abnormalities, establishing family relationships and in forensic investigations.

13.3 The cell cycle

Every time a cell divides to form new cells it goes through a complex series of changes which is called the cell cycle, whether the cell is a newly fertilised egg or a skin cell that may have divided many times in a person's life. The cell cycle is a complex process composed of an **interphase** followed by **mitosis** and **cytokinesis**.

13.3.1 Phases in the cell cycle

The main phases in a cell cycle (→ Fig. 13.4) are:
- **interphase**. This is the longest and most active stage of a cell's lifetime during which the cell grows then carries out preparation for mitosis (cell division) (**G1 – first growth phase**). When a cell is preparing for cell division, it duplicates its contents including DNA (**S – synthesis phase** and **G2 – second growth phase**)
- **mitosis** (**M**). The cell's DNA is shared between two daughter cells (→ Fig. 13.8). The mitotic division takes a relatively short time
- **cytokinesis**. The cell membrane constricts around its middle and pinches off the two new daughter cells which contain identical genetic information.

The whole cell cycle takes approximately 24 hours, with mitosis accounting for about an hour. A cell that is cultured in laboratory conditions can undergo about 80 cell cycles before it dies, but in physiological contexts, the cell's function and environment determine how often it divides. For example, stem cells in skin, bone marrow and intestinal mucosa divide continuously, while neurons never divide.

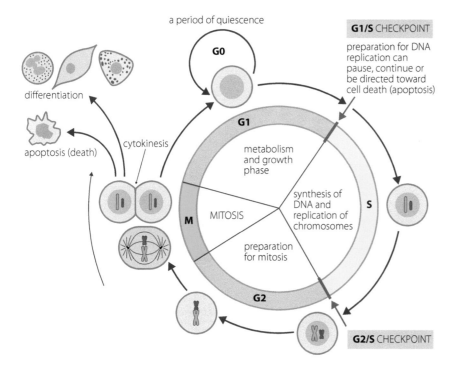

Fig. 13.4 Cell cycle.

13.3.2 Checkpoints in the cell cycle

Checkpoints (**restriction points**) occur at the end of the G1 and G2 phases. These are decision points in the cell cycle where its internal state is examined. Each checkpoint therefore determines a cell's fate – whether it will be allowed to divide, stay specialised and alive but not divide, or to die.

The checking processes exist as a safeguard because each cell must be able to deal with DNA damage in a way that ensures that **mutations** – changes in DNA sequence – are not passed on to their daughter cells.

G1 checkpoint

The G1 checkpoint determines whether cell processes are taking place in the right order.
- If conditions at G1 are favourable, including cell size, nutrient availability, growth factors and the DNA has integrity (is undamaged), the cell progresses to the S phase, which is the next stage of the cycle.
- If internal sensors detect failures, e.g. DNA damage or other defects, then the transition to the S phase is stopped.

S phase

During the S phase, the cell's DNA is replicated (copied) and the cell becomes irreversibly committed to producing daughter cells.
DNA replication is the process by which an identical copy of the DNA molecule is made before mitosis – the type of cell division that produces new cells for growth and replacement of worn-out or damaged cells. This enables DNA to pass from one cell to its daughter cells and from one generation to the next (→ Fig. 13.5).

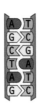 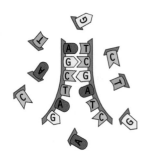 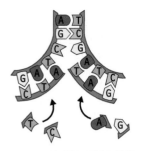 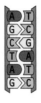

stage 1 - UNCOILING
The DNA molecule uncoils

stage 2 - UNZIPPING
The base pairs uncouple allowing the two strands of DNA to separate to create a 'Y' shape called a replication 'fork'

The two separated strands will act as templates for making the new strands of DNA

stage 3 - BASE PAIRS RE-FORM
The bases in each strand unite with one of the free nucleotides in the cytoplasm to form base pairs (A with T, C with G)

stage 4 - TWO IDENTICAL DNA MOLECULES ARE FORMED

Once all bases are matched up (A with T, C with G), the two new DNA molecules are identical with each other and with the original DNA molecule

Fig. 13.5 Replication of DNA results in two identical copies and takes place during the S phase of the cell cycle.

Control by enzymes

The process of DNA replication is controlled by enzymes, e.g. polymerase and telomerase.

DNA polymerase is the enzyme that normally carries out the unzipping function as it slides along the molecule in one direction only. If there is an error, DNA polymerase is able to cut out the wrong nucleotide and replace it with a correct one (→ Box 13.2).

Telomerase is the enzyme which counteracts the shortening of telomeres and may even lengthen them. A **telomere** is the section of DNA found at the end of a chromosome which protects the end and ensures that each cycle of DNA replication is completed. It consists of a sequence of bases – TTAGGG – that is usually repeated about 3000 times. Every time the DNA replicates a telomere is removed, until eventually the cell stops dividing and undergoes apoptosis – a process called **senescence** that is associated with ageing (→ Box 13.3).

G2 checkpoint

At the G2 checkpoint, the cell pauses while the DNA structure is checked for damage or incomplete replication. If the cell can repair any damaged DNA, it will be allowed to progress to cell division by mitosis. If a damaged cell cannot be repaired it will be eliminated by apoptosis. These examination and repair steps are important, because if irreparable damage to DNA is detected at either checkpoint, the cell should restrict division and arrest the cycle (→ Box 13.4).

Apoptosis

Apoptosis (programmed cell death) is a sequence of events that eliminates cells without releasing harmful substances that destroy surrounding tissues. This process plays a crucial role in maintaining the health of the body by eliminating old, damaged, unhealthy or unwanted cells. About one million cells are produced each second, and about the same number are removed by apoptosis. But when apoptosis does not work correctly:

- too many cells are eliminated, resulting in disorders such as Alzheimer's, Huntington's and Parkinson's diseases; or
- cells are not eliminated, which can result in cancer. Cancer develops when damaged cells contain mutated genes that either accelerate cell division or prevent apoptosis. As a mass of cancerous cells grows, it can develop into a tumour (→ 15.10).

13.4 Chromosomes

Chromosomes are composed of tightly coiled DNA and become visible when a cell is actively dividing (→ M phase in Fig. 13.4). There are a total of 46 chromosomes in human cells and they form the complete set known as the human genome.

Diploid and haploid. The 46 chromosomes in each cell is the **diploid** number (diploid 46). Of these chromosomes, 23 came from the father and 23 from the mother. Half the diploid number is known as the **haploid** number, in the case of humans haploid 23 – as found in eggs and sperm.

Box 13.2 In the laboratory, sections of DNA can be made using a **polymerase chain reaction** (PCR), which is key to DNA sequencing, genetic recombination and cloning investigations.

Box 13.3 The amount of the enzyme **telomerase** in cells normally falls as people age – except in germ cells. Cancer cells have larger amounts of telomerase which seems to enable them to keep on dividing uncontrollably.

Box 13.4 Study of the checking and repair processes that take place at the **cell checkpoints** has provided insights about regulation of the cell cycle (and the function of stem cells). Many of the genes and proteins that influence the phases of the cell cycle are now identified. When gene expression is altered by DNA damage, it is often associated with the accumulation of oncogenes and increased tumour formation (→ 15.10.1).

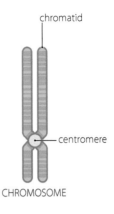

chromatid

centromere

CHROMOSOME

Fig. 13.6 Two chromatids linked by a centromere that result from the replication of a chromosome.

Chromosomes exist in pairs

- one chromosome from each pair is inherited from the father, and
- one chromosome from each pair is inherited from the mother.

Autosomes. Of the 23 pairs of chromosomes, 22 pairs are called autosomes and do not differ in length or differ between the sexes. The remaining two chromosomes (pair 23) are known as sex chromosomes.

Sex chromosomes. Both males and females have an X chromosome:
- in females the X chromosome is paired with another X chromosome, making a female XX
- in males the X chromosome is paired with a much shorter Y chromosome, making a male XY.

Chromatids. Before replication, a chromatid is a single DNA molecule. After the chromosome replicates (→ Fig. 13.5), each identical copy is called a chromatid and is linked to the other at the centromere (→ Fig. 13.6).

Centromere. Since the centromere has a characteristic locus (position) on each chromosome, it helps with identification of the different chromosomes. The centromere's function is part of the mechanism for signalling to cell cycle machinery that the spindle attachments have formed correctly during mitosis, and it is safe for cell division to proceed.

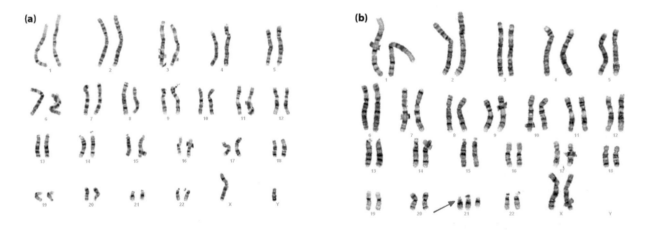

(a)

(b)

Fig. 13.7 (**a**) Normal male karyotype (XY); (**b**) female with trisomy 21 (an additional copy of chromosome 21), characteristic of Down syndrome.

Box 13.5 Examples of chromosome abnormalities:
- **gross deletions** – when a part of a chromosome or a sequence within the DNA has been lost during interphase of the cell cycle
- **duplications (amplification)** – when new genetic material is generated, often through errors of DNA replication or repair machinery.

13.4.1 Karyotyping

The human cell contains two sets of chromosomes, one set inherited from each parent. The chromosome complement within a cell nucleus is called a **karyotype**. Karyotyping is the process of separating the chromosomes from a cell when they become visible during cell division, then:
- matching them in pairs, according to their length (homologous pairs)
- arranging them in order from the largest (numbered 1) to the smallest (numbered 22) to make identification easier
- the 23rd pair – the sex chromosomes – are placed last (→ Fig. 13.7)
- the chromosomes are photographed so they can be examined by a cytogeneticist for abnormalities (→ Box 13.5).

13.4.2 Mitosis

Mitosis is a type of cell division that results in two identical daughter cells each having the same number of chromosomes as the parent nucleus, which is 46 (the diploid number). It is the process that enables a fertilised egg to produce all the cells required for **growth and development** of the body, the repair of damaged tissues and the continuous replacement of hair, skin and blood cells (→ Fig. 13.8).

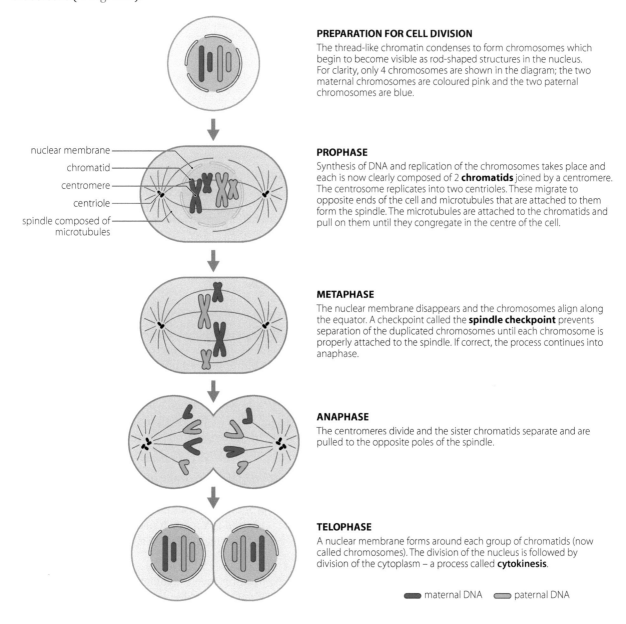

PREPARATION FOR CELL DIVISION
The thread-like chromatin condenses to form chromosomes which begin to become visible as rod-shaped structures in the nucleus. For clarity, only 4 chromosomes are shown in the diagram; the two maternal chromosomes are coloured pink and the two paternal chromosomes are blue.

nuclear membrane
chromatid
centromere
centriole
spindle composed of microtubules

PROPHASE
Synthesis of DNA and replication of the chromosomes takes place and each is now clearly composed of 2 **chromatids** joined by a centromere. The centrosome replicates into two centrioles. These migrate to opposite ends of the cell and microtubules that are attached to them form the spindle. The microtubules are attached to the chromatids and pull on them until they congregate in the centre of the cell.

METAPHASE
The nuclear membrane disappears and the chromosomes align along the equator. A checkpoint called the **spindle checkpoint** prevents separation of the duplicated chromosomes until each chromosome is properly attached to the spindle. If correct, the process continues into anaphase.

ANAPHASE
The centromeres divide and the sister chromatids separate and are pulled to the opposite poles of the spindle.

TELOPHASE
A nuclear membrane forms around each group of chromatids (now called chromosomes). The division of the nucleus is followed by division of the cytoplasm – a process called **cytokinesis**.

maternal DNA   paternal DNA

Fig. 13.8 Mitosis. For simplicity, only two of the 23 pairs of chromosomes are shown.

13.4.3 Meiosis

Meiosis (reduction division) is a type of cell division that occurs only in the production of **gametes** – sperm and eggs (→ Fig. 13.9). During meiosis, cell division takes place twice (the 1st and 2nd divisions) to produce four daughter cells that are haploid because their number of chromosomes is

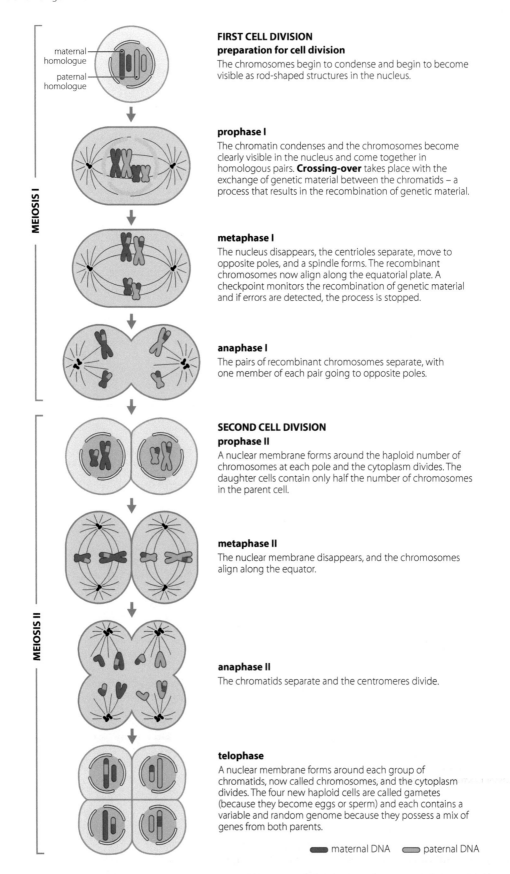

FIRST CELL DIVISION
preparation for cell division
The chromosomes begin to condense and begin to become visible as rod-shaped structures in the nucleus.

prophase I
The chromatin condenses and the chromosomes become clearly visible in the nucleus and come together in homologous pairs. **Crossing-over** takes place with the exchange of genetic material between the chromatids – a process that results in the recombination of genetic material.

metaphase I
The nucleus disappears, the centrioles separate, move to opposite poles, and a spindle forms. The recombinant chromosomes now align along the equatorial plate. A checkpoint monitors the recombination of genetic material and if errors are detected, the process is stopped.

anaphase I
The pairs of recombinant chromosomes separate, with one member of each pair going to opposite poles.

SECOND CELL DIVISION
prophase II
A nuclear membrane forms around the haploid number of chromosomes at each pole and the cytoplasm divides. The daughter cells contain only half the number of chromosomes in the parent cell.

metaphase II
The nuclear membrane disappears, and the chromosomes align along the equator.

anaphase II
The chromatids separate and the centromeres divide.

telophase
A nuclear membrane forms around each group of chromatids, now called chromosomes, and the cytoplasm divides. The four new haploid cells are called gametes (because they become eggs or sperm) and each contains a variable and random genome because they possess a mix of genes from both parents.

maternal DNA   paternal DNA

Fig. 13.9 Meiosis. For simplicity, only two of the 23 pairs of chromosomes are shown.

reduced by half, i.e. 23 single chromosomes instead of the normal diploid state of 46 chromosomes (→ Telophase in Fig. 13.9).

Meiosis first cell division begins when the chromosomes come together in homologous pairs (→ Box 13.6). Homologous chromosomes are pairs of chromosomes, one from each parent, that are similar in length, gene position, and centromere location. Although the position of the genes on each homologous chromosome is the same, the genes may contain different alleles – alternative forms of the gene (→ 13.6.6). Meiosis first division is very similar to mitotic division in that two daughter cells are formed, each with a full complement of chromosomes. The main difference is that meiosis first division takes a much longer time and there is a 'crossing over' of genetic information between the actual chromosome pairs before division (→ Fig. 13.10).

Box 13.6 Human **oocytes** in primary follicles (→ 12.4.4) can remain in the recombinant state of metaphase 1 for many decades. This is because oocytes form during embryonic development of the ovary and the cohesion of the crossover state is maintained for decades. Ovulation triggered by the luteinising hormone (LH) resumes the process of meiotic division.

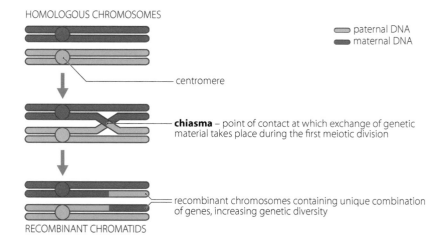

Fig. 13.10 Crossing over of genetic material.

HOMOLOGOUS CHROMOSOMES

paternal DNA
maternal DNA

centromere

chiasma – point of contact at which exchange of genetic material takes place during the first meiotic division

recombinant chromosomes containing unique combination of genes, increasing genetic diversity

RECOMBINANT CHROMATIDS

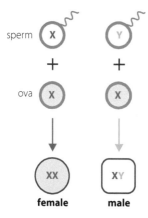

Fig. 13.11 Sex determination.

Restoration of the diploid state

Meiosis produces the sex cells – sperm and eggs – each with a haploid set of chromosomes. The diploid state is restored at the moment of conception when a sperm fertilises an egg (→ Fig. 13.11). All the information that specifies a new individual is now contained within the 23 pairs of chromosomes in the **fertilised egg**. Whether the individual is male or female depends on whether the egg containing an X chromosome is fertilised by a sperm containing an X or a Y chromosome (→ Box 13.7).

Box 13.7 Fertilisation – the union of an egg and a sperm – usually takes place in the fallopian tube and results in the formation of a zygote (fertilised egg). There are several stages in the process, called **egg activation**, that results in the first cell division by mitosis, which is the beginning of development of the embryo which will eventually develop into a new human being.

13.5 Genes

A **gene** is part of a chromosome that contains the genetic code (instructions) for making a specific protein. A **protein** is made up of a chain of **amino acids**, and the gene codes for which type of amino acid goes where in the chain to produce the protein (→ Fig. 13.13).

There are some 19 000–20 000 different genes in the human genome. A segment of DNA which makes a gene consists of hundreds or thousands of nucleotide bases; it is the order in which the nucleotides are arranged that makes each gene different from other genes (→ Box 13.8).

Box 13.8 Although most genes contain the instructions for making a protein, some provide instructions for making transfer RNA and ribosomal RNA, which are chemical cousins of DNA. These types of RNA help assemble amino acids into functioning proteins such as enzymes (→ 20.12).

13.5.1 Functions of genes

The **function of a gene** is to govern the order in which amino acids are arranged to build a particular type of protein molecule with a specific shape and size that becomes either:

- a **structural protein** that forms part of the cell, e.g. the actin in muscle cells or collagen in connective tissue
- a **functional protein** with a role in the life of the cell, e.g. receptor or enzyme (→ Box 13.9)
- a **special protein** such as a hormone, antibody, clotting factor or blood group factor.

13.5.2 How proteins are made

Proteins are not made in the cell nucleus but are assembled in the cell cytoplasm by small structures called **ribosomes**. The segment of DNA that codes for a protein does not move out of the cell nucleus, but a copy of that segment is made and moves from the nucleus to the cytoplasm. The copy is made from RNA (ribonucleic acid). RNA differs from DNA as it contains uracil (U) as a base instead of thymine.

13.5.3 Ribonucleic acid

Ribonucleic acid (RNA) is a molecular chain of nucleotides but differs from DNA in consisting of a single strand (→ Fig. 13.12).

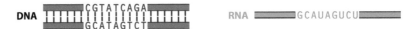

Fig. 13.12 Comparison between double-stranded DNA and single-stranded RNA.

Types of RNA

There are a number of types of RNA that perform vital roles in the coding, decoding, regulation and expression of genes. Three important forms are:

- **messenger RNA** (mRNA) which is synthesised from DNA in the nucleus by a process called transcription, moves into the cytoplasm and engages with the ribosome which translates the base sequence on the mRNA
- **transfer RNA** (tRNA), which is also made in the nucleus, moves to the ribosomes in the cytoplasm where it transfers amino acids to the ribosome
- **ribosomal RNA** (rRNA) is found only in the ribosomes where it links amino acids together for protein synthesis (→ Box 13.10).

13.5.4 Gene expression

Gene expression is the process by which information from a gene is used in the synthesis of proteins (→ Box 13.11). The two key stages that are involved when a gene makes a protein are:

- **transcription** – takes place in the nucleus when RNA polymerase (an enzyme) copies (transcribes) a segment of DNA (a gene) to make a single strand of mRNA, which moves into the cytoplasm (→ Fig. 13.13a)
- **translation** – takes place in a ribosome when the information in mRNA is 'decoded' to build a polypeptide by arranging the amino acids in the correct order for that particular protein (→ Fig. 13.13b).

Box 13.9 There are about 2000 different enzymes in a cell, each with its own part to play in the cell's metabolism. If even one of these enzymes is missing or fails to function properly, it can have a drastic effect on development or health.

Box 13.10 Types of RNA not mentioned here play a regulatory role in cells, e.g. catalysing biochemical reactions and acting as switches for expression of genes. These forms are therefore called **non-coding RNA**.

Box 13.11 Although a cell has a complete set of genes, only about 1% of these genes are **expressed** – switched on – at any one time. The other genes are expressed when required.

13.5.5 Central dogma of biology

The **central dogma of molecular biology** describes the flow of genetic information in cells from DNA to mRNA to protein, thus:

DNA $\xrightarrow{\text{(transcription} \to \text{Fig. 13.13(a))}}$ **RNA** $\xrightarrow{\text{(translation} \to \text{Fig. 13.13(b))}}$ **protein** ($\to$ Fig. 13.12).

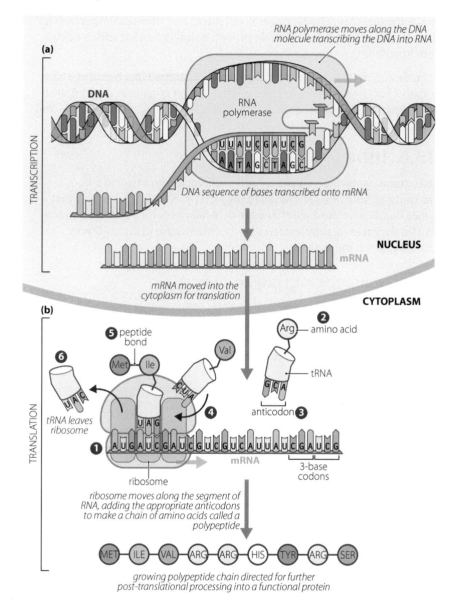

Fig. 13.13 How a gene encodes the assembly of a protein: (**a**) transcription (**b**) translation.

❶ Codons of mRNA are being decoded by the ribosome
❷ Incoming amino acids bind to tRNA
❸ Anticodon prepares to line up and bind with the mRNA codon
❹ tRNA docks with the codon within the ribosome
❺ Peptide bond forms and elongates the chain
❻ Outgoing tRNA is released from the ribosome and goes off to collect another amino acid

13.5.6 Mitochondrial DNA

Although most DNA is packaged in chromosomes within the nucleus, mitochondria also have a small amount of their own DNA (**mtDNA**) that contains 37 genes. Thirteen of these genes provide instructions for making enzymes involved in oxidative phosphorylation and the release of energy in the cells. The remaining genes provide instructions for making molecules called transfer RNA (tRNA) and ribosomal RNA (rRNA). These types of RNA help assemble protein building blocks (amino acids) into functioning proteins.

Mitochondrial DNA is inherited through the maternal line because when a sperm fertilises an egg, its mitochondria are left outside in the midpiece of the sperm tail and discarded. When the fertilised egg starts to divide and replicate, the mitochondria also replicate.

13.6 Inheritance

Inheritance is the mechanism by which characteristics (traits) are transmitted from one generation to the next (→ Box 13.12). The way that genes combine to produce characteristics follows certain patterns, which can be shown in its simplest form by the inheritance of the ability, or inability, to roll the tongue.

Box 13.12 Inheriting one of each pair of chromosomes from the father and one from the mother explains why a person inherits characteristics from each parent, and why siblings, grandparents and other family members may resemble each other in various ways.

13.6.1 Genotype and phenotype

Genotype refers to the genes possessed by an individual – one set inherited from the father and one from the mother. **Phenotype** refers to an individual's observable characteristics – height, shape, appearance, behaviour – which are determined by the interaction between genotype and environmental factors (→ Box 13.13).

Box 13.13 The theory of inheritance was introduced by an Austrian monk, **Gregor Mendel** (1822–1884), based on his work with pea plants. Mendel reasoned that heredity depends on discrete units of inheritance, which we now call genes, and he derived the principles that still form the basis of genetic inheritance.

13.6.2 Monogenetic inheritance

Monogenic inheritance occurs when a trait is passed from parents to their children by the expression of a single gene (**allele**). Single-gene modes of inheritance are relatively uncommon and typically follow one of the following patterns:

- **autosomal dominant** – expressed when a single copy of the gene (allele) is present (→ Box 13.14)
- **autosomal recessive** – expressed only when two alleles are present
- **X-linked** – the gene is transmitted on the X chromosome
- **mitochondrial** – the gene is transmitted on DNA mitochondria and inherited maternally.

Box 13.14 Autosomal is the term used to describe DNA which is inherited from any of the pairs of chromosomes numbered 1–22, as opposed to the sex chromosomes (→ Fig. 13.7).

13.6.3 Polygenetic inheritance

Polygenetic inheritance is the cumulative effect of many genes, e.g. height, weight, and skin colour, because they are determined by two or more alleles. For example, more than 20 are thought to contribute to intelligence.

13.6.4 Multifactorial inheritance

Multifactorial inheritance refers to inheritance that includes a combination of genes from the parents and interactions with the environment, e.g. arthritis, diabetes, heart disease, obesity, Alzheimer's disease and cancer.

13.6.5 Mechanism of inheritance

Two sets of chromosomes are inherited, one set from each parent. Therefore, two sets of genes – known as **alleles** – are inherited. The alleles match together in pairs, one from each parent, occupy the same position (locus) on their respective chromosomes and affect the same characteristic (→ Fig. 13.14).

13.6.6 Alleles

Alleles are alternative forms of the same gene (→ Box 13.15). Although they occupy the same locus on the chromosomes, they can have varying effects, e.g. the various alleles for eye colour – brown, blue, green or hazel.

Homozygous alleles refer to a pair of alleles that have the same effect, e.g. two alleles encoding for blue eyes.

Heterozygous alleles refer to a pair of alleles that have different effects, e.g. one allele encodes for blue eyes and the other encodes for brown eyes.

Dominant alleles mask the effect of recessive alleles and produce the same effect whether two alleles are present or only one. For example, if a child inherits an allele for brown eyes from the father and an allele for blue eyes from the mother, the child will have brown eyes because the brown allele is dominant to the blue allele. It is the expression of the dominant allele that determines the person's phenotype.

Recessive alleles do not have an effect when they are paired with a dominant allele, because they only have an effect when there are two recessive alleles within an individual's genome (→ Box 13.16).

Co-dominant alleles have equal dominance in a heterozygous person.

13.6.7 Inheritance of tongue-rolling alleles

Some people (rollers) can roll their tongue so that the sides curl up, but others cannot (non-rollers). The ability to roll the tongue is due to a dominant allele (T), so:
- rollers possess either one dominant allele and one recessive allele (Tt) or two copies of the dominant allele (TT) (→ Fig. 13.15)
- non-rollers possess two recessive alleles for tongue-rolling (tt).

13.6.8 Examples of environmental influences on genes

Genes are not only responsible for inherited characteristics such as eye colour; they also guide how cells function throughout life and can be switched on and off in response to the internal or external environment, e.g.:
- **growth genes** and hence the weight of a baby developing *in utero* are affected by the environment in the uterus, including the mother's levels of glucose, lipids and chemicals from cigarette smoke
- **training** to increase athletic performance stimulates the genes that regulate the stem cells in bone marrow to increase production and enhance the oxygen-carrying capacity of blood
- **infection** by a pathogenic agent stimulates the genes of the appropriate B lymphocytes (→ 14.5.3) to increase the production of specific antibody molecules.

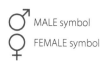
MALE symbol
FEMALE symbol

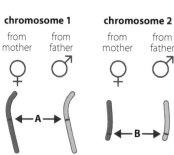

Fig. 13.14 Genes occur in pairs of alleles.

Box 13.15 Alleles for the brown and black forms of melanin which determine darker skin tone and hair colour are more commonly distributed amongst people who have their ancestry near the equator. Recessive mutations for red hair, fair skin and freckles are more common amongst those who have ancestry from nearer the North Pole.

Box 13.16 Monogenic diseases are often inherited through a recessive allele that occurs when an individual inherits two recessive alleles for that disease. Examples are cystic fibrosis (→ 13.8.2) and thalassaemia (→ 13.8.3).

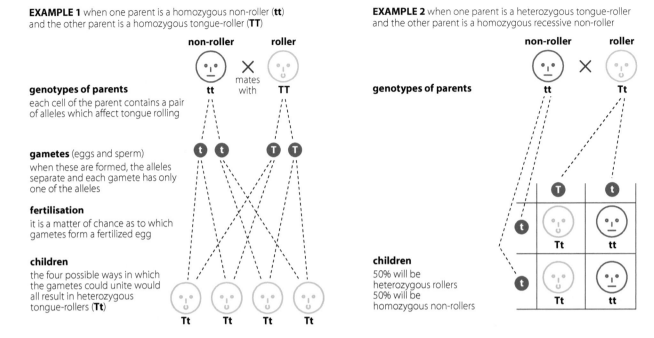

EXAMPLE 1 when one parent is a homozygous non-roller (**tt**) and the other parent is a homozygous tongue-roller (**TT**)

EXAMPLE 2 when one parent is a heterozygous tongue-roller and the other parent is a homozygous recessive non-roller

genotypes of parents
each cell of the parent contains a pair of alleles which affect tongue rolling

gametes (eggs and sperm)
when these are formed, the alleles separate and each gamete has only one of the alleles

fertilisation
it is a matter of chance as to which gametes form a fertilized egg

children
the four possible ways in which the gametes could unite would all result in heterozygous tongue-rollers (**Tt**)

genotypes of parents

children
50% will be heterozygous rollers
50% will be homozygous non-rollers

Fig. 13.15 Diagrams to illustrate the inheritance of tongue-rolling. Example 2 is the punnet square method.

13.7 Mutations

A **mutation** is a change in the genetic material of a cell brought about by a range of mechanisms including inaccurate replication, errors in translation or transcription, or DNA damage via exposure to environmental factors such as excess sunlight. The change can be as large as an entire chromosome or as small as a single nucleotide in one gene (→ Box 13.17).

Box 13.17 Mutations can be beneficial when they provide the genetic material for natural selection and survival of the fittest, but they may also result in chromosomal abnormality or genetic disease.

Box 13.18 Prader–Willi syndrome is caused by a rare genetic defect on chromosome number 15. Symptoms may include restricted growth and short stature, lack of secondary sexual development, learning difficulties, challenging behaviour, a constant desire to eat and obesity.

13.7.1 Chromosome mutations

A **chromosome mutation** occurs when there is a change in the number of chromosomes or in the structure of a chromosome. Mutations usually arise due to an error in cell division and are often harmful to the individual, e.g. Prader–Willi syndrome (→ Box 13.18).

13.7.2 Changes to the chromosome structure

Different types of chromosome mutations most often arise in germinal cells (ovary or testes) during meiosis or by mutagens such as radiation. This kind of mutation may impact on the entire chromosome, resulting in altered numbers or changes in structure and include:

- **translocation** – a piece of chromosome detaches then moves to a new position on another chromosome
- **deletion** – genetic material breaks off from anywhere on the affected chromosome
- **duplication** – extra copies of genes or DNA sequences are produced on the chromosome
- **inversion** – a broken segment, which may include the centromere, of a chromosome is reversed and inserted back into the chromosome
- **isochromosome** – the centromere does not divide properly so an isochromosome contains either two short arms or two long arms.

Chromosome mutations affect protein production by changing the genes on the affected chromosome; some are not harmful but others may contribute to developmental difficulties or death. Examples of disorders associated with chromosome mutations include:

- **Down syndrome** which arises because the individual has three copies of chromosome 21– an example of **trisomy**, which is the presence of an extra chromosome in each cell
- **Klinefelter syndrome** which arises when a male inherits two copies of the Y chromosome and thus is XYY (a trisomy)
- **Turner syndrome** which arises when one of the X chromosomes in a female is missing or incomplete, and thus is XO (→ Box 13.19).

13.7.3 Point mutations

Point mutations (**single gene mutation**) alter the structure of a gene. They arise when a change in a single gene has occurred following the alteration of one base pair in the DNA sequence. The mutation can be due to mistakes made during DNA replication (→ Fig. 13.5) or exposure to environmental factors such as radiation.

To function correctly, each cell depends on thousands of proteins to do their jobs in the right places at the right times. By changing a gene's instructions for making a protein, the point mutation can sometimes cause the protein to malfunction or to be missing entirely. When a mutation occurs to a protein that plays a critical role in the body, it can cause disease. For example, sickle cell anaemia is the result of a single point mutation in the gene for haemoglobin, resulting in abnormal red cells (→ 13.8.3). If the mutation occurs in the embryo it may disrupt development and result in miscarriage.

Over 4000 human disorders are caused by inherited single gene defects on the autosomes (chromosomes that are not the sex chromosomes).

13.7.4 Sex-linked inherited conditions

Sex-linked inherited conditions result from a mutant allele located on either the X or the Y chromosome, which are different shapes and do not share the same genes (→ Box 13.20). Haemophilia is an example of an inherited sex-linked disease passed on the X chromosome from mothers to their sons. Boys and men with haemophilia lack the gene which makes factor VIII – a protein essential for blood clotting (→ Box 13.21).

Genetic explanation for haemophilia

The inheritance of the faulty recessive allele for factor VIII is located on the X chromosome, but not the Y chromosome.
- Females have two X chromosomes. X-linked traits are inherited in the same way as autosomal traits, thus women do not express the recessive allele for haemophilia, although they can be **carriers** of the haemophilia allele (d).

The genotype of mothers can therefore be:
- **XX** – no haemophilia, or
- **XXd** – no haemophilia, but will be a carrier with a 50% chance of passing the d allele to her offspring in every pregnancy.

The father's sperm determines the gender of all offspring, which are either XX (girl) or XY (boy).

Box 13.19 Turner syndrome is characterised by short stature, non-functioning ovaries, puffiness (lymphoedema) of the hands and feet, skeletal abnormalities, heart defects, high blood pressure and kidney problems.

Box 13.20 Two well-known X-linked traits are red–green colour blindness which is much more common in males, and haemophilia which occurs almost exclusively in males but is inherited from females.

Box 13.21 Haemophilia is a disorder in which the blood's ability to clot is severely reduced, causing the sufferer to bleed severely from even a slight injury, external or internal. It also follows dental and general surgery unless clotting factors are given beforehand.

In the example shown below (→ Fig. 13.16) the mother possesses the haemophilia allele on her X chromosome:

- the **carrier mother** has the haemophilia allele (XXd) and the potential to pass it on in her ova (eggs) to 50% of her offspring in any pregnancy
- the **father** does not have the haemophilia allele because his X chromosome has the normal blood-clotting allele
- **sons** have a 50% probability of inheriting the haemophilia allele from the maternal X chromosome, and this will be expressed
- **daughters** inheriting the haemophilia allele would not have the disease. However, there is a 50% probability that they are carriers.

In an affected family there may be children who possess the haemophilia allele and children without it. It is also possible for all the children in the family to inherit the normal allele or all to inherit the haemophilia allele (→ Box 13.22).

Box 13.22 Acquired (rather than inherited) forms of haemophilia are rare forms of the disease that are not present at birth but can develop suddenly at any stage in the lifespan of a person who does not have a family history of haemophilia. For the majority of people who are affected, **acquired haemophilia** is the result of inappropriate antibody production – an autoimmune condition that prevents blood from clotting. Sometimes acquired haemophilia is associated with bone marrow problems, tumours and cancers, some medications or vitamin K deficiency.

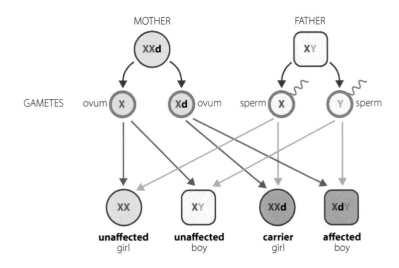

Fig. 13.16 Sex-linked inheritance for haemophilia from a carrier mother.

Carriers of the haemophilia allele

If the father's X chromosome has the allele for haemophilia, all daughters would be carriers (called obligate carriers) of the disorder. However, daughters would not necessarily have haemophilia; this is because the normal blood clotting allele from the mother is dominant so code from the haemophilia allele will not be expressed. Daughters would only have haemophilia if both of their X chromosomes were affected.

13.8 Examples of genetic disorders

13.8.1 Carriers

Box 13.23 Inheritance of **recessive alleles** for a disease differs from that of dominant alleles (e.g. Huntington's) because two recessive alleles are required to have an effect and cause the disease.

The possession of a **recessive allele** for a genetic disorder which does not have an effect makes a person a **carrier** for that allele. The allele may be passed on to future generations and will only have an effect and be expressed if it pairs up with a similar recessive gene, e.g. cystic fibrosis is an example of a recessive gene; another example is albinism (→ Box 13.23).

13.8.2 Cystic fibrosis

Cystic fibrosis (CF) is an inherited, autosomal recessive disorder that develops in a child who inherits two copies of the mutated allele – one from each parent (→ Box 13.24).

The CF gene affects the exocrine glands – those that discharge their secretions through a duct that opens onto a surface either inside or outside the body, with the following effects:

- **lungs**: mucus in the airways of the lungs is too thick to be transported up to the pharynx by the cilia lining the trachea, and bacteria that are trapped in the respiratory tract increase the risk of respiratory infections
- **digestive tract**: the thick layer of sticky mucus lining the digestive tract slows and reduces absorption of lipids and other nutrients. Lipids are an important source of energy and the lack of fat-soluble vitamins increases the risk of deficiency diseases
- **digestion**: mucus blocks the ducts that carry bile and pancreatic juice to the duodenum, which hinders the digestion of fats and other nutrients, making the stools bulky, fatty and malodorous (→ Box 13.25)
- **insulin production** is affected, leading to a specific form of diabetes called **cystic fibrosis-related diabetes**
- **fertility**: in women, the thick cervical mucus obstructs the entry of sperm; in men, the vas deferens can be blocked by thick secretions and a section of the duct is often congenitally absent
- **salty sweat** (→ Box 13.26).

Management of cystic fibrosis

CF usually becomes apparent in the first year of life but is sometimes not diagnosed until later (→ Box 13.27). There is currently no cure but many treatments are available to manage the disorder, including:

- **physiotherapy** to help with the removal of mucus from the lungs
- **exercises** to maintain good posture and full movement of the muscles and joints around the shoulders and chest
- **physical activity** to prevent deterioration of the lungs, e.g. running, swimming, football, tennis
- **medication**, which could include:
  - bronchodilators to relieve tightness and shortness of breath
  - antibiotics to treat or control persistent infection
  - steroids to reduce inflammation in the airways
- **DNAase** (deoxyribonuclease) – medicine that breaks down mucus and makes it easier to clear
- **Creon (pancreolipase)** – a mixture of digestive enzymes that is taken at mealtimes to help with digestion.

13.8.3 Haemoglobinopathies

Haemoglobinopathies are a group of inherited diseases in which there is an abnormality in the production of haemoglobin (→ Fig. 5.3). They are single-gene disorders, usually inherited as autosomal co-dominant characteristics, examples being sickle cell anaemia and thalassaemia. Antenatal programmes consist of identifying and counselling couples who carry the relevant alleles, with the aim of offering options that would enable them to have a healthy family.

Box 13.24 About 10 000 people in the UK have cystic fibrosis and one in 25 people in the UK **carry** the faulty recessive gene for the disease.

Box 13.25 Before meals, people with cystic fibrosis can take pancreatic enzymes in capsule form to aid digestion.

Box 13.26 The **sweat test for cystic fibrosis** measures the amount of chloride in sweat because people with CF can have 2–5 times the normal amount. In the test, the skin is stimulated to produce enough sweat to be absorbed into a special collector and then analysed. An early sign of the disease is salt (sodium chloride) on the skin that can be noticeable when a baby is kissed.

Box 13.27 About one in ten children with cystic fibrosis are diagnosed before, or shortly after birth due to a condition called **meconium ileus (CF fibrosing colonopathy)**. The first stool is even thicker and stickier than usual (sometimes described as putty-like), causing an obstruction of the bowel. If the meconium cannot be dispersed, the baby may need surgery.

Sickle cell anaemia

Sickle cell anaemia arises from an inherited **point mutation** that changes the sequence of the DNA in the gene responsible for producing the haemoglobin molecule. The mutation causes the red cells to become sickle-shaped when deprived of oxygen (→ Fig. 5.11). The sickle cells are rapidly removed from the bloodstream, leading to anaemia and jaundice; they can also become trapped in capillaries and in the joints, causing pain. It is estimated that 7% of the world's population (420 million) are carriers of the mutated gene on chromosome 16, mainly affecting people of African ancestry (→ Box 13.28).

Thalassaemia

Thalassaemias are caused by a different type of inherited mutation in the genes that encode haemoglobin; they are characterised by a decrease or complete absence of one of the two polypeptide chains – α (alpha) or β (beta) – of the haemoglobin molecule (→ Fig. 5.3).

- Normal individuals have two active alpha (α)-globin genes on both copies of chromosome 16 and two active beta (β)-globin genes on both copies of chromosome 11
- More than 200 mutations of these genes have been identified
- Carriers of the mutations are generally healthy individuals; they have the thalassaemia trait and are at risk of having children with thalassaemia.

Mutations for β-thalassaemia are carried by an estimated 85 million people, being more prevalent in people of Mediterranean ancestry. Alpha (α-) thalassaemia is rarer but with greater prevalence in south-east Asia, Africa and India.

The disorders are inherited in an **autosomal recessive pattern** and result in reduced haemoglobin content of erythrocytes and anaemia, causing fatigue, shortness of breath, pallor and weakness; there may also be problems with iron (Fe) overloading.

The disorders are named according to the globin chain that is defective. Homozygosity (of one or more alleles) or compound heterozygosity (a different mutation in each allele) will result in different disorders and so clinical classification of thalassaemia is determined according to severity (phenotype) or genotype (the type of mutation), which can be quite variable:

- individuals with one or two non-functional α-globin genes are usually asymptomatic but may need to be protected from iron supplementation, which could be detrimental for them
- beta thalassaemia major is the most severe type of defect of the β-globin chain and the only potential 'cure' is transplantation of haematopoietic (bone marrow) stem cells
- beta thalassaemia intermedia
- alpha thalassaemia major and haemoglobin H disease are caused by a dysfunction of α-globin genes.

13.8.4 Huntington's disease

Huntington's disease (HD) is an inherited neurodegenerative disorder with adult onset, usually in people in their 30s or 40s. As the disease progresses, affected people have increasing difficulties that include uncontrolled movement (chorea), personality changes, irritable and impulsive behaviour,

Box 13.28 The **sickle cell trait** confers some resistance to the malaria parasite. This gives heterozygotic individuals – those with a single sickle cell gene – a selective advantage in environments where malaria is present.

It appears that infected sickled red blood cells are actually a hostile environment for the parasite and prevent the disease from taking hold.

and problems with thinking and planning. Huntington's disease is caused by mutation (H) in either of an individual's alleles for a gene called *Huntingtin* (also called the *HTT* and *HD* gene); all humans have two copies of this gene and it codes for a protein called huntingtin that has multiple physiological functions.

Huntington's disease is normally inherited in an **autosomal dominant** pattern (→ Fig. 13.17), but about 10% of cases are the result of new mutations. The faulty gene (a repeated trinucleotide sequence) is genetically dominant; mutation in either allele results in synthesis of an altered, defective version of the protein (called mutant huntingtin; mHTT) which damages neurons and causes pathological changes in brain structure and behaviour of affected people over time.

The parts of the brain most affected include the cerebral cortex and basal ganglia – areas responsible for movement, learning, thinking, planning and motivation, and there is no cure for HD. As the disease progresses, people who are affected become less able to care for themselves, so the multidisciplinary team all contribute to providing care.

Genetic pedigree

A pedigree analysis is a study of inheritance patterns between different generations of the same family. Healthcare professionals gather data from an individual who is requesting genetic advice. Information is collected in the form of a family tree, which uses recognised international symbols to make it easier to recognise relationships and disorders within the family (→ Box 13.29). The aims of pedigree analysis are to determine the mode of inheritance and the probability of an affected offspring; an example is provided that shows inheritance of Huntington's disease (→ Fig. 13.17).

Box 13.29 Pedigree diagrams are visual charts that depict a family history and the pattern of inheritance of a specific trait. They are often used by healthcare professionals who are trying to determine the chances of a person carrying an inherited disease. They use a standard set of symbols, where squares represent males and circles represent females. Parents are shown by horizontal lines, while vertical lines lead from parents to offspring. Birth order is noted from left to right.

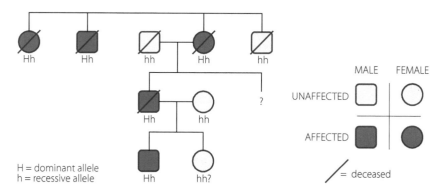

Fig. 13.17 Genetic pedigree showing three generations of a family affected by Huntington's disease.

The genetic pedigree in Fig. 13.17 shows an **autosomal dominant** pattern of inheritance. The disease does not skip generations and there are no unaffected carriers. Affected children will always have an affected parent; when the parent is heterozygous, i.e. with a dominant and a recessive allele in the genome, then approximately half of the children will be affected.

13.9 Clinical applications

13.9.1 Human Genome Project

The Human Genome Project (HGP) was an international scientific research project that began in 1988 to determine the entire sequence of genes on all the human chromosomes. It was completed in 2003 and the human genome, which is a genetic blueprint for building a human being, is known to be composed of about 3 billion nucleotide base pairs forming about 22,000 genes distributed between the 23 pairs of chromosomes.

13.9.2 The 100,000 Genomes Project

The aim of this UK project was to create a new genomic medicine service for the NHS to transform the way that healthcare is given. The project aims to sequence **100,000 genomes**. DNA sequencing is the process of determining the precise order of the four bases (A, G, C and T) in a strand of DNA (→ 13.2). Participants in the project were NHS patients with a rare disease (→ Box 13.30) and their families, and patients with cancer. Combining genomic sequence data with medical records will enable new and more effective treatments to be developed.

13.9.3 Personalised medicine

Genomic healthcare and personalised medicine is a new approach to the management of patients who have a specific condition. Genomic information provides healthcare professionals with a clear basis on which they can group patients according to:

- their predicted risk of disease
- their fundamental biology – DNA, RNA or protein – which can confirm disease
- mutations associated with specific diseases, e.g. *BRCA1* and *BRCA2* mutations and familial breast cancer.

Diagnosis, treatment conditions and medication can then be tailored to each person.

Pharmacogenomics

Pharmacogenomics combines pharmacology (the science of drugs (→ 18.1)) and genomics (the study of genes and their functions) which means that drug prescriptions can be tailored to a person's unique genome, e.g. the use of monoclonal antibodies to treat some cancers (→ 14.7.2).

Genetic screening and testing

Genetic screening is only offered to populations who are deemed to be 'at risk' from a particular disorder; for example, screening for cystic fibrosis amongst all newborns. **Genetic testing** is when an individual is tested for one particular disorder. Testing that individual will only result in a positive or negative result for that particular disorder and will not give results for all possible genetic disorders.

Box 13.30 Williams syndrome is an example of a rare developmental disorder. It occurs when a region of chromosome 7 containing 25 genes is deleted. The syndrome is characterised by cardiovascular disease, developmental delays and learning disabilities. These occur side by side with verbal ability, a highly social personality and an affinity for music.

Key points

1. The human genome (genotype) is the complete set of genetic instructions in the nucleus of every cell.
2. A gene is a segment of deoxyribonucleic acid (DNA) that contains the code for a protein.
3. When it is expressed, a gene is transcribed into a single strand of messenger ribonucleic acid (mRNA) which moves from the nucleus into the cytoplasm where it is translated by the ribosome to synthesise a protein.
4. Every time a cell divides to form two identical daughter cells, it passes through a tightly regulated sequence of changes – called the cell cycle – whose main phases are interphase, mitosis and cytokinesis.
5. Meiosis is a special form of cell division that results in the creation of gametes (germ cells) – sperm and eggs.
6. Inheritance is the mechanism by which characteristics and traits are transmitted from one generation to the next.

Test yourself! Go to *www.lanternpublishing.com/AandP* and try the questions to check your understanding.

CHAPTER 14
IMMUNITY

Immunity is the body's ability to resist infection by pathogens that are always present in the environment. Babies would have no chance of surviving to old age without the protection of their immune system, which consists of natural barriers and the complex network of cells, tissues and organs that work together to defend the body against disease.

14.1 Immunity

Immunity is either **innate** (present at birth) or **adaptive** (acquired), the main difference being that **innate immunity** depends on natural barriers, inflammation and a variety of white cells to provide rapid response protection against all pathogens, whereas **adaptive immunity** depends on one type of white cell – lymphocytes – that takes time to develop and provides highly focused and specific responses to individual pathogens and to the memory of them (→ Fig. 14.1; → Box 14.1).

Box 14.1 Immunity is the reaction of white cells to pathogenic microorganisms. The white cells – phagocytes, natural killer cells and lymphocytes – reach every part of the body. Although separated from each other, they communicate and cooperate to mount an immune response by releasing and responding to signalling molecules called cytokines (→ 14.3.2).

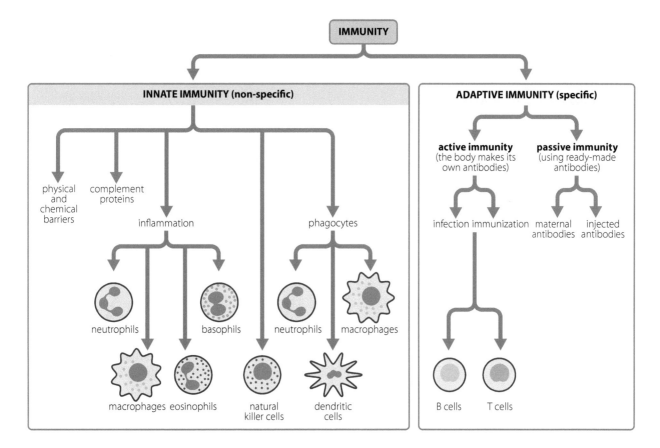

Fig. 14.1 Summary of immunity.

14.2 First line of defence

The first line of defence against infection is also known as the **non-specific immune system**, 'non-specific' because its physical and chemical barriers (→ Table 14.1) defend the body against all pathogens (→ Fig. 14.2). If these barriers are breached and pathogens gain entry, they meet the **second line of defence** – the **innate response** – which includes inflammation and the activity of phagocytes and natural killer cells. These provide immediate defence against pathogens but do not confer long-lasting immunity (→ Fig. 14.3). The **third line of defence** depends on **adaptive immunity** and lymphocytes to provide long-term immunity (→ 14.5).

Table 14.1 Physical and chemical barriers in the body

Physical barriers	Chemical barriers
Unbroken skin is waterproof and an abrasion-resistant epithelium which provides some protection against microorganisms and damage	**Lysozymes** are enzymes that destroy bacterial cell walls in secretions such as tears, sweat, saliva, mucus and vaginal fluid
Mucous membranes line the cavities inside the body, and the mucus they produce protects the underlying tissues	**Hydrochloric acid** in gastric juice kills ingested bacteria
Coughing reflex prevents a build-up of mucus in the lungs	**Microbiota,** including skin and gut flora, live on or in the human body
Blink reflex protects the eyes	**Cerumen** (earwax) protects and lubricates the ear canal

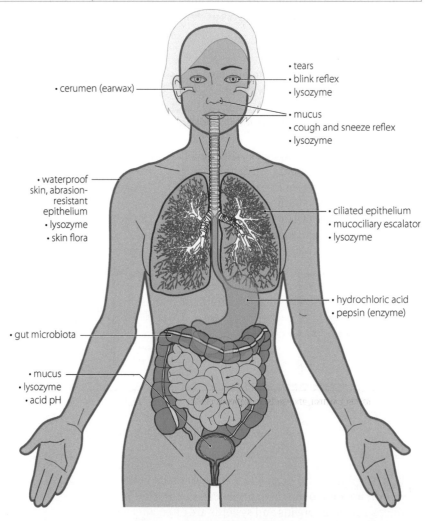

Fig. 14.2 Physical and chemical barriers protecting the body from infection.

14.3 Second line of defence

The second line of defence is the **innate response**. It provides an early, rapid and effective means of recognising and reacting to 'non-self' particles, meaning particles that do not belong to the body, including bacteria and other pathogenic microbes. The response is rapid because the white cells are all in place before a person comes into contact with the pathogens, so they are able to destroy them rapidly and promote healing (→ Box 14.2).

14.3.1 Pathogens

In its oldest and broadest sense 'pathogen' is anything that can produce disease. The term now usually means an infectious agent, e.g. bacterium, virus, fungus and protozoan. Most pathogens, sometimes called 'germs', are microscopic entities that cannot be seen by the naked eye. Nevertheless, each has its own particular characteristics that can be determined by laboratory examination, and if causing illness, each produces its own distinctive symptoms and signs.

Protection by the immune system against a pathogen can be:
- **total** – when pathogens entering the body are destroyed
- **incomplete** – when the body does not develop enough immunity to prevent a disease, but sufficient to make it less severe
- **absent**, or **insufficient** to prevent the disease.

14.3.2 Cytokines

Cytokines are signal molecules – the biochemical messengers involved in immunity and inflammation (→ Box 14.3). They are secreted by white cells of the immune system and act by binding to specific receptors on their target cells and evoking a response:
- an **autocrine effect** occurs when a cytokine acts on the cell in which it is produced
- a **paracrine effect** occurs if the cytokine acts locally
- an **endocrine effect** occurs when the cytokine enters the bloodstream and affects the function of distant cells.

Cytokines include:
- **histamine** – a vasodilator that widens blood vessels and increases blood flow (→ Box 14.4); it is released in large amounts when the skin and mucous membranes are damaged, causing itching and pain
- **interferons** – inhibit replication of viruses
- **interleukins** – a large group of protein molecules that regulate many aspects of the inflammatory response
- **prostaglandins** – substances that participate in a wide range of functions such as the contraction and relaxation of smooth muscle, the dilation and constriction of blood vessels, control of blood pressure, and involvement in inflammation
- **lymphokines** – signal the production of increased numbers of lymphocytes and macrophages
- **tumour necrosis factors** (**TNF**) – a family of signal molecules with diverse roles, e.g. inducing the inflammatory response.

Box 14.2 The innate response is particularly important in babies during the vulnerable time after the maternal antibodies have ceased to have an effect (→ 14.7.2) and before the third line of defence – the adaptive immune system and its antibodies – has had time to develop.

Box 14.3 When the body is fighting a pathogen, cytokines instruct immune cells, e.g. macrophages, to travel to the area and stimulate them to produce more cytokines – a positive feedback loop (→ 1.4.2).

Box 14.4 Histamine is one of the chemical agents produced during reactions to stings and urticaria (nettle rash, hives). **Antihistamine** medication is prescribed to reduce the reaction or for people who have allergies (→ 14.9.1).

Box 14.5 Inflammation and
infection are often confused because
they commonly exist together.
However, **inflammation** can
occur without infection, whereas
infection is always accompanied by
inflammation.

Box 14.5 Inflammation and
infection are often confused because
they commonly exist together.
However, **inflammation** can
occur without infection, whereas
infection is always accompanied by
inflammation.

Box 14.6 Chemotaxis is the
response of white cells to chemical
signals (cytokines). The white cells
move along the lining of the blood
vessels and through spaces in the
capillary wall into the tissues in
response to a gradient of chemical
concentration. **Positive chemotaxis**
occurs if the movement is towards
a higher concentration of the
chemical; **negative chemotaxis**
occurs if the movement is in the
opposite direction.

14.3.3 Inflammatory response

The **inflammatory response** happens very rapidly, with the affected tissue
becoming red, hot, painful and swollen, maybe with some loss of function
(→ Box 14.5). Inflammation occurs when tissues are damaged by:

- infection by pathogens and bacterial toxins (→ Fig. 14.3)
- injury and trauma (wounds), e.g. abrasions (cuts and bruises), burns and
  surgery
- foreign bodies, e.g. splinters, dirt, sutures, stings
- hypersensitive reactions to substances in the environment, e.g. hay fever,
  eczema, asthma and dermatitis.

Damaged tissue and the entry of microbes release prostaglandins and
histamine from mast cells. These signal molecules trigger:

- **heat and redness (erythema)** or darker colouration caused by dilation of
  the blood vessels and the increased blood flow to the area
- **swelling** – the result of vascular leakage (**oedema**); as the blood vessels
  dilate, they become more permeable, allowing fluid to leak from the
  capillaries into the tissue spaces
- neutrophil activity – white cells which migrate from blood into the tissues
  by chemotaxis (→ Box 14.6) and engulf pathogens and other foreign
  particles
- macrophage activity – white cells which engulf and digest the microbes
  and dead cells, enabling the process of healing to begin
- **pain**, making the individual aware of the situation
- loss of function of the affected part, possibly limiting movement.

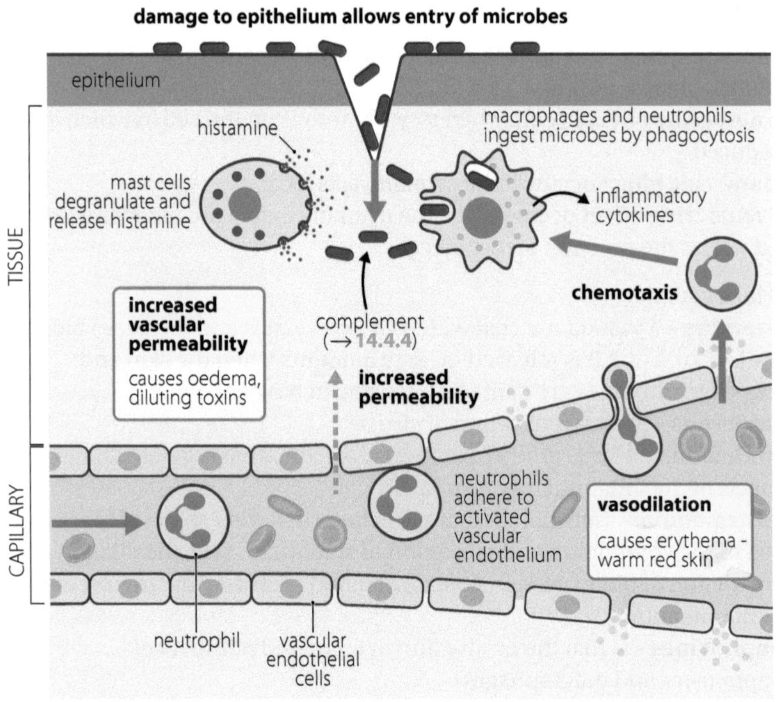

Fig. 14.3 Inflammatory response.

Healing

Without inflammation, tissue will not heal because the increased activity of phagocytic cells is required to clear away dead tissue, harmful pathogens and their toxins. After this has happened, damaged cells are replaced by new ones, new blood vessels are formed (**angiogenesis**), and normal function of the tissue can be restored (→ 3.5.1). Because the components that contribute to the inflammatory response are capable of eliminating and destroying pathogens, they also have the potential to damage the surrounding healthy tissue.

14.3.4 Chronic inflammation

Chronic (prolonged) inflammation can impair healing and may result in the accumulation of macrophages. Clusters of these white cells, called **granuloma**, may surround resistant organisms such as *Mycobacterium tuberculosis* and become the source of infection at some time in the future (→ Table 14.2).

A wide range of diseases are associated with **chronic inflammation**:
- autoimmune disease, e.g. rheumatoid arthritis (→ 14.9.3) and systemic lupus erythematosus (→ 16.6)
- persistent injury or infection, e.g. tuberculosis or chronic pancreatitis (→ Box 14.7)
- prolonged exposure to noxious agents, e.g. asbestosis, silicosis
- pressure ulcers (→ 3.5.2).

Box 14.7 Pancreatitis is characterised by inflammation of the pancreas. This gland produces two types of secretions – digestive juices and digestive hormones. When infected, the pancreas becomes inflamed and the digestive juices can be trapped within the swollen gland where they begin to 'digest' it. This disorder can become acute or chronic, and may be life-threatening. It is more common in men and 80–90% of cases are associated with alcohol misuse or gallstones.

Table 14.2 Differences between acute and chronic inflammation

	Acute inflammation (e.g. from an insect bite)	Chronic inflammation (e.g. from an ulcer)
Reaction time	fast reaction (minutes/hours)	progressive
Signs/symptoms	redness, discolouration, heat, pain	painful, open wound
Effect	short-term	long-term
Tissue injury	mild	severe
Time to heal	quickly	slowly

14.3.5 Fever

Fever (pyrexia; febrile response) is a rise in body temperature above the normal range of 36.5–37.5°C due to an increase in the **temperature set point** – the level at which the body attempts to maintain its temperature. This usually triggers shivering and a feeling of cold despite an increase in body temperature. Once the body temperature has increased to a new, higher, temperature set point, the person feels hot and may begin to sweat.

Fever is the natural response to many infections and is usually related to the innate response. It is also a common response to sepsis (→ 16.5.1, item 4). The trigger for fever is usually either:
- **cytokines** and/or **pyrogens** (fever-inducing agents) because they increase the temperature by shifting the temperature regulatory set point upwards, or

Taking it Further
Temperature is one of the basic physiological observations taken by healthcare professionals when assessing patients' wellbeing.

You can find out more in online Chapter 17.

- the presence of **pathogens** which cause an upward shift in the temperature regulation set point as an aid to the healing process, promoting the creation of an environment that is unfavourable for heat-sensitive pathogens.

However, prolonged periods of very high body temperatures that are beyond the normal range can put cells and tissues under severe thermal stress by altering membrane stability and protein functions.

14.4 Phagocytes

Inflammation is a protective immune response that attracts phagocytes to an injured area by chemotaxis (→ Box 14.8). Once there, white cells engulf and destroy bacteria, cellular debris and foreign particles not normally found in the body, by a process called **phagocytosis** – the process of engulfing particles with the aim of destroying them (→ Fig. 5.6). The two principal phagocytes that have a special ability to recognise bacteria are:
- **neutrophils** – engulf bacteria and destroy them
- **macrophages** – engulf bacteria and digest them to produce antigen fragments (→ Fig. 14.6) that are presented to helper T cells (→ 14.4.5).

14.4.1 Neutrophils

Neutrophils are the most abundant phagocytic cells normally found in the bloodstream and they seek out and kill bacteria. When they are activated by cytokines (chemical signals) from a site of infection or trauma, they follow the chemical trail along a concentration gradient towards the source. They stop at the site of infection by using receptors on the plasma membrane to adhere to the endothelial cells that line the inside of blood vessels (→ Fig. 14.3). The neutrophils then move out of the blood vessels and into infected or inflamed tissues and, after engulfing and digesting a number of pathogens, they die and form **pus** (→ Box 14.9).

14.4.2 Macrophages

Macrophages ('large eaters') are giant scavenger cells derived from monocytes. They are most often found in connective tissue, where they search by amoeboid (crawling) movements for potential pathogens. In addition to their role as phagocytes, macrophages have many other functions including **antigen presentation** (→ Fig. 14.4).

14.4.3 Natural killer cells

Natural killer (NK) cells are lymphocytes which have no B- or T-cell markers (→ Fig. 14.1), and which do not depend on the thymus for their development. They are considered to be part of the innate response as they seek out and attack tumour cells and body cells infected with viruses. The NK cells kill by inducing apoptosis (→ Box 14.10). When NK cells arrive at a site of infection they secrete cytokines to attract macrophages to act as reinforcement.

14.4.4 Complement proteins

Complement proteins are a special group of proteins, sometimes just referred to as **complement**. They are part of the innate immune system and function in inflammation, cell lysis (destruction) and a process called **opsonisation**, which marks a pathogen and attracts phagocytes.

- Complement proteins are produced in the liver and circulate in an inactive form in the blood and interstitial fluid.
- When activated, the complement proteins enhance the ability of phagocytes and antibodies to eliminate pathogens and damaged cells from the body.

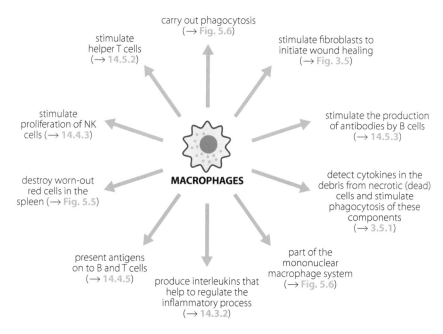

Fig. 14.4 Some of the functions of macrophages.

Activation of complement proteins

Several different pathways lead to the following effects (➔ Fig. 14.5).

❶ **Opsonisation** is a process in which complement proteins tag pathogens and attract phagocytes which will kill and eliminate them.

❷ The **membrane attack complex** (**MAC**) is a channel through a membrane structure typically formed on the surface of pathogen cell membranes as a result of the activation of the host's complement protein cascade. When the complex is inserted into a bacterial cell membrane, it causes **lysis** (cell death).

❸ Complement proteins play a crucial part in the **inflammatory response** by stimulating the release of histamine from mast cells and the chemotaxis of macrophages and neutrophils.

❹ When **antibodies** bind to antigens they form immune complexes that become coated in complement which helps to keep them soluble so they can be cleared by phagocytes in the liver.

❺ **Natural killer cells** are cytotoxic cells that secrete substances that rapidly induce apoptosis (cell death) in tumour- and virus-infected cells.

Complement control proteins

The complement system is tightly regulated, which is achieved by **complement control proteins** that are also circulating in blood and sometimes on the surface of cells. Their function is to protect the body's own tissues from being targets for complement attack. However, it is increasingly recognised that abnormalities of the complement control system play a role in many disorders which have an immune component including arthritis,

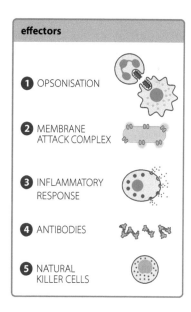

Fig. 14.5 Activated complement has several effects.

multiple sclerosis, glomerulonephritis, inflammatory bowel disease, lupus and transplant rejection.

14.4.5 Antigen-presenting cells

Antigen presentation is the link between innate and adaptive immunity as it involves both macrophages and lymphocytes (helper T cells). An **antigen-presenting cell** is a macrophage or dendritic cell that can 'present' an antigen (a microbe or fragments of a microbe) to a T-cell lymphocyte (→ Fig. 14.6):

❶ A macrophage encounters an antigen.
❷ The antigen is engulfed...
❸ ... and is processed inside the cell.
❹ The antigen is split into fragments which are combined with special proteins on the surface of the cell known as major histocompatibility complex (MHC) receptors which help the immune system to recognise the difference between the body's own cells and foreign substances.
❺ The MHC–antigen complexes move to the surface of the cell and the macrophage 'presents' them to T lymphocytes.

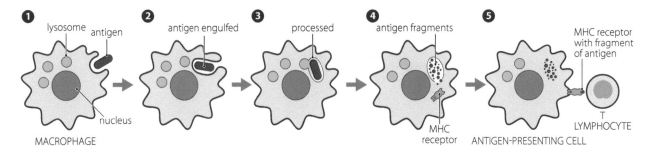

Fig. 14.6 Presentation of an extracellular antigen to a lymphocyte.

14.4.6 Dendritic cells

Dendritic cells get their name from projections called dendrites that extend outwards from the cytoplasm. They are found in lymphoid tissue and in tissue that has contact with the external environment, e.g. skin and mucous linings.

Dendritic cells are sometimes called professional antigen-presenting cells because they are continuously sampling their surroundings to capture invading antigens, processing them internally, and then presenting antigen fragments on their cell surface in a form that can stimulate the T cells. Dendritic cells also:

• contribute to the formation of B-cell memory by producing cytokines that promote B-cell differentiation
• play a crucial part in the adaptive immune response because their main function is to present antigens to inactive or naive lymphocytes, thus inducing a primary immune response (→ 14.6.2)
• play a part in maintaining immune tolerance.

14.4.7 Immune tolerance

Immune tolerance is key to the way in which the immune system responds and learns to tell the difference between cells which are 'self' (belonging to the body) and 'non-self' cells.

Examples of immune tolerance

- Most people do not mount an immune reaction to the commensal bacteria that live on skin and in the digestive tract.
- Many tumours are capable of inducing immune tolerance as they grow, so that they avoid being eliminated by the immune system.
- The immune system of a pregnant woman is tolerant of the growing foetus – an individual that is genetically distinct from the mother – and so it is not usually rejected.

14.4.8 Reaction to ectoparasites

Ectoparasites are parasites that live on or in the skin, not within the body, e.g. fleas, lice, ticks and the itch mites that cause scabies (→ Fig. 3.7). They are successful because they have immense capacity to evade the human body's immune response when they feed on the host's blood. The phagocytes that destroy these ectoparasites, or attempt to do so, are two types of white cell:

- **eosinophils** found in the lining and covering surfaces within the body
- **basophils** that circulate in the bloodstream and move into the tissues when needed.

These phagocytes are found in high numbers at sites of ectoparasite infection and secrete **histamine** – the vasodilator which increases blood flow to tissues and causes itching, and **heparin** – a substance which acts as anticoagulant and helps to defend against parasites.

14.5 Third line of defence

The third line of defence is **adaptive** (active) **immunity**. It is activated when the body uses lymphocytes to produce a specific response to a specific antigen. The term **antigen** means **anti**body **gen**erator, and is therefore any substance that stimulates the generation (production) of antibodies (→ 14.6), e.g. bacteria, viruses, pollen, peanuts, stings, snake venom and antibiotics. Adaptive immunity is:

- **specific** because it can distinguish between antigens and respond differently to each one, the antigen being a substance the body recognises as being foreign (non-self) or dangerous
- **adaptive** because it has **memory** and can produce a faster response on re-exposure to the antigen.

Sometimes antigens are part of the body's own tissues, a condition which is known as **autoimmunity** (→ 14.9.3).

14.5.1 Lymphocytes

Lymphocytes circulate in the bloodstream and lodge in the lymph nodes – places where pathogens and other antigens are filtered from the lymph as it passes through them (→ Fig. 5.30). They are small white cells with a nucleus that fills most of the cell and, like all white cells, they originate from stem cells in the bone marrow. Stem cells divide continuously to produce immature lymphocytes that either mature inside the bone marrow as **B cells**, or leave for the thymus gland where they mature into **T cells**. A key difference between them is that B cells produce antibodies, whereas T cells do not, but both lymphocyte types collaborate to destroy antigens.

14.5.2 T lymphocytes

There are a number of types of T lymphocytes (**T cells**) and each can be identified as being different from other lymphocytes because of the marker proteins and glycoproteins on their surface, which provide them with a 'signature' or 'fingerprint'. The two major groups depend on the presence of either CD4$^+$ or CD8$^+$ markers on their surface.

CD4$^+$ T cells are the **'helper' T cells** as they interact with macrophages and other antigen-presenting cells and secrete cytokines to lead an immune response and antibody production by B cells. In most cases, close interaction between the helper T cell and the B cell is required for full activation of the B cell after antigen binding has taken place (→ Box 14.11).

CD8$^+$ T cells are the **cytotoxic cells** that seek out, recognise and kill other cells in the body that have been attacked by viruses or become malignant, primarily defending the body against viral diseases and cancer. Activated CD8$^+$ T cells secrete cytokines such as **tumour necrosis factor** (TNF) and **interferon** which have anti-tumour and anti-viral actions (→ 14.3.2). Their second function is to form a close attachment with their target cells and secrete cytotoxic granules which contain a protein called **perforin** that is similar to complement. It forms pores in target cells, thus killing them.

14.5.3 B lymphocytes

B lymphocytes (**B cells**) are the white cells that produce antibodies. They are produced in the bone marrow as naive B cells – B cells that have not yet been exposed to an antigen. Once exposed to an antigen, the naive B cell either becomes a:

- **plasma cell** that secretes antibodies, or
- **memory** B cell.

How B cells produce antibodies to destroy antigens

Naive B cells circulate in the bloodstream and lymph nodes until they come into contact with an antigen that binds precisely to the antibody molecule by a 'lock-and-key' mechanism. The binding process activates the B cell to clone (by mitosis) and change into a **plasma cell** which produces and secretes many identical antibody molecules (→ Box 14.12). Antibodies circulate in the bloodstream where they can bind to other molecules of the same antigen, then either:

- form an immune complex that stimulates phagocytosis (→ Fig. 14.7a)
- stimulate mast cells to degranulate and release histamine (→ Fig. 14.7b)
- attract cytotoxic natural killer (NK) cells which induce the death of the target cell (→ Fig. 14.7c)
- activate complement to destroy the antigen (lysis) (→ Fig. 14.7d).

Ultimately the B cells and antibody production ensure that the antigen is cleared from the body.

Memory B cells

Some of the B cells differentiate into **memory cells** that may persist in the circulation and lymph nodes for many years. Memory cells 'learn' to make a particular type of antibody in response to each different antigen. If there is a second exposure to the antigen, they divide rapidly and produce many more B cells (→ Fig. 14.10) which can rapidly produce the right type of antibody against the specific infection.

Box 14.11 CD4$^+$ cells are a form of T lymphocyte that are extremely important in detecting pathogens and interacting with antigen-presenting cells (→ 14.4.5) to lead the attack against infections. There are many different families of CD4$^+$ cells, each of which can fight a specific pathogen.

Unfortunately, CD4$^+$ cells are themselves attacked by the HIV virus, leading to a fall in numbers detected in a blood cell count and reduced immunity, resulting in acquired immune deficiency syndrome (AIDS).

Box 14.12 B lymphocytes are **naive** before they become activated by the antigen presentation process. It leads to multiplication and proliferation to form a clone of plasma cells. These are cells dedicated to making and secreting high amounts of a specific antibody into the bloodstream.

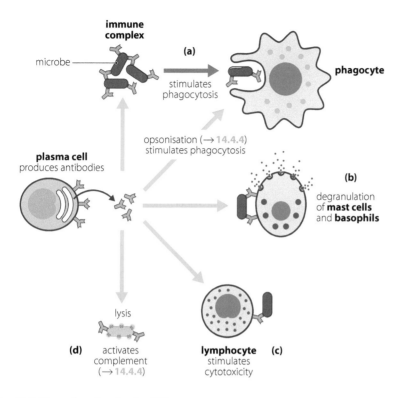

Fig. 14.7 The action of antibodies (Ab).

14.6 Antibodies

Antibodies (**Ab**) are **immunoglobulins** – molecules of glycoprotein produced by plasma B cells. They form an essential part of the immune response by specifically recognising and binding to particular antigens and aiding in their destruction (→ Box 14.13).

The general structure of an **antibody** molecule includes two large peptides called the **heavy chains** and two small peptides called the **light chains** (→ Fig. 14.8). The base region of the heavy chains is called the Fc region and the different molecular structure of this part of the antibody molecule allows them to be divided into five different subclasses.

Although the general structure of all antibodies is very similar, a small region – the **hypervariable region** – at the tip of the antibody is extremely variable, allowing millions of antibodies with slightly different tip structures to exist. Each of these variants – **antigen-binding sites** – can bind precisely in a lock-and-key fashion to a different antigen, and the enormous diversity of antibodies allows the immune system to specifically recognise an equally wide variety of antigens.

14.6.1 Immunoglobulins

Immunoglobulins (**Ig**) are glycoproteins with sites that bind to antigens. A specific antibody is produced to combat each different antigen, e.g. the antibody for measles is not quite the same as the antibody for any other disease. The five subclasses of Ig are (→ Fig. 14.9):

Immunoglobulin A (**IgA**) are found in high concentrations in mucous membranes, particularly those lining the respiratory, urogenital and

Box 14.13 Immunoglobulin tests measure the level of antibodies in the blood and provide information about the functioning of the immune system, especially relating to infection or autoimmune disease. Immunoglobulin replacement therapy can be life-saving treatment for certain immunodeficiency disorders (→ 14.9.4).

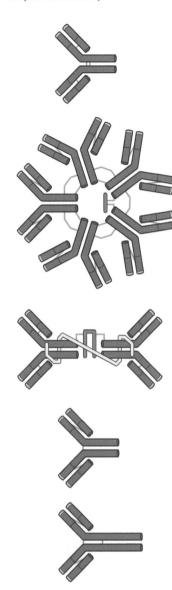

Fig. 14.9 Immunoglobulins.
The basic structure of antibodies is a monomer (single Ig unit) but they can form dimers (two units), tetramers (four units) and pentamers (five units).

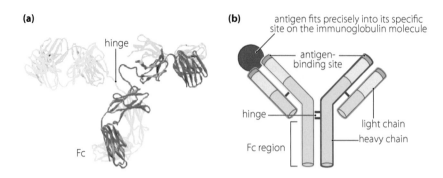

Fig. 14.8 Antibody structure (**a**) the immunoglobulin molecule much-folded into a Y shape; (**b**) the generalised Y-shaped structure of an antibody.

gastrointestinal tracts, as well as in saliva, tears and breast milk. IgA antibodies protect mucous membranes from invading pathogens.

Immunoglobulin G (IgG) – most abundant type of antibody found in body fluids. It protects against bacterial and viral infections. As it is able to cross the placenta, it provides protection to the unborn baby.

Immunoglobulin M (IgM) – found mainly in the blood and lymph and fights new infections. Its shape means that it can create insoluble immune complexes. Immune complex formation is a means of inactivating antigens and rendering them harmless.

Immunoglobulin E (IgE) – associated mainly with allergic reactions and also protects against parasitic infections.

Immunoglobulin D (IgD) – exists on the surface of B cells and can bind to antigens in extracellular fluid, thus playing a part in activation of B cells.

14.6.2 Summary of antibody production

The **immune response** is the response of the immune system to antigens – bacteria, viruses and other foreign substances such as vaccines (→ Box 14.14). The plasma cells involved in the process of antibody production and secretion are activated B cells (→ Fig. 14.10).

❶ The **primary response** by lymphocytes starts with exposure to the antigen.

❷ Antibodies are produced that can bind specifically to the antigen molecules. The process of antibody production involves several steps including antigen presentation, binding to naive B cells, and proliferation to form a clone of plasma cells. During this time the antigen(s) may cause signs and symptoms of disease in the body.

❸ The level of antibodies in the blood rises and they can bind precisely to antigens, identifying their presence to other components of the immune system such as phagocytes and complement.

❹ Antibody levels rise to a peak 7–10 days after exposure to the antigen. Symptoms begin to decline – a sign that the immune system is acquiring immunity against the antigen, but some plasma cells remain as **memory cells**.

❺ The **secondary response** occurs when the same antigen is encountered at a later date, which leads to the activation of previously generated memory cells and results in a much more rapid response with greater amounts of antibody.

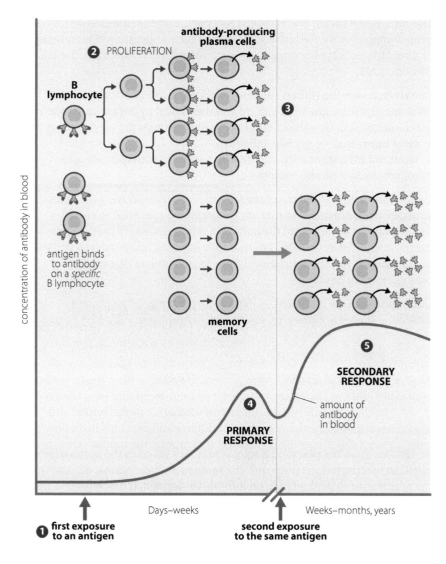

Fig. 14.10 Primary and secondary immune response.

14.7 Immunisation

Immunisation (vaccination; inoculation) uses vaccines to stimulate the process of adaptive immunity. Some vaccines are given in two or three doses, with intervals between to build up more and more antibodies (→ Fig. 14.10). A booster dose may be needed after a time to maintain the immunity.

14.7.1 Vaccines

A **vaccine** is a special preparation of antigenic material that is used to produce active immunity to a specific disease by stimulating the production of antibodies.

Live attenuated vaccine is made from a form of a particular bacterium or virus that has been made harmless. It stimulates the body to produce antibodies without causing the symptoms of infection and usually gives long-lasting protection, e.g. measles and mumps vaccines.

Box 14.14 Vaccines are antigenic preparations that should produce strong, measurable immunity that protects people with the minimum of side-effects.

The most common method of administering vaccines is by injection, but influenza vaccine can be given by nasal spray, and polio vaccine is given by mouth.

Box 14.15 Live attenuated vaccines usually need to be refrigerated to stay potent, so they may not be suitable for use in countries that lack widespread refrigeration.

Box 14.16 Conjugate vaccines are used in babies because immature immune systems often have difficulty in recognising certain antigens, so ordinary vaccines may not be effective for some diseases. The conjugation of the antigen with a protein creates a substance that is more easily recognisable by the white cells in the blood, resulting in a stronger immune response. Two important vaccines in child healthcare are the pneumococcal conjugate vaccine (PCV) and the meningococcal conjugate vaccine (MCV).

Box 14.17 Breast milk contains all the nourishment that a young baby needs for growth and development, and it is delivered to the baby without the risk of contamination by pathogens. Breastfed babies are therefore at lower risk of infections than bottle-fed babies, especially those that cause vomiting and diarrhoea. Worldwide, many millions of babies die from gastroenteritis, particularly those who are bottle-fed.

Box 14.18 The neonatal immune system differs from that of an adult. Although mature and functional lymphocytes are present:
• their repertoire of antibodies and B cells is restricted
• their T cell population is biased toward helper T cells, with a relative deficiency of cytotoxic T cells that seek out virally infected and defective cells (→ 14.5.1).
By the age of 4 years, 40% of infants have achieved adult levels of important antibodies.

Live attenuated vaccines are not given to people whose immune system has been damaged or weakened, e.g. those who have undergone chemotherapy or have HIV, because these vaccines may cause a mild case of the disease (→ Box 14.15).

Inactivated vaccine (killed vaccine) is obtained from bacteria or virus particles which are grown in culture and then killed by heat or formaldehyde that renders them non-infectious. Inactivated vaccines are used to prevent:
• **viral infections** – e.g. polio, influenza
• **bacterial infections** – e.g. diphtheria, pertussis (whooping cough), tuberculosis, typhoid, cholera.

Genetically-engineered vaccines are produced by modifying the genetic structure of an organism so that it is programmed into making vaccines that contain only the part of the pathogen that is necessary to stimulate the production of antibodies. For example, hepatitis is caused by a virus but hepatitis B vaccine is produced from yeast (a unicellular fungus) by reprogramming its genes.

Conjugate vaccine is created by joining a weak antigen to a protein molecule. These vaccines are usually used to immunise babies (→ Box 14.16).

14.7.2 Passive immunity

Passive immunity gives short-term protection acquired from ready-made antibodies obtained by maternal transfer or from antiserum preparations.

Maternal transfer

Antibodies cross the **placenta** from the mother's blood to the unborn baby's blood so that the baby is born with the same protection against diseases that the mother has either had or been immunised against. If breastfed, the baby continues to receive antibodies in colostrum and **breast milk** because the baby's stomach wall is permeable enough to allow these protein molecules to pass through without being digested (→ Box 14.17).

These antibodies circulate in the baby for several months and then gradually disappear, giving time for the baby's immune system to develop and mature. By the age of 3 months, the baby is better able to make its own antibodies; this is generally the recommended time to begin immunisation (→ Box 14.18).

Antiserum

Passive immunity is obtained by the injection of **antiserum**, which is blood serum containing ready-made antibodies. This type of immunity provides only short-term protection but is useful for treating or preventing some diseases, e.g. tetanus, hepatitis and rabies, and preventing Rh damage of the foetus by injections of anti D (→ 5.9). Similarly, the antibodies in antivenom can prevent or reverse most of the effects of snakebite.

Immunotherapy

Immunotherapy uses industrially produced immunoglobulins known as **monoclonal antibodies** (**MABs**) as a way of stimulating the patient's immune system in:
• cancer therapy to target malignant cells
• therapy for autoimmune disorders such as Crohn's disease, rheumatoid arthritis and multiple sclerosis.

14.8 Transplants and rejection

Transplantation is the implanting of a tissue or organ from one person (the donor) into another (the recipient), e.g. kidney transplant or a blood transfusion (→ Box 14.19). Its success depends on the degree of compatibility between the recipient's and donor's immune system.

Tissue typing (**HLA typing**) is carried out before a transplant operation using **human leucocyte antigens** (HLA). These are 'markers' used by the immune system to recognise which cells belong in the body and which ones do not. Each person possesses many HLA markers, half inherited from their father and half from their mother.

Matching HLA markers between donors and recipients is important for successful transplant outcomes. The process of testing for HLA markers is more complicated than blood group matching (→ 5.8). The cross-match between the donor's and recipient's tissues is usually not perfect so the aim is to match 8–10 of the markers (→ Box 14.20).

Immunosuppressant drugs are used to suppress the recipient's immune system to prevent it from attacking and rejecting the transplant. Corneal transplants are an exception because the cornea has no blood supply and transplants are rarely rejected. The same principle applies to transplants between identical twins.

Types of rejection

All transplant recipients have some degree of rejection, which is why anti-rejection drugs are necessary.
- **Hyperacute rejection** occurs a few minutes after the transplant when the antigens are completely unmatched, e.g. when donor and recipient's blood groups are incompatible.
- **Acute rejection** may occur any time from the first week after transplant and surgery to 3 months afterwards.
- **Chronic rejection** takes place over many years. The body's constant immune response against the new organ slowly damages the transplanted tissues or organ.
- **Graft-versus-host disease (GvHD)** is a complication that can occur after a bone marrow or stem cell transplant when the newly transplanted donor cells attack the recipient's body. GvHD can be acute or chronic, and the symptoms can range from mild to severe.

14.9 Immune disorders

The immune system provides powerful responses that maintain homeostasis by protecting the body from invading pathogens and foreign substances, and by ensuring that they are rapidly and efficiently eliminated from the body. However, these responses also have the potential to become immune disorders when the immune system is induced to mount exaggerated responses (**hypersensitivity** → 14.9.1) or to destroy the body's own tissues (**autoimmunity** → 14.9.3).

14.9.1 Allergy

An allergy is a detrimental immune reaction to a substance to which the body has become hypersensitive. In some families there may be an inherited predisposition to hypersensitivity to one or more allergens. Although allergic

Box 14.19 A blood transfusion is a transplant of blood from a donor to a recipient and so cross-matching must take place to enhance compatibility. A transfusion reaction is rare but is a sign that the recipient is rejecting donated blood.

Box 14.20 Human leucocyte antigen (HLA) system refers to the proteins (antigens) encoded by the HLA genes located on chromosome 6. These proteins occur on the plasma membrane of human cells, and each is unique to an individual except in the case of identical twins. Therefore any transplanted tissue which possesses different HLA marker types is perceived as a dangerous invader by the immune system and is attacked and rejected.

Box 14.21 Babies are more likely to develop **allergies** when there is a history of eczema, asthma, hay fever or food allergies in the family. Therefore, it is recommended that babies in these families are breastfed exclusively for the first six months.

When weaning starts, foods that can trigger allergic reactions should be introduced one at a time so that any adverse reaction can be spotted. Many children outgrow their allergies, but a peanut allergy is generally lifelong.

Box 14.22 Antihistamine medication blocks the actions of histamine and is effective in reducing the symptoms of seasonal allergies such as hay fever symptoms – watery eyes, itchy skin and runny nose.

Box 14.23 Treatment for autoimmune disorders depends on the disease, but in most cases requires the inflammation to be reduced. Corticosteroids or other drugs that reduce the immune response are sometimes prescribed.

Immunosuppressants are drugs that suppress the immune system. Because immunity is lowered during the treatment, the patient has an increased risk of infection.

Box 14.24 Symptoms of **coeliac disease** are:
- diarrhoea, maybe with a strong unpleasant smell
- bloating and flatulence
- abdominal pain
- weight loss and tiredness due to malnutrition
- poor growth in children.

Box 14.25 Symptoms of **Addison's disease:**
- low energy and weakness
- low blood pressure
- dark pigmentation of the skin.

reactions are often mild, they can also be very serious and affect different areas of the body at the same time. Allergic reactions can be triggered by:
- pollen – causes hay fever and rhinitis
- dust mites – cause asthma
- bee stings – cause inflammation
- foods, e.g. eggs, wheat, nuts, seeds, fish and shellfish.

Effects of histamine

Histamine is one of the signal molecules (→ 14.3.2) released by mast cells as part of the inflammatory response and allergic reaction, causing the typical symptoms of itching, sneezing, wheezing and swelling (→ Box 14.22). **Mast cells** are derived from basophils and are located in connective tissue in the skin, nose, lungs, the linings of the stomach and intestine, and many other sites. Symptoms of their activation include tingling or itching in the mouth, itchy, red skin perhaps with a rash, swelling of the face, mouth, throat or other areas of the body, difficulty in swallowing, wheezing and shortness of breath (→ Box 14.21).

14.9.2 Anaphylaxis

Anaphylaxis is a severe and potentially life-threatening allergic reaction, most commonly triggered by foods, insect stings and medications. Symptoms can include:
- skin reactions such as hives, flushed skin, or paleness
- swollen tongue or lip and difficulty in swallowing
- abdominal pain, nausea, vomiting or diarrhoea
- runny nose and sneezing
- a weak and rapid pulse and circulatory shock (→ 16.5).

14.9.3 Autoimmune disease

Autoimmune disorders can affect many parts of the body and they develop when the immune system inappropriately attacks healthy cells. The first symptoms are usually fatigue, muscle aches, a low grade fever and inflammation, followed by flare-ups when the symptoms get worse, and remissions when the symptoms either improve or disappear. As some autoimmune diseases have similar effects, it can be difficult to determine the cause, but they tend to run in families and more often affect women (→ Box 14.23).

There are more than 80 types of autoimmune diseases including:
- **rheumatoid arthritis** – a disease of the synovial lining of the joints, making them swollen, painful and stiff
- **multiple sclerosis** – a demyelinating disease that affects the conduction of nerve impulses to and from the brain and spinal cord (→ 9.12.1)
- **type 1 diabetes** – the immune system attacks the cells in the islets of Langerhans in the pancreas that produce insulin (→ 16.1.2)
- **lupus** – a complex disorder (→ 16.6)
- **coeliac disease** (→ Box 14.24) and **Crohn's disease** (→ 7.9.1) are examples of disorders in which the immune system inappropriately attacks the digestive tract, resulting in inflammation and malabsorption of food
- **Hashimoto's disease (thyroiditis)** – chronic inflammation of the thyroid gland which most often affects women and leads to hypothyroidism (→ Box 11.17)
- **Addison's disease** – when the immune system attacks the adrenal glands, reducing the production of adrenaline and the steroid hormones cortisol and aldosterone (→ Box 14.25).

14.9.4 Immunodeficiency disorders

Immunodeficiency disorders occur when part of the immune system is missing or defective and the body's ability to fight infection is impaired. An affected person will have frequent infections that are generally more severe and last longer than is usual.

Primary immunodeficiency disorders

These are rare genetic disorders present at birth. Those affected are very susceptible to infectious diseases because the immune system is virtually absent (→ Box 14.26).

Secondary immunodeficiency disorders

These are acquired after birth, e.g. acquired immune deficiency syndrome (AIDS). AIDS is the final stage of infection by the human immunodeficiency virus (HIV) that occurs when the body can no longer fight life-threatening infections (→ Box 14.27). With early diagnosis of HIV and effective treatment, most people with the virus will not go on to develop AIDS.

Effects of stress on the immune system

Long-term stress or depression, or short-term stress caused by life experiences including bereavement or examinations, can lead to reduced immunity and vulnerability to infectious and autoimmune diseases, which overwhelm the existing response to pathogens. The hormones produced by the adrenal glands (→ 11.7), particularly the stress hormone **cortisol** (→ Box 14.28), play an important role in regulating the immune system. If cortisol levels become too low or too high, this may lead to regular infections, chronic inflammation, autoimmune disorders or allergies.

14.9.5 Immunosenescence

Immunosenescence refers to the gradual deterioration of immune functions that occurs as people get older. T lymphocytes tend to become less responsive to antigens and their numbers begin to fall. A consequence of reduced T-cell function is that it takes longer to mount an antibody response. This means that elderly people can become more susceptible to infection, and also helps to explain the increased incidence of cancers (→ 15.10).

Immunosenescence can be partly explained by cumulative oxidative damage to cells leading to:
- decline in the ability of stem cells in bone marrow to produce new immune cells
- falling numbers of phagocytic cells
- reduced numbers of B lymphocytes and antibodies
- deficiency in production of T lymphocytes
- a higher risk of infection, autoimmune disease and cancers.

Box 14.26 Severe combined immunodeficiency disease (**SCID**) is sometimes known as "bubble baby disease" because its victims are extremely vulnerable to infectious diseases and so have to live in an infection-free 'bubble'. Inherited defects lead to absence of lymphocyte function and this results in severe susceptibility to infections, which is potentially fatal. Innovative treatments such as stem cell transplantation can be life-saving.

Box 14.27 HIV virus attacks the CD4+ cells; when an infected person's CD4+ cells drop to very low levels, the ability to fight disease is lost.

Box 14.28 Many students are familiar with examination stress which includes tension, worry and dread of failure before taking tests or assessments. Although some pressure can improve performance, too much anxiety can impair concentration and memory, leading to poor academic results.

Cortisol is necessary for normal function of the immune system but the relationship between stress, cortisol and immunity is a complex one. The onset of stress is usually accompanied by high levels of cortisol, which is thought to affect the immune system by suppressing inflammation, inhibiting production of some cytokines and preventing the proliferation of T cells.

Key points

1. Immunity is either innate (present at birth) or adaptive (acquired) and depends on complex interactions between cells, tissues and organs that cooperate to defend the human body against disease.
2. Innate immunity depends on non-specific but very rapid responses including inflammation and fever (pyrexia) that provide the first line of protection against pathogens and foreign substances.
3. Adaptive immunity is specific, mediated by lymphocytes and coordinated by a sub-group known as T cells.
4. Adaptive immune responses are activated through the process of antigen presentation; antigens – fragments of foreign material such as bacteria and viruses – are presented to the immune system in a specific way by macrophages and dendritic cells.
5. B lymphocytes make antibodies that can bind with specific antigens; the antigens are then eliminated.

Test yourself! Go to *www.lanternpublishing.com/AandP* and try the questions to check your understanding.

CHAPTER 15
DISEASE

Disease refers to any condition that impairs the normal functioning of the body. Because many of the disease groups have been dealt with in other parts of the book, this chapter concentrates mainly on infectious disease and cancer, with the aim of developing awareness of the key principles that highlight differences between normal physiological processes and disturbed homeostasis.

15.1 Epidemiology

Epidemiology is the study and analysis of the distribution and determinants of health, wellbeing and disease conditions in defined populations. It includes causation, transmission, investigation of outbreaks, screening and use of statistics to better understand how disease progresses and disturbs homeostasis.

Epidemics

An **epidemic** occurs when a disease spreads rapidly and infects a large number of people; it becomes a **pandemic** when an outbreak of infectious disease crosses international boundaries. Epidemics are more likely to occur with a virulent strain of the disease that spreads easily and where the population is in a poor state of health with little or no immunity to that disease (→ Box 15.1).

Endemic and sporadic disease

A disease is **endemic** if it is always present in a particular part of the world, e.g. malaria in the tropics, or if it affects people right across the globe, e.g. diabetes and schizophrenia. Disease is **sporadic** if it occurs in different places or different times with no known connection between the outbreaks.

15.1.1 Pathology

Pathology is the study of disease. Many diseases are recognised and most belong to one of eleven major groups (→ Fig. 15.1).

Box 15.1 The 1919 influenza **pandemic** swept the world and killed an estimated 50 million people, one-fifth of the world's population. Within months, it had killed more people than any other illness in recorded history.

A cluster of cases of pneumonia of unknown cause emerged in China in December 2019, and at the time of writing, the COVID-19 pandemic is a public health emergency of international concern.

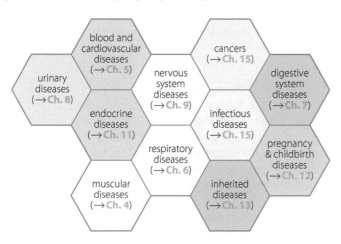

Fig. 15.1 Major groups of disease, with reference to the chapter in which they are discussed.

15.1.2 Disease, disorder and morbidity

Disease, **disorder** and **morbidity** are often used interchangeably but in some situations each of these terms is considered preferable; a person who is affected may also use illness and sickness as synonyms for these terms.

Disease – medical conditions that are associated with specific symptoms and signs. The term most commonly refers to infectious diseases but is also used for non-infectious diseases including cancer and genetic disease (→ Box 15.2).

Disorder – in medicine, a disorder is a functional abnormality and the term may be used to distinguish physical disorders from infectious diseases; *Chapter 16* examines some examples of multisystem disorders. The term **mental health disorder** is commonly used in preference to mental illness or mental disease as it is considered more value-neutral and less stigmatising; examples of these disorders are described in *Chapter 9*.

Morbidity – 'morbid' means 'sick' or 'unhealthy' and, when used medically, indicates the presence of disease.

Co-morbidity – two or more diseases existing together, e.g. people who have diabetes and also hypertension and heart disease (→ 16.8).

15.1.3 Disease terminology

Symptoms are evidence of disease noticed by an affected individual, e.g. inflammation, pain, rash or fever.

Signs are objective evidence of disease that can be observed by a health professional, e.g. changes in breathing patterns, pulse rate, skin colour, temperature or blood parameters. Signs from laboratory testing might include results from urine and stool samples, biopsy or imaging (→ Ch. 17).

Syndrome – the combination of several signs and symptoms that are characteristic of a particular disease or disorder, e.g. Down syndrome.

Diagnosis – the process of determining the nature of a disease by clinical consideration of the patient's signs, symptoms and **medical history** – the record of the medical events and problems a person has previously experienced. A diagnosis may also include blood tests, scanning or other investigations (→ Ch. 17).

Prognosis – an assessment of the future course and outcome of a patient's disease based on knowledge of the course of the disease in other patients and the general health, age and gender of the patient.

Nature of a disease

Depending on the type of disease, it can be:
- **acute** – short-term, e.g. influenza
- **chronic** – long-term or constantly present, e.g. diabetes, hypertension
- **progressive** – gets worse; degenerates over time so that the function or structure of the affected tissues or organs will increasingly deteriorate, e.g. dementia, Parkinson's disease
- **localised** – affects only one part of the body, e.g. athlete's foot or an eye infection
- **disseminated** – spreads to other parts of the body, e.g. fibromyalgia
- **systemic** – affects the entire body, e.g. lupus erythematosus or hypertension

Box 15.2 According to the World Health Organization (WHO), the most common **diseases** in the world are:
- coronary heart disease (coronary artery disease)
- stroke
- infections of the lower respiratory tract, e.g. influenza, pneumonia
- chronic obstructive pulmonary disease
- cancers of the trachea, bronchus and lung
- diabetes
- dementias including Alzheimer's
- diarrhoeal diseases
- tuberculosis
- cirrhosis.

- **malignant** – becomes life-threatening if not treated, e.g. cancer
- **refractory** – resists treatment
- **flare-up** – refers to either the recurrence of symptoms or an onset of more severe symptoms, e.g. Crohn's disease, rheumatoid arthritis
- **in remission** – lessens in severity or temporarily disappears
- **stable** – does not get any worse.

15.1.4 Factors that contribute to disease

Development of a disease in an individual (**the host**) usually depends on the presence or absence of risk factors. A **risk factor** is any condition that increases the likelihood of development of disease or injury in that person, e.g. the health of the host, the environmental conditions, and the virulence of the agent (→ Fig. 15.2).

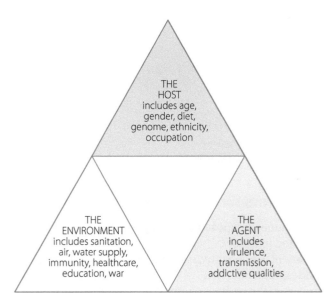

Fig. 15.2 Risk factors that contribute to disease.

15.2 Pathogens

Pathogens are microorganisms (microbes) that cause infectious disease, mainly bacteria, viruses, fungi, protozoa and prions.

Portals of entry into the body

The skin normally provides an effective barrier to most pathogens, but a break in the skin and openings such as the mouth, nose and urogenital tract enable them to gain access to the body and infect the tissues (→ Fig. 15.3).

15.2.1 Conditions for growth of pathogens

Different pathogens require different environmental conditions for survival and when in an environment that allows them to grow and multiply, they can cause disease. Infected tissues will then be prevented from functioning normally, which disturbs homeostasis. Some pathogens produce toxins that travel in the bloodstream and harm other parts of the body.

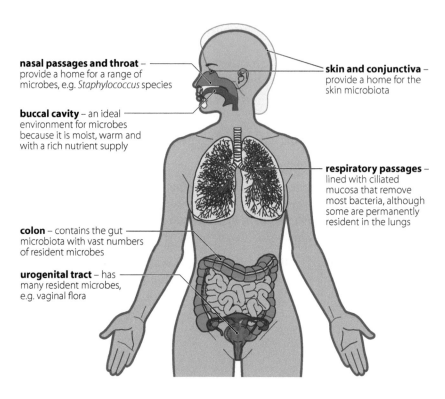

nasal passages and throat – provide a home for a range of microbes, e.g. *Staphylococcus* species

buccal cavity – an ideal environment for microbes because it is moist, warm and with a rich nutrient supply

colon – contains the gut microbiota with vast numbers of resident microbes

urogenital tract – has many resident microbes, e.g. vaginal flora

skin and conjunctiva – provide a home for the skin microbiota

respiratory passages – lined with ciliated mucosa that remove most bacteria, although some are permanently resident in the lungs

Fig. 15.3 Portals of entry for pathogens.

15.2.2 Risk factors for infectious diseases

People are continuously exposed to many pathogens, but the risk of becoming infected increases when:

- the environment is unhealthy, e.g. contaminated drinking water, poor air quality, widespread infection
- large numbers of the pathogens enter the body and overwhelm the immune system
- the disease is virulent, i.e. has a rapid, harmful effect (→ Box 15.3)
- the body's resistance is impaired because of a low level of immunity, personal stress, poor nutrition or poverty
- people who are very young or very old, as they have less resistance to infection.

15.3 Infection

Infection is the invasion and multiplication of pathogenic microbes that are not normally present within the body. An infection may:

- be subclinical, i.e. cause no symptoms
- cause symptoms of disease
- remain localised
- spread throughout the body in the blood or lymphatic systems.

Microbes that live naturally in the body are not considered infections, e.g. gut microbiota – the microorganisms that live in the mouth, stomach and intestines.

Box 15.3 Virulence is a term used to quantify the severity or potential for harm of a disease.

Virulence factors are molecules produced by pathogens that avoid the body's usual defence mechanisms and become attached to the host's cells, causing disease.

15.3.1 Chain of infection

The chain of infection is the sequence of events which has to happen for a pathogen to pass from one person to another. Since each link has a unique place, breaking the chain of infection disrupts an outbreak or epidemic (→ Fig. 15.4).

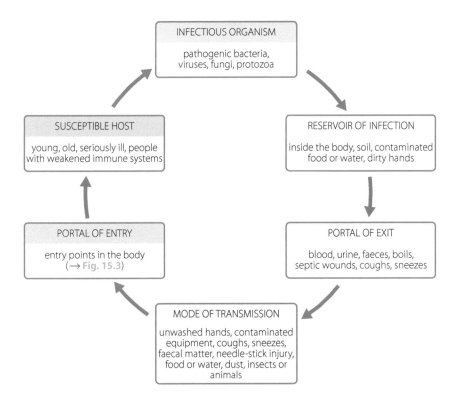

Fig. 15.4 Chain of infection.

15.3.2 Breaking the chain of infection

Infectious diseases can be controlled and reduced by conditions that disrupt the chain of infection (→ Fig. 15.4). These include:

- **elimination of the reservoir of infection**. Examples include pasteurisation of milk, which destroys the bacteria that cause tuberculosis, and the successful worldwide vaccination campaign to eradicate smallpox
- **control of the vector**. A vector is an organism that does not cause disease itself but which spreads infection by conveying pathogens from one host to another; for example, mosquitoes are the vectors for several diseases including malaria, West Nile virus and dengue fever
- **precautions by carriers**. Known carriers of disease should adhere to hand-washing protocol and not take employment in the catering industry (→ Box 15.4)
- **isolation** of infectious patients and **quarantine** of people who have been in contact with the disease, e.g. Ebola
- **antibiotics** and other forms of medication (→ Ch. 18).

Box 15.4 'Typhoid Mary', an Irish immigrant, was a chronic, symptom-free **carrier** of typhoid bacteria who made her living as a cook in and around New York in the early 1900s, and infected about 50 people with typhoid fever.

Asymptomatic carriers of typhoid, such as Typhoid Mary, may be apparently healthy people who have survived a bout of the disease but continue to shed bacteria – in this example it was *Salmonella typhii* in her faeces and urine.

Other diseases for which there can be asymptomatic carriers include HIV, chlamydia, COVID-19 and Epstein–Barr virus (→ Box 5.78).

Elimination of pathogens

Exposure to ultraviolet rays in sunlight or to **boiling water** for a few hours can kill a large number of bacteria, but some bacterial spores can withstand prolonged boiling, e.g. *Clostridium botulinum*, which causes botulism – a very severe form of food poisoning.

Germicides are chemicals used to destroy pathogens. Generally:
- **antiseptics** are used to destroy or inhibit the growth of pathogens on the skin
- **disinfectants** kill most bacteria, bacterial spores and viruses. They are therefore used to sterilise items that touch intact skin but do not penetrate the tissues, e.g. bed linen. Disinfectants are also used to sterilise equipment and drains.

Sterilisation can be achieved in an autoclave or by gamma irradiation. Any article or equipment receiving either of these treatments is sterile – free from microorganisms.

15.3.3 Infection control

Standard precautions for infection control are designed for the protection of both healthcare workers and their patients (➔ Box 15.5).

Hand washing

Research shows that washing hands is the single most important action that prevents transmission of disease. Pathogens are transmitted by touching another person (direct contact) or a surface that is contaminated in the home, in workplaces and all other settings (➔ Box 15.6).

Faecal–oral transmission

To prevent hand-to-mouth transmission of bacteria, hands should always be washed immediately:
- after visiting the toilet, changing babies' nappies, blowing the nose and sneezing
- after contact with body fluids, e.g. – vomit, blood, saliva, semen
- before preparing food and eating
- after handling rubbish bags and bins, cleaning cloths, pets and pet food.

Soap

Liquid soap is best or bars of soap in containers that allow free drainage. Soap creates a slippery environment where bacteria can slide off skin. Antibacterial washes are not usually necessary in everyday settings and they can contribute to spreading antibacterial resistance.

Hand sanitisers

When soap and water are not readily available or the hands are not visibly soiled, hand sanitisers are the preferred option.

Personal protective equipment

Personal protective equipment (PPE) such as gowns, gloves, masks, goggles, and respirators should be worn as appropriate by healthcare professionals and others when handling body fluids, to form a barrier to protect the skin, respiratory tract, mucous membranes and clothing from microorganisms.

Box 15.5 Within the world of healthcare, the risks of infection increase significantly, so infection prevention is essential to help to reduce the risks of hospital-acquired infection (HAI).

Box 15.6 *Effective* **hand washing** is the best way anybody can protect themselves from common infections such as food poisoning or influenza. When it is performed correctly, hand washing reduces the number of microorganisms on hands, which helps to reduce their transfer between people.

Social distancing

Social distancing is a term applied to certain actions taken to stop or slow down the spread of a highly contagious disease, e.g. during outbreaks of norovirus in healthcare settings or workplaces. This includes encouraging people to stay at home, banning visits to hospital wards and reducing workplace gatherings or where people come into contact with others who may carry pathogens.

15.4 Transmission of infectious disease

Infectious diseases are also known as **communicable diseases** or **transmissible diseases** because they can be transmitted from one person to another by a number of routes (→ Box 15.7).

Carrier. This is a person who harbours infectious pathogens without ill effects. They may be unaware that they are a carrier for diseases such as typhoid, hepatitis and AIDS and do not show any symptoms of the disease.

Contagious diseases. These are transmitted by contact. Many skin diseases are contagious, e.g. ringworm, impetigo, chickenpox, gonorrhoea, herpes and Ebola. They can spread by:
- **direct contact** – touching an infected person or their body fluids
- **indirect contact** – touching articles such as bedding, towels, handkerchiefs and toys that can carry disease-causing organisms Non-living objects that can transmit disease are called **fomites** and are associated particularly with hospital-acquired infections and may contribute to development of resistance.

Droplet infection. Microscopic droplets sprayed from an infected person during sneezing, coughing or talking can be inhaled by people close by. Alternatively, droplets may dry rapidly and be carried some distance in an air current to infect people further away. Diseases of the respiratory tract, e.g. the common cold and influenza, and the so-called infectious diseases of childhood, such as measles and whooping cough, are often spread by droplet infection.

Contaminated water. Polluted drinking water or poor sanitation is a source of waterborne diseases, e.g. typhoid and cholera.

Contaminated food. Food that has not been properly cooked or stored can be a source of food poisoning. Food can also be contaminated by hands that have been in contact with faeces (**faecal–oral route**).

Wounds. Pathogens can enter the body when the skin is broken by cuts, grazes and open sores. Diseases spread via wounds include tetanus, rabies, septicaemia and methicillin-resistant *Staphylococcus aureus* (MRSA).

Dormant spores. Some types of pathogen can survive as spores for a long time in dust, dirt or soil, e.g. tetanus and anthrax. Infection occurs when spores enter the body through a break in the skin. Once inside the body, the spores germinate into bacteria, which then multiply.

Inadequate sterilisation. When instruments or equipment such as catheters and needles are not properly sterilised, pathogens could spread from infected patients to others, e.g. hepatitis and AIDS. Diseases also spread amongst communities of drug users in this way.

Box 15.7 Knowing the ways in which microorganisms spread between people is the basis for effective prevention of infection by nurses and other healthcare professionals and caterers. Each disease has characteristics that are determined by the pathogen and the way it spreads. The various routes described here are not mutually exclusive, as some infections spread from carrier to susceptible host by more than one route.

15.4.1 Pattern of infectious disease

Most infectious diseases follow a typical progression, starting with a reservoir of pathogens and ending with an infected host (→ Fig. 15.5).

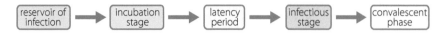

Fig. 15.5 The usual pattern of infectious disease.

When a sufficiently large number of pathogens get past the body's portals of entry there is an **incubation stage** – the time between their entry and the appearance of signs and symptoms. The incubation stage varies with different diseases, e.g. three days for diphtheria, one to three months for viral hepatitis, and more than a year for leprosy.

The **latency period** is the time between infection and the ability of the disease to spread to another person. This may precede or be simultaneous with the appearance of symptoms, or follow them. Some viruses exhibit a prolonged dormant phase.

The **infectious stage** is the time during which the pathogens can be transmitted to others. Depending on the disease, the patient can be infectious during the incubation stage or during the illness itself.

Convalescence is the time during which the symptoms disappear and the patient regains strength.

15.5 Bacteria

Bacteria (singular bacterium) are everywhere – in air, water, food, and on the outside and inside of the body (→ Box 15.8). They can be grouped into bacteria that are:
- **harmless to humans**, which refers to most species of bacteria
- **pathogenic** and cause disease or illness in their hosts
- **essential**, e.g. those that live in the colon and those that produce vitamin K
- **useful**, e.g. for food production – bread, cheese, beer, wine – and the production of antibiotics and other medicines such as insulin
- **commensal** – living on or within a person, deriving food or other benefits without hurting or helping the host, e.g. skin microbiota (skin flora) and gut microbiota (gut flora → Box 15.9).

15.5.1 Types of bacteria

There are many, many different species of bacteria and they range in size from 0.5–1.5 μm, which makes them visible through a microscope (→ Fig. 15.6). Each species has its own particular shape, size and optimum conditions in which it can survive, grow and reproduce (→ Table 15.1).

15.5.2 Structure

A bacterium consists of a single cell enclosed in an envelope (→ Box 15.10). There is no nucleus, the activities of the cell being controlled by a coiled strand of DNA and plasmids (→ Fig. 15.7). Substances necessary for life are absorbed through the envelope and unwanted substances are excreted in the opposite direction.

Box 15.8 Archaea and **bacteria** are two domains of living organisms that belong to the **prokaryotes** – single-celled organisms that lack a membrane-bound nucleus, and evolved at an early stage of evolutionary history. Humans belong to a third domain – **eukaryotes** – that have cells separated by membranes and clearly defined compartments within them.

Box 15.9 The colon contains tens of trillions of microorganisms, including at least 1000 different species of bacteria.

Box 15.10 Bacteria possess a rigid cell wall envelope that is essential to their survival. Some antibiotic medications, e.g. penicillins and cephalosporins, act by inhibiting synthesis of the cell wall.

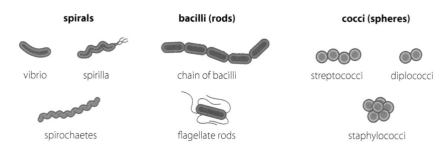

Fig. 15.6 Some examples of three types of bacteria.

Table 15.1 Characteristics of some types of bacteria

Bacterial group	Appearance	Examples of diseases
Spirochaetes	Spiral, coiled	Leptospirosis, Lyme disease
Cocci	Spherical or oval; often joins with others to form specific patterns	*Staphylococcus* – normally present on the skin and harmless, but can cause boils and abscesses and respiratory problems *Streptococcus* – throat infections, impetigo, sinusitis, conjunctivitis, meningitis, peritonitis, endocarditis and sepsis
Bacilli	Rod-shaped, some with flagella	Listeria, botulism, *Clostridium difficile*, salmonella *Escherichia* – UTIs, GI disease *Pseudomonas* – pneumonia and UTIs
Vibrio	Curved, comma-shaped; typically have two chromosomes	Cholera, gastroenteritis, sepsis
Mycoplasmas	Small, highly variable	Many are commensals but some cause pneumonia and genital infections
Rickettsiaceae	Variable	Typhus
Chlamydiaceae	Typically spherical, oval or rod-shaped	Sexually transmitted infections, respiratory tract infections, pneumonia and ocular infections in the newborn

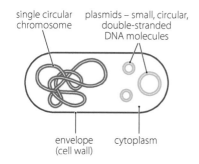

Fig. 15.7 Bacterium.

Taking it Further
You can find out more in online Chapter 17 about ways in which bacteria are grown in culture and identified.

15.5.3 Bacterial growth

Bacterial growth refers to an increase in cell numbers, not to the increase in size of an individual bacterial cell, and takes place by the asexual method of binary fission (→ Fig. 15.8). When the conditions for growth are favourable, some bacteria can reproduce approximately every twenty minutes. In the course of 24 hours, one bacterium can multiply to produce a **colony** – a group of many millions of bacteria.

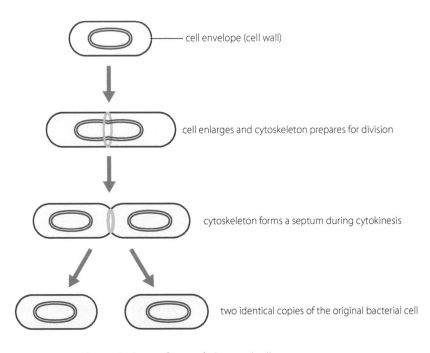

Fig. 15.8 Reproduction by binary fission of a bacterial cell.

Box 15.11 A serious outbreak of cholera in London's Soho in 1854 was a mystery. At that time, germ theory was not yet understood and cholera was believed to be spread by miasma (an unpleasant smell or vapour). Dr John Snow did not accept this and, by plotting cases of cholera on a map of the area, he was able to identify a water pump in Broad Street as the source of the disease. He had the handle of the pump removed, the pump was shut down, and cases of cholera immediately began to diminish. However, Snow's theory of disease was not widely accepted until Louis Pasteur published his 'Germ Theory' in 1861.

15.5.4 Conditions for bacterial growth

Water

Water is essential for bacterial growth. Most bacteria are capable of living in water and some can thrive in polluted water (→ Box 15.11).

Temperature

Many bacteria grow best in moderate temperatures of 25–38°C, a range which includes normal body temperature of around 37°C. Temperatures above 60°C kill most bacteria, but spores can survive in boiling water, some surviving for years. Freezing kills many bacteria, but some survive and become active again when the temperature rises. An example of this is *Listeria monocytogenes*, commonly found in unpasteurised milk and cheeses, and which can contaminate ready-to-eat meals and other foods, causing food poisoning.

Oxygen

Bacteria vary in the way they obtain energy:
- **aerobic bacteria** require oxygen to make the ATP (adenosine triphosphate) that provides energy for survival and growth (→ 19.11)
- **anaerobic bacteria**, e.g. the bacteria that produce foul-smelling gases in the colon, will not grow in the presence of oxygen
- **facultative anaerobes** use oxygen to obtain energy when it is available, but switch to anaerobic respiration when oxygen is absent.

Nutrients

All bacteria need a source of energy and matter in the form of **nutrients** to live (→ 19.12). Although some bacteria can carry out photosynthesis to create energy, many (called heterotrophs) obtain energy from organic (carbon-based) molecules, while others can generate their own energy from inorganic sources (autotrophs). Each species differs in its specific need for trace elements.

pH

Most bacteria prefer a neutral pH of 7.35–7.45, which includes the average pH of blood of 7.41. The low pH of hydrochloric acid in the stomach kills most ingested bacteria.

Sunlight

The ultraviolet rays in direct sunlight can kill bacteria or slow down their growth.

15.5.5 Biofilms

Biofilms form when colonies of free-living bacteria stick to each other and to surfaces and form a slimy, gooey matrix made of polysaccharide that is resistant to the action of antibiotics and disinfectants. Biofilms have been connected to food-borne disease and hospital-acquired infections, e.g. *Pseudomonas aeruginosa* and *Streptococcus pneumoniae*, which are often difficult to eradicate. Other diseases that are caused by biofilms include gingivitis and periodontal disease, catheter-related infections and inner ear infections. Plaques of biofilm can form on the surface of catheters, medical implants, dentures and wound dressings. Less commonly, biofilms have been associated with endocarditis (inflammation of the endocardium) and Legionnaire's disease, caused by *Legionella* bacteria.

> **Taking it Further**
> Antibiotic drugs inhibit the growth of bacteria.
>
> You can learn more about their action and antibiotic resistance in online Chapter 18.

15.5.6 Bacterial spores

Spores are dormant forms of bacteria that are highly resistant to destruction by environmental and chemical stressors including high temperatures, freezing, ultraviolet radiation, dehydration and household disinfectant agents. The formation of spores, which often happens when bacteria are short of nutrients, enables them to survive in water and soil for a very long time (→ Box 15.12).

Spore-forming bacteria dangerous to human health include:
- **Clostridium perfringens**, which can cause gas gangrene – a fast-spreading and potentially life-threatening form of **necrosis** (death of body tissue) that releases bubbles of gas at the site of infection
- **Clostridium difficile (C. diff)**, which can cause colitis – a form of antibiotic-associated diarrhoea. It follows antibiotic treatment that has allowed the presence of *C. diff* to disturb the normal population of the bacteria that are resident in the colon.

> **Box 15.12 Spores** can be destroyed by incineration at very high temperatures (800–1100°C) and by autoclaving – exposing them to pressurised steam at 121°C for 15–20 minutes.
>
> Disposal of infectious clinical waste that poses a hazard to humans who come in contact with it is subject to complex legal regulations and requires special attention to protect human health and the environment.

15.6 Viruses

Viruses are non-living particles, much smaller than bacteria, ranging in size from 10–300 nanometres (nm), and impossible to see except with an electron microscope. Each **virion** (virus particle) consists of a strand of nucleic acid, either DNA or RNA, surrounded by a protein coat. RNA viruses are also known as **retroviruses** (→ Fig. 15.9).

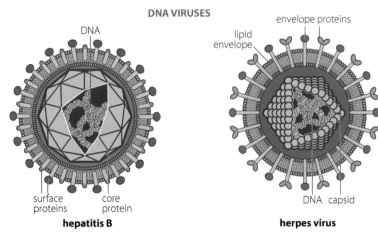

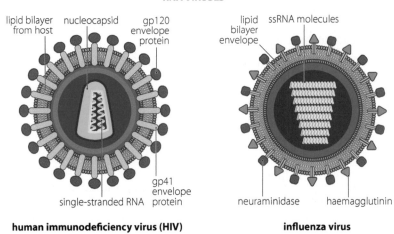

Fig. 15.9 Examples of DNA and RNA viruses.

15.6.1 Mechanism of viral infection

Viral infection involves the incorporation of its genetic material (DNA or RNA) into a host cell, replication of that material, and the release of the new virus particles. The stages include:

1. **attachment** – the virus attaches itself to a host cell
2. **penetration** – the virus penetrates the plasma membrane and injects its genetic material into the host cell
3. **replication** – viral genetic material is incorporated into the host cell's genetic material, induces it to replicate the viral genome and produces multiple copies of the virus particle
4. **release** – the newly-created virus particles are released from the host cell, either by causing the cell to break apart, waiting for the cell to die, or by budding off through the cell membrane (→ Box 15.13).

15.6.2 Viral latency

Some viruses may have a dormant phase when they 'hide' in the body in an inactive state and become active later. For example, the herpes virus causes chickenpox and after the body has recovered from the initial infection, the virus may remain dormant in the nerve cells for many years, and then cause herpes zoster (shingles) (→ Table 15.2).

Box 15.13 Louis Pasteur (1822–95) is the famous microbiologist after whom the process of pasteurisation – the process of using heat to eliminate pathogens from milk and juices – is named. He could not identify a means of transmission for the disease rabies and speculated that tiny agents that were too small to be seen through a microscope could be responsible for the disease. Subsequently he was proven correct when the electron microscope was invented in the latter half of the 20th century and it was found that rabies is transmitted by a type of RNA virus.

Table 15.2 Examples of viral diseases

Disease	Body parts affected	Mode of transmission
Chickenpox	Skin	Contact
Glandular fever	Lymph glands in neck	Saliva
Hepatitis A	Liver	Food, water, contact
Hepatitis B	Liver	Body fluids
Influenza	Respiratory tract	Airborne droplets
Measles	Repiratory tract, skin	Airborne droplets, contact
Mumps	Swollen parotid glands	Airborne droplets
Norovirus	Stomach, intestines	Food contaminated by unwashed hands, contact
Polio	Intestine, brain, spinal cord	Food, water, contact
Rhinitis (common cold)	Upper respiratory tract	Airborne droplets, contact
Smallpox	Skin, blood	Airborne droplets, contact
Yellow fever	Liver, blood	Mosquitoes
Ebola	Whole body	Body fluids, contaminated articles

15.6.3 Defence against virus attack

The immune response to virus infection depends mainly on CD8+ T lymphocytes. They can recognise the presence of viral proteins on virus-infected tissue cells and trigger the apoptosis process as an attempt to prevent viral replication. In addition, CD8+ T cells stimulate the production of interferons.

Interferons

Interferons are cytokines (→ 14.3.2), and as their name implies, are able to interfere with the production of new virus particles. They are produced by infected cells and bind to the plasma membrane of neighbouring cells, warning them of attack, encouraging them to stop growing and focus on defence mechanisms. These include the synthesis of hundreds of proteins that stop the disease process.

Certain symptoms of viral disorders, including fevers and muscle aches, are the result of interferon actions.

15.7 Virus-linked diseases

Some types of virus may play a role in triggering the onset of diseases including chronic fatigue syndrome, meningitis, subacute sclerosing panencephalitis, coeliac disease and some forms of cancer.

15.7.1 Meningitis

Meningitis is inflammation of the meninges caused by a virus or, less often, by bacteria. Symptoms are linked to damaged nerve cells and can develop in any order, although some neurological signs may not appear:
- **babies and toddlers** – fever, cold hands and feet, pale, blotchy skin (non-blanching rash), photophobia (sensitivity to light), stiff neck, refusing food, vomiting, fretful and showing a dislike of being handled

- **children and adults** – fever, cold hands and feet, vomiting, drowsiness, confusion and irritability, muscle pains, photophobia (sensitivity to light) and rash.

Unless meningitis is diagnosed and treated quickly, especially bacterial meningitis, death can occur rapidly, particularly in children.

15.7.2 Chronic fatigue syndrome

Chronic fatigue syndrome (CFS) is also known as **ME** (**myalgic encephalomyelitis**) and it typically occurs after a viral infection. It is a complex condition with fever, aching, chronic fatigue and depression. These symptoms are so severe that they limit a person's ability to carry out ordinary daily activities (→ Box 15.14).

15.7.3 Subacute sclerosing panencephalitis

Subacute sclerosing panencephalitis (SSPE) is a type of encephalitis that may follow an attack of **measles** if the virus remains passively inside brain cells. There is usually a delay of 5–10 years after the measles infection before symptoms are seen. Children under 2 years of age who catch measles are more vulnerable to SSPE because their immune system is immature. SSPE can have a rapid onset if caught by the infant around the time of birth.

15.7.4 Coeliac disease

Infection with retrovirus, a common but otherwise harmless virus, can sometimes trigger an abnormal immune response to gluten that leads to **coeliac disease**, a painful autoimmune condition that damages the villi of the small intestine (→ 7.6.3).

15.7.5 Cervical cancer

Cancer of the cervix is associated with infection of some types of **human papillomavirus** (**HPV**) that causes genital warts. The DNA in the virus mixes with the cell's DNA, triggering changes that make the cells grow and multiply. There are more than 100 different types of of human papillomavirus. Many are harmless, but some types of HPV can cause abnormal changes to the cells of the cervix, which can eventually lead to cervical cancer (→ Box 15.15).

15.8 Fungal infection

Diseases caused by fungi are called **mycoses**. They can be caused either by single-celled yeasts, e.g. *Candida albicans*, or a network of thread-like filaments (hyphae) that live on, or in, the tissues, e.g. ringworm. People are at greater risk of fungal infections when they are taking strong antibiotics for a long period of time because antibiotics kill not only the infecting microbes, but healthy ones as well. This alters the balance of the normal microbiota in the mouth, vagina, colon and other portals of entry, and provides an opportunity for the growth of fungal infections (→ Box 15.16).

Cutaneous mycoses (**dermatophytes**) are caused by fungi that require keratin (→ Box 3.2) for growth and live in the keratinised layers of the skin, hair and nails, e.g. ringworm. **Tinea** (ringworm) is a common and highly infectious skin infection that has several forms:
- tinea pedis (**athlete's foot**) (→ Box 15.17)
- tinea capitis (**scalp ringworm**) that often results in bald patches on the head

Box 15.14 The cause of CFS is unknown but suggestions include:
- a viral or bacterial infection
- problems with the immune system
- an imbalance of hormones
- psychiatric problems, e.g. stress and emotional trauma
- a genetic component, as the condition is more common in some families.

Box 15.15 In the UK, the HPV vaccine is being offered to adolescents aged 12–13 years of age to protect against two types of HPV virus that are responsible for more than 70% of cervical cancers.

Some transgender people and men who have sex with men are also eligible for the vaccine in England.

Box 15.16 Individuals with weakened immune systems, including people with HIV/AIDS and those under treatment with steroids or chemotherapy, are at increased risk of developing infections. People with diabetes also tend to develop infections.

Box 15.17 Tinea pedis. The creases on the feet provide a warm, dark, moist environment that is ideal for tinea pedis to live and multiply. This fungus also thrives in swimming pools, showers and changing rooms. It spreads easily by direct contact and can be passed from person to person through contaminated towels, clothing and surfaces. It is prevented by keeping the skin clean and dry, as well as by maintaining good hygiene.

- **tinea versicolor** that causes small patches of skin to become scaly and discoloured and is a common condition, especially in young people; the areas most often affected include the trunk, neck, upper arms and back.

Systemic mycoses are fungal infections that spread to many organs via the bloodstream, e.g.:
- **cryptococcosis** infections cause meningitis if they spread to the brain
- **aspergillosis** is a fungal disease of the lungs
- **candidiasis** infections are caused by a type of yeast (*Candida albicans*).

15.8.1 Candida

Candida albicans is an opportunistic pathogen that can multiply in warm, moist conditions, causing **thrush** of the mouth and vagina, nappy rash and intertrigo (→ 3.5.2). More than 70% of the population have this organism living harmlessly as **commensals** (→ 15.5) in the digestive tract, having been passed from mother to infant during labour and then remaining as part of the infant's microbiota. However, when *Candida* overgrows and out-competes other commensals, this organism can invade tissues and cause **candidiasis**, particularly in people whose immune system is compromised. There are several forms of this disease:
- **Vulvovaginal candidiasis** affects 75% of women at least once in their life; some have recurrent episodes of rash, itchiness, burning, and discharge that looks like cottage cheese; men can also contract candidiasis
- **Oropharyngeal candidiasis** forms white plaques on mucous membranes in the mouth and throat, which cause soreness when eating
- **Invasive candidiasis** develops when the fungus enters the bloodstream and then has the potential to infect every organ in the body.

15.9 Parasitic infections

A parasite is an organism that lives on or in a host. This group includes:
- commensals – the skin and gut microbiota (→ 15.5)
- parasites that live on the skin (→ 3.6)
- parasites that invade organs or systems, resulting in infections.

15.9.1 Vectors

Vectors are organisms that transmit parasitic diseases to humans, e.g.:
- mosquitoes spread **malaria**, **dengue fever** and **elephantiasis** (→ Fig. 15.10)
- dogs can spread **toxocariasis** in their faeces (→ Fig. 15.11)
- tropical water snails spread **schistosomiasis** (bilharzia)
- ticks can spread **Lyme disease** (→ Fig. 15.12).

15.9.2 Risk factors for parasitic infections

Parasites are transmitted in a number of ways, e.g. contaminated water and food, waste matter, soil, blood, sexual contact and vectors. Anyone can acquire a parasitic infection but people at greater risk are those who:
- have a weakened immune system or already have another illness
- lack clean, treated drinking water
- swim in lakes, rivers or ponds where waterborne parasites are common
- have contact with soil containing the faeces of infected humans or animals
- live or travel in tropical or sub-tropical regions of the world. Although parasitic infections exist in all parts of the world they are a major health problem in tropical and sub-tropical regions, caused mainly by protozoa and helminths (worms).

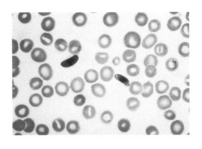

Fig. 15.10 Blood smear containing *Plasmodium* parasites (darker purple crescents).

15.9.3 Protozoan infections

Protozoa are single-celled organisms that can live and multiply inside the body, e.g.:

- **malaria** is caused by the *Plasmodium* parasite that spreads between humans via the bites of mosquitoes who have previously had a blood meal from an infected person (→ Fig. 15.10)
- **trichomoniasis** is a sexually transmitted infection spread by the *Trichomonas vaginalis* parasite
- **Chagas' disease** is caused by a trypanosome transmitted by blood-sucking protozoans; it often leads to cardiomyopathy (chronic disease of the heart muscle) and heart failure. This disease kills more people than any other parasitic disease in Latin America.

15.9.4 Helminth infections

Helminths include flatworms, tapeworms, thorny-headed worms and roundworms.

- *Ascaris lumbricoides* is a roundworm that can grow up to 35 cm in length, usually causing no symptoms; it infects one-sixth of the world's population.
- **Toxocariasis** is caused by parasitic roundworms commonly found in the intestine of dogs and cats (→ 15.9.5).
- **Schistosomiasis**, also known as bilharzia, is a tropical disease caused by parasitic flatworms (→ 15.9.6).

15.9.5 Toxocariasis

Toxocariasis is an infection caused by larvae of the dog roundworm *Toxocara canis* (→ Fig. 15.11). It usually affects children 2–7 years old, particularly those who put things in their mouths or who have contact with dogs that are are not wormed regularly. Infected dogs release eggs in their faeces and, if ingested, the eggs hatch into larvae in the small intestine, usually causing no symptoms and dying within a few months. In rare cases, the larvae migrate to the liver, lungs, eyes or brain, causing severe symptoms including breathing difficulties, seizures and blindness.

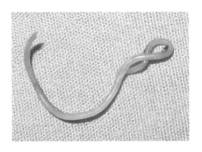

Fig. 15.11 *Toxocara canis*. Adult worms measure 9–18 cm.

15.9.6 Schistosomiasis

Schistosomiasis is a tropical disease caused by parasitic flatworms and spread through contact with contaminated water. Their eggs are released into water in the faeces and urine of infected people and they hatch to infect freshwater snails where they grow and develop. On leaving the snails, the parasite can infect a new human host by burrowing through skin, eventually settling in deeper organs of the digestive and excretory systems. After a few weeks, they can begin to lay eggs and the cycle continues. This disease affects more than 250 million people worldwide and is second only to malaria in terms of economic impact.

15.9.7 **Lyme disease**

Lyme disease is an illness caused by the bite of an infected tick and named after the town in the USA where it was first described. The ticks are tiny creatures about the size of a pinhead that feed by biting the skin and sucking blood (→ Fig. 15.12). *Borrelia* bacteria are passed from the tick into the skin, where they multiply and travel in the bloodstream to other parts of the body, affecting the skin, joints, nerves and heart.

15.10 Cancer

Cancer is not just one disease but a collection of many diseases and a leading cause of death worldwide (→ Box 15.18). Each person's cancer is different with a unique combination of genetic changes. Some of these can be inherited from parents, some by exposure to certain substances from the environment, and some may be the result of the cancer itself because as cancer develops, it damages local tissues and causes inflammation.

Cancer begins when one cell or a group of cells multiplies more rapidly than is necessary, producing an excess number of cells that typically form a swelling called a tumour or growth. A tumour can be:
- **benign** – contained within a thick fibrous capsule; it grows slowly and does not destroy the tissue in which it originates, or spread to other sites
- **malignant** – tends to grow quickly, spreads to other tissues and organs, and threatens life or wellbeing (→ Table 15.3)
- **primary** – at the original site where it first developed
- **secondary** (**metastatic**) – spread from the primary tumour to other sites (→ Box 15.19).

Not all cancers are solid tumours, as they can affect the production of blood cells (→ 15.10.5).

Metastasis

Metastasis is the development of secondary malignant growths at a distance from a primary site of cancer. A feature of cancer is that cells can break away, travel through blood or lymph and invade other tissue, forming new tumours by metastasis. In order to do this, the cells must escape by moving through the extracellular space and penetrating blood or lymph vessel walls. They then settle in a new space, acquire nutrients, and survive in this different environment.

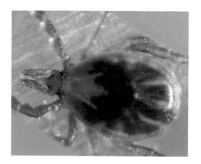
Fig. 15.12 Ticks transmit Lyme disease. Adult ticks measure 2–3.5 mm although an engorged tick may be as much as 10 mm in length.

Box 15.18 Worldwide, the most common causes of death from cancer are lung, liver, colorectal (bowel), stomach and breast.

Box 15.19 When a primary skin cancer, e.g. melanoma (→ 15.10.5, item 4) spreads to form a metastatic tumour in the skeleton, the secondary tumour is called **metastatic bone cancer**, not bone cancer, because it will have cellular and molecular features of the original skin cancer cells.

Table 15.3 Summary of the differences between benign and malignant tumours

	Benign	**Malignant**
Mitoses (cell divisions)	Few	Many
Growth rate	Slow	Rapid
Localisation	Strictly local, often encapsulated	May spread
Infiltrative /invasive	No metastasis	Frequent metastases
Recurrence after treatment	Rare	Common
Prognosis	Good, unless in critical area, e.g. brain	Poor if untreated

15.10.1 Genetics of cancer

Cancer is a complex disease that can arise in almost any part of the body when an error occurs in gene expression – the way that cells divide, grow and develop. Errors made while a cell is copying its DNA and before it divides may result in many of the cancer-causing mutations which affect some of the core signalling processes (→ 13.3.2) within the cell. Mutations are sometimes known as the 'drivers' of cancer and can affect oncogenes, tumour suppressor genes and DNA repair genes.

Proto-oncogenes code for the hundreds of intracellular components that encourage normal cell growth and internal signalling processes. If mutations arise in these genes, they can become oncogenes.

Oncogenes are genes that have the potential to cause cancer. When mutations occur in a cell's genes, most normal cells undergo apoptosis. But if the mutations turn the genes into activated oncogenes, these can stop apoptosis and allow the mutated cell to survive and proliferate instead. Most oncogenes require an additional factor before they can cause cancer, e.g. mutations in another gene, or environmental factors such as a viral infection or smoking. The incidence of cancer rises dramatically with age and is related to a build-up of the risk factors over a lifetime (→ Box 15.20).

Tumour suppressor genes normally function to inhibit cell proliferation and act as 'brakes' to slow cell division and stop the formation of tumours (→ Box 15.21). But when mutations occur in tumour suppressor genes and result in uncontrolled cell division, tumour formation can occur.

DNA repair genes are responsible for fixing and repairing DNA that has become damaged. If these genes become mutated, then cells start to accumulate errors in their DNA and can become cancerous.

15.10.2 Progression of cancer

In healthy tissue, cells mature into very specific types, each of which performs a specialised function in the tissue and has a predictable relationship with neighbouring cells, e.g. muscle cells work together to contract. When these cells become old or damaged they die – apoptosis (→ 13.3.3), and are replaced by new ones. The rate of replacement is subject to homeostatic regulations that determine whether new cells are required and the space available. But when mutations occur and result in cancer cells, these cells stop obeying 'the rules' and behave differently. Examples of abnormal cell behaviour are:

- **hyperplasia** – cells ignore the signals that normally stop mitosis or trigger apoptosis (→ Box 15.22)
- **dysplasia** – cells lose the special features of the tissue in which they are growing and become abnormal
- ***in situ* cancer** – cells become genetically unstable and evolve by accumulating new mutations
- **invasive cancer** – cells evade the immune system and stop it from killing them; they also induce nearby cells to form blood vessels to supply them with the nutrients they need for growth and the formation of a tumour
- **cancer cells** that have the ability to migrate to distant parts of the body (→ Fig. 15.13).

Box 15.20 Since the 1970s, dozens of **oncogenes** have been identified in human cancer, and many chemotherapy drugs target the proteins encoded by the oncogenes.

Box 15.21 An example of a tumour suppressor gene is the *p53* gene. This gene inhibits the cell cycle, allowing time for DNA to be repaired; the *p53* gene also triggers apoptosis of mutated cells (→ 13.3.2).

Box 15.22 Hyperplasia is the enlargement of an organ or tissue caused by an increase in the reproduction rate of its cells, often as an initial stage in the development of cancer.

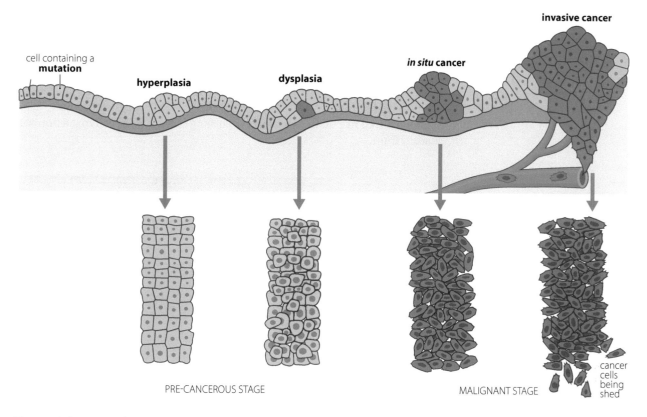

Fig. 15.13 Progression from a pre-cancerous stage to increasingly abnormal stages to malignancy.

15.10.3 Risk factors for cancer

It can be difficult to know whether a cancer results from a spontaneous mutation or is encouraged by environmental factors. A **carcinogen** is defined as any substance or agent that is capable of promoting cancer, but the **risk** of developing cancer depends on many different factors, including the individual's genetic make-up and the length and intensity of their exposure to:

- tobacco smoke
- low fruit and vegetable diet
- a high body mass index
- lack of physical activity
- certain bacteria, e.g. *Helicobacter pylori*
- some viruses, e.g. hepatitis B and C, human papillomavirus, Epstein–Barr virus.
- alcohol misuse
- asbestos
- urban air pollution
- ionising radiation

> **Taking it Further**
> Diet appears to play an important part in the prevention of cancer.
>
> You can find out more about a healthy, balanced diet in online Chapter 19.

15.10.4 Signs and symptoms of cancer

Changes in the body that may (or may not) indicate early stages of cancer include persistent coughs, indigestion, unusual bleeding or discharge, changes in the colour and/or size of moles, sores that do not heal easily, unusual patches of white tissue and lumps in tissue – all of which should be reported to health professionals for investigation.

As a tumour grows and swells it causes symptoms that include pain (which is often feared), weight loss (cachexia) and weakness, often as a result of substances and toxins released by the tumour cells. Since cancers often secrete substances that inhibit the immune system, people who have cancer often demonstrate immune system deficiency.

Diagnosis of cancer is by **histological tests** (microscopic examination of tissue samples) and by detection of 'biomarkers' such as the proteins and hormones made by the cancer cells.

15.10.5 Categories of cancers

Over 200 different types of cancer have been identified, which can be grouped into five main **categories** according to the type of cell that a tumour starts from.

1. Carcinoma

Carcinoma is the most common type of cancer which is formed by epithelial cells (→ 2.5.1) that cover both the external and internal surfaces of the body (→ Box 15.23). They are often named after the type of tissue in which they originate:

- **adenomas** form in epithelium that secretes fluids or mucus, so this group includes breast, colon and prostate cancers
- **squamous cell carcinomas** originate in tissues made of flattened cells such as those that form the lining of lungs, kidneys or intestines (→ Box 15.24)
- **transitional cell carcinomas** form in the special type of epithelium that is found in the lining of the ureters and bladder.

Box 15.23 More than half of new cases of cancer in the UK in 2014 were carcinomas of the breast, prostate, lung or bowel.

Box 15.24 In the UK, lung cancer is rare in people under 40 but rises sharply with age, being most commonly diagnosed in people aged 70–74.

2. Sarcoma

Sarcomas can form in the soft connective tissues of the body and include cancers of muscle, tendons and ligaments, blood and lymph vessels and adipose tissue.

3. Leukaemia

Leukaemia is the name given to cancers that originate in bone marrow where blood cells are formed (→ 2.4.1). Unlike other types, these are not solid tumours but very large numbers of abnormal white cells. A reduction in numbers of normal white cells means that it becomes harder to control bleeding, fight infections and deliver oxygen to body organs and systems.

4. Lymphatic system cancers

- **Lymphoma** begins in T or B lymphocytes and abnormal ones build up in lymph vessels and nodes as well as other tissues.
- **Melanoma** is a type of cancer that specifically originates in melanocytes – the cells which are specialised to make the pigment melanin. Although they most usually form in skin, melanomas can also form in other areas of pigmentation, e.g. choroid of the eye.
- **Multiple myeloma** is a cancer that originates in plasma cells (→ 14.5.3) which can form tumours all through the body.

5. Central nervous system cancers

- **Glioma** refers to a broad category of cancers that begin in glial cells (→ 2.5.5). They can be further identified according to the type of glial cell in which the tumour starts, e.g. astrocytic cell tumours start in the astrocytes.

- **Neuroendocrine cancers** form in cells that release hormones into blood, so this kind of tumour may secrete very large amounts of the hormone, causing a very wide range of signs and symptoms.

15.10.6 Treatment for cancer

A significant proportion of primary cancers can be successfully **treated** by surgery, radiotherapy or chemotherapy, and many cancers have a good chance of being cured if they are detected and treated early. Nevertheless, metastases (secondary cancers) are a major cause of death from cancer. 70% of all cancer deaths happen in low- or middle-income countries where access to adequate cancer care may be problematic (→ Box 15.25).

Box 15.25 Cancer is the fastest growing disease worldwide with an estimated 12 million people diagnosed with cancer each year.

Cell cycle and cancer treatment

For health professionals, understanding of the **cell cycle** (→ Fig. 13.4) is important in cancer treatment because some therapies work best when cells are actively dividing, e.g.:
- **radiation therapy** seems to be most effective when cells are undergoing cell division in the M phase
- some **chemotherapy drugs** work by attacking cells in a particular phase of the cell cycle such as G1, S or G2 phase (→ 13.3.1)
- **checkpoint inhibitors** – a form of immunotherapy that activate anti-tumour immunity thus enabling T cells to seek out and attack the cancer cells.

Key points

1. Disease refers to any condition that impairs normal function of one or more organs of the body.
2. Epidemics occur when disease spreads rapidly through a population, becoming pandemic if the disease crosses international boundaries.
3. Pathogens are microorganisms that cause infectious disease – bacteria, viruses, fungi, parasites and prions.
4. The chain of infection refers to the way pathogens are transmitted from one person to another; thus infection control is about disrupting the chain to reduce the spread of infectious (communicable) disease.
5. Cancer refers to a collection of non-communicable diseases that can arise in almost any part of the body when errors occur in gene expression.

Test yourself! Go to *www.lanternpublishing.com/AandP* and try the questions to check your understanding.

CHAPTER 16
MULTISYSTEM DISORDERS

Unlike diseases that normally have a predominant effect on only one system, multisystem disorders affect the physiological function of a number of organs or the whole body. There are many examples, and only a few are explored in this chapter to illustrate some of the features of these complex conditions.

The disorders in this chapter were chosen because they are complex and are commonly encountered in healthcare practice, namely diabetes, stress, lupus, metabolic syndrome and obesity.

16.1 Diabetes

Diabetes is a metabolic disorder causing fatigue, excessive thirst and the production of large amounts of urine. There are different forms of the disease, the most common being diabetes mellitus (→ Box 16.1).

16.1.1 Diabetes mellitus

The level of glucose in the blood is normally kept within the homeostatic range by two hormones – insulin and glucagon (→ Fig. 1.7). The normal blood glucose range is:
- 3.5–5.5 mmol/L before meals
- less than 8 mmol/L, two hours after meals.

Insulin produced in the pancreas enables glucose to move into the body's cells by facilitated diffusion (→ 2.2.2). When glucose is inside cells, it can be broken down by cell respiration to produce energy (→ 6.6.5).

Diabetes mellitus develops when not enough glucose can enter the body's cells because either:
- the pancreas has little or no ability to produce insulin (**type 1 diabetes**), or
- the body's cells develop insulin resistance and no longer respond to the insulin produced by the pancreas (**type 2 diabetes**) (→ Box 16.2).

Characteristic signs of diabetes mellitus are:
- **glucosuria** ('sugar in the urine') occurs when the level of glucose filtered into the nephrons exceeds their capacity to reabsorb it and leads to
- **polyuria** – the production of abnormally large volumes of urine
- **excessive thirst** to replace the large volume of water excreted in urine
- **fatigue** due to lack of energy because cells can no longer use glucose effectively for energy production
- **weight loss** (→ Box 16.3).

16.1.2 Type 1 diabetes

Type 1 diabetes is an autoimmune disorder (→ 14.9.3) characterised by destruction of beta cells in the islets of Langerhans of the pancreas (→ Fig. 11.9), resulting in little or no secretion of insulin. It accounts for

Box 16.1 Diabetes mellitus is a chronic disorder resulting from defects in insulin production or its action on the body. The disorder ultimately leads to elevated blood glucose levels, causing serious health complications that contribute to premature death if not treated properly.

Taking it Further
You can find out more in online Chapter 20 about the way the human body uses energy for the enormous number of metabolic reactions needed to maintain homeostasis.

Box 16.2 The signs of **type 1 diabetes** develop over a matter of weeks. The signs of **type 2 diabetes** may go unnoticed for several years.

Taking it Further
Testing the amount of glucose in blood and urine is an important aspect of diagnosis and management of diabetes; see online Chapter 17.

Box 16.3 Type 1 diabetes is associated with weight loss because fats and protein in the body are used for energy production in place of the glucose lost in urine; the depletion of body reserves can result in fatigue.

about 5% of all diabetes and is usually diagnosed between infancy and 40 years of age. It is not usually inherited but some genetic factors may predispose certain individuals to develop this type of diabetes.

Management of type 1 diabetes

A plan for the management of type 1 diabetes is designed for each individual according to their age and level of activity, the aim being to keep glucose levels in the blood within a normal range to reduce the risk of the long-term complications associated with the disorder. The plan involves:

- **insulin** administered either by regular injections or an insulin pump; some insulins are short-acting, while others have a longer action
- **controlling the diet**, especially meal timings, quantity and type of carbohydrate intake and other nutrients
- **physical activity** – any type of physical exercise that is regular and enough to give slight shortness of breath (→ Box 16.4)
- **regular monitoring** of blood glucose levels.

16.1.3 Type 2 diabetes

Most people with diabetes have **type 2**, with the severity of the disorder varying from slight to severe. The amount of available insulin is inadequate for the body's needs because either:

- the pancreas may be producing normal or increased levels of insulin but the body has become **resistant** to it; some people develop a high resistance and with others there is only slight resistance, or
- the pancreas retains some ability to produce insulin, but the amount is **insufficient** for the body's needs (→ Box 16.5).

People most at risk of developing type 2 diabetes

Type 2 diabetes is more likely to develop in people who:

- are over 40 (or over 25 if South Asian); in the past, type 2 diabetes was rare in people under the age of 65 but, as it is strongly associated with obesity, it is increasingly being seen in children, adolescents and young adults
- are of South Asian, black African or African Caribbean origin
- have a close family member with diabetes
- take medication for schizophrenia, bipolar illness or depression
- are overweight, with a waist size over 80 cm (31.5 inches) for women, 94 cm (37 inches) for men, or 89 cm (35 inches) for South Asian men.

Management of type 2 diabetes

Lifestyle factors such as obesity, poor diet and lack of physical activity are known to be important risk factors in the development of type 2 diabetes. Initial management is therefore by dietary changes with a regular pattern of meals, and by increasing the amount of exercise taken, because active muscles use up more glucose for energy than do resting ones. If diet and exercise are not effective in reducing blood glucose levels, then antidiabetic medication may be prescribed, e.g. metformin tablets or insulin. The same regular monitoring of **blood glucose** levels may need to be carried out as in type 1 diabetes (→ Box 16.6).

Box 16.4 Recommended guidelines: adults should aim to be active daily. Over a week, activity should add up to at least 2.5 hours of moderately intense activity in bouts of 10 minutes or more; one way to approach this is to do 30 minutes on at least 5 days a week.

Children should have at least 60 minutes of physical activity every day.

Box 16.5 Incretins are gastrointestinal hormones that stimulate the pancreas to release insulin after a meal has been eaten which, in turn, results in the reduction in blood glucose levels. They are currently being evaluated as potential drugs for therapeutic management of diabetes, but there is some concern over safety.

Box 16.6 Self-monitoring of blood glucose levels is an important way of maintaining **glycaemic control** in people who are taking insulin – those who have type 1 diabetes and some who have type 2. Many people will do this at home and it can help them to judge how effectively they are meeting treatment goals, and to adjust daily insulin doses according to dietary intake and physical activity levels.

16.2 Pathophysiology associated with diabetes mellitus

Uncontrolled or poorly controlled diabetes increases the risk of heart attack and stroke and can damage the blood vessels and nerves, and is the reason for:

- regular monitoring of blood glucose levels; some diabetics may need to carry out self-testing several times a day
- regular health checks (→ Box 16.7).

16.2.1 Examples of blood glucose variations

Hypoglycaemia

Hypoglycaemia (a 'hypo') means low blood sugar and occurs when the blood glucose level falls, usually to under 4 mmol/L. People with type 1 diabetes are more at risk of a 'hypo' than those with type 2, and it can happen if:

- too much insulin or other medication has been taken
- a meal or snack is delayed or missed
- not enough carbohydrate has been eaten
- more strenuous exercise has been taken than is usual
- alcohol has been consumed without food.

Warning signs of a 'hypo' are:

- hunger
- shaking
- pallor
- irritability
- rapid heartbeat
- tingling in the lips
- sweating
- dizziness and confusion.

If left untreated, the patient might eventually become unconscious and would then need a glucagon injection to raise blood glucose levels. 'Hypos' can be particularly dangerous when taking alcohol without food because the liver is less able to release glucose stored as glycogen and the blood glucose level may quickly fall dangerously low.

Prolonged severe **neonatal hypoglycaemia** in babies can cause long-term neurological damage (→ Box 16.8).

Hyperosmolar hyperglycaemic state

A hyperosmolar hyperglycaemic state (HHS) occurs in people with diabetes and those with profound beta cell dysfunction (→ 11.6) who experience very high blood glucose levels, often over 40 mmol/L. It can develop over several weeks through a combination of illness and dehydration. The symptoms are thirst, nausea, vomiting, dry skin, disorientation and, in later stages, drowsiness and a gradual loss of consciousness (→ Box 16.9).

Treatment to correct dehydration and bring the blood glucose down to an acceptable level is achieved through vigorous fluid management, which aims to restore blood volume and then to reduce the hyperglycaemia. This is accomplished most effectively within an intensive care setting.

Box 16.7 It is recommended that people with diabetes mellitus have a yearly **screening test** on their blood lipids (cholesterol test), blood pressure, kidney function, eyes and eyesight, feet and weight.

Taking it Further
People who have diabetes may need to test their blood glucose levels several times every day. Find out more about this and other physiological observations in online Chapter 17.

Box 16.8 Risk factors for **neonatal hypoglycaemia** include:
- preterm (less than 37 weeks' gestation)
- low birthweight (<2.5 kg)
- 'large for dates' (>4.5 kg)
- maternal diabetes mellitus (all types).

Box 16.9 Normally glucose is filtered by the glomeruli of the nephrons in the kidneys and then completely reabsorbed by facilitated diffusion into the bloodstream by cells in the proximal tubule (→ 8.2.2). In people who are **hyperglycaemic**, the volume of filtered glucose exceeds the kidney's capacity to reabsorb it and the excess spills over into urine. Since glucose is an osmotically active molecule, water tends to follow it, thus the urine volume increases and the person becomes exceedingly dehydrated and thirsty.

Box 16.10 Diabetic ketoacidosis (DKA) is a potentially life-threatening complication. Signs evolve over about 24 hours and include vomiting, **Kussmaul breathing** (a deep gasping, laboured breathing pattern), diuresis (excessive production of urine) and loss of consciousness. Blood testing shows low pH (acidosis) due to ketone bodies, accompanied by hyperglycaemia. If DKA is diagnosed early, it can be treated with extra insulin, glucose and fluid. If left untreated, it can be fatal.

Box 16.11 '-opathy' denotes a disease or disorder.

Box 16.12 Peripheral neuropathy can lead to 'diabetic holiday foot syndrome'. When people with diabetes go on holiday they may wear sandals, or walk barefoot on sand or sharp stones, and be unaware of any damage to their feet; this can lead to the development of ulcers. People with diabetes are more likely to be admitted to hospital with a foot ulcer than with any other complication of diabetes, and may need to have a limb amputated later due to gangrene.

16.2.2 Diabetic ketoacidosis

Most cases of diabetic ketoacidosis (DKA) occur in people with type 1 diabetes when there is a severe lack of insulin in the body. This means that glucose cannot be used for energy and so fat or body tissues provide an alternative energy source. Ketones (keto acids) are the waste product of this process and as they build up, they will cause the body to become acidic, hence the name 'acidosis'. Ketones can be detected by urinalysis and a warning sign of DKA is the smell of ketones on breath, usually likened to the smell of pear drops. Other symptoms include passing large amounts of urine, thirst, vomiting and abdominal pain (→ Box 16.10).

16.2.3 Diabetic neuropathy

Diabetic neuropathy (→ Box 16.11) is long-term damage to the nerve fibres, which develops when high blood glucose levels are present over several years; it affects nerves to different parts of the body:

- **peripheral neuropathy** is the most common type of diabetic neuropathy and usually starts with loss of feeling or pain in the feet. Foot injuries or sores may therefore not be noticed by the person, which can lead to ulcers and infections; peripheral neuropathy can eventually spread up the legs and then to the hands and arms (→ Box 16.12)
- **proximal neuropathy** causes pain in the thighs, hips or buttocks and leads to weakness in the legs
- **focal neuropathy** results in the sudden weakness of one nerve or a group of nerves anywhere in the body, causing muscle weakness or pain
- **autonomic neuropathy** is due to damage of the autonomic nerves (→ 9.8) that supply involuntary muscles involved in digestion, bowel and bladder function, sexual response, perspiration, heart and blood pressure control, lungs and eyes. Autonomic neuropathy can also cause hypoglycaemia unawareness, a condition in which people no longer experience the warning symptoms of low blood glucose levels.

16.2.4 Diabetic nephropathy

In some people with long-term diabetes, the basement membrane of the glomeruli in the kidneys (→ Fig. 8.3) becomes damaged, which allows excessive amounts of protein to leak into the urine, followed by gradual decline of function that can lead to kidney failure.

16.2.5 Diabetic retinopathy

Long-term diabetes can damage the blood vessels in the eye, leading to haemorrhage into the retina. The condition can be detected by careful eye examination before it causes deterioration in vision – hence the need for regular eye screening. Diabetes is also associated with increased risk of glaucoma and cataract.

16.3 Other forms of diabetes

16.3.1 Gestational diabetes

Pregnancy changes the way the mother's body handles nutrients including glucose and if diabetes develops it can be diagnosed at 20–24 weeks' gestation. Poorly-controlled diabetes in the mother means that her blood glucose levels lie outside the homeostatic range, that the growing foetus is being over-fed and becomes large for its gestational age. This situation increases the risk of complications during delivery, and the likelihood of the child also developing diabetes in later life is higher.

Gestational diabetes is usually diagnosed by antenatal blood tests during weeks 24–28 in women who did not have diabetes before they became pregnant, and it frequently goes away after the baby is born. At this stage, it often causes few signs or symptoms (→ Box 16.13).

16.3.2 Cystic fibrosis-related diabetes

Cystic fibrosis (CF) is characterised by lung infections and inflammation (→ 13.8.2). **Cystic fibrosis-related diabetes** (CFRD) is a special form of diabetes that develops when thick sticky mucus accumulates in the pancreas and blocks the pancreatic ducts, leading to the formation of cysts and inability to produce insulin. Although CFRD is rare in children under ten years old, some 50% of people with CF will develop the disorder by the time they are 30, and it is particularly prevalent in women.

16.3.3 Diabetes and the risk of dementia

There is evidence that diabetes and Alzheimer's may be linked in some way that is not yet fully understood. Recent research has discovered that:
- insulin is produced by the brain as well as the pancreas
- people who have insulin resistance, in particular those with type 2 diabetes, appear to have an increased risk of suffering from Alzheimer's disease; this is estimated to be 50–65% higher than in people who do not have diabetes
- many people with type 2 diabetes have deposits of a protein called amyloid beta in their pancreas which is similar to the protein deposits found in the brain tissue of Alzheimer's sufferers (→ Box 16.14).

16.3.4 Diabetes insipidus

Diabetes insipidus (DI) is a rare disease where the body loses too much fluid through urination. Antidiuretic hormone (ADH) is produced in the hypothalamus of the brain (→ 11.3.1) and plays a key role in regulating the amount of fluid in the body. The presence of ADH helps to retain water, but in DI, less ADH is produced than required, or the kidneys are insensitive to it. Large quantities of pale-coloured urine are excreted, causing a great thirst and a significant risk of dangerous dehydration.

16.4 Stress

Stress is the adverse reaction to perceived pressure when that pressure exceeds the individual's ability to cope. Although stress is not a disease it can increase the risk of several major causes of premature mortality, including heart disease, cancer, hypertension, diabetes, respiratory disorders and suicide.
- **Acute stress** is a physiological, psychological and emotional response to a frightening event, e.g. anxiety about injections or surgery which can trigger a 'fight, flight or freeze' reaction (→ 11.7.1); after the threat is over, the body returns to homeostasis
- **Chronic stress** is triggered by a range of events that lead to long-term physical and psychological ill health (→ Box 16.15).

Box 16.13 If **gestational diabetes** becomes apparent in the first trimester, it is likely that diabetes was present before the pregnancy. Maternal diabetes is a risk factor for neonatal hypoglycaemia (→ 16.2.1).

Box 16.14 Research studies are showing that type 2 diabetes can be a **risk factor** for Alzheimer's disease, vascular dementia and other forms of dementia (→ 9.12.4). This may be because dementia is caused by destruction and death of nerve cells that appears to be partly related to insulin resistance.

The management and care of people affected by both diabetes and dementia can present health professionals with both clinical and ethical challenges, and coordinating their care can be extremely complex.

Box 16.15 Life events are experienced uniquely by each individual, and **stressors** may include: death of a loved one, imprisonment, wedding, divorce or separation, examinations, becoming seriously ill, arrival of a first baby, identity theft, starting a new job or being fired, commuting delays, moving home or other housing issues, fire or flood, losing a mobile phone, terrorist threats, road rage and accidents, going on holiday, caring responsibilities and social media. In general, each of these events is perceived as being less stressful by men than by women.

16.4.1 Chronic stress

The hypothalamic–pituitary–adrenal axis (→ Fig. 11.10) plays a key role in the stress response. When a person is exposed to long-term stress, the levels of **cortisol** (→ 11.7.2) are high, which makes the body more susceptible to a variety of disorders (→ Box 16.16). Depending on the individual, chronic stress can result in:

- **headaches**, **mood swings** and **sleep problems** (→ Box 16.16)
- **impaired cognitive abilities** including shortened attention span, reduced performance and memory
- **hypothyroidism** due to the failure of the thyroid gland to produce enough thyroxine, resulting in weight gain and depression
- **hyperglycaemia** with symptoms similar to those of untreated diabetes – increased thirst, the need to urinate frequently and tiredness
- **hypertension** due to repeated episodes of high blood pressure and the stimulation of the nervous system to produce large amounts of vasoconstrictor hormones such as adrenaline
- **digestive upsets**, e.g. diarrhoea, vomiting or worsening of an irritable bowel
- **peptic ulcers**
- **panic attacks**, **anxiety** or **depression**.

Box 16.16 Cortisol circulating around the body can help people to remain alert, which enhances their reaction time and means they can react more rapidly to changes. When accompanied by a boost in adrenaline levels, blood flow to the brain can be improved, which can enhance memory and cognition while reducing pain. This is an important response for survival in dangerous situations. If cortisol levels remain high for a prolonged period of time, risk factors for disease begin to threaten wellbeing.

Chronic stress and immunity

The presence of high levels of cortisol in the body over a long time:

- **lowers immunity** because the number of lymphocytes becomes reduced and the risk of chronic infections increases
- **damps down the inflammatory response** (→ 14.3.3) and wound healing takes longer
- **increases the likelihood of autoimmune diseases** – the immune system attacks healthy cells (→ 14.9.3).

Management of stress

There is no quick cure for stress or a single treatment that works for everyone. Non-medication therapies can be effective, e.g.:

- **physical exercise and activities** that can trigger a positive and energising outlook on life
- **relaxation techniques** that relieve physical and mental tension, e.g. meditation, yoga, acupressure, reiki, music therapy and mindfulness (→ Box 16.17)
- **cognitive behavioural therapy** (CBT; 'talking therapy') can help to manage stress by changing thoughts and behaviours (→ 9.14).

Box 16.17 Mindfulness is about quiet reflection, focusing on awareness of the present moment and noticing feelings and emotions.

16.5 Circulatory shock

Circulatory shock, usually referred to simply as **shock**, is a condition associated with extreme physical collapse that occurs due to the failure to maintain adequate blood pressure and tissue oxygenation (→ Box 16.18). Obvious physical signs of **hypoperfusion** (decreased blood flow through the organs) and **hypoxia** (deficiency of oxygen) are:

- rapid shallow breathing
- rapid, thready (very fine) pulse
- confusion or loss of consciousness
- cold, sweaty, pallid skin
- dilated pupils
- low urine output.

Box 16.18 Circulatory shock is a life-threatening condition due to the inadequate flow of blood. It should not be confused with acute stress reaction which may also be referred to as 'a shock'.

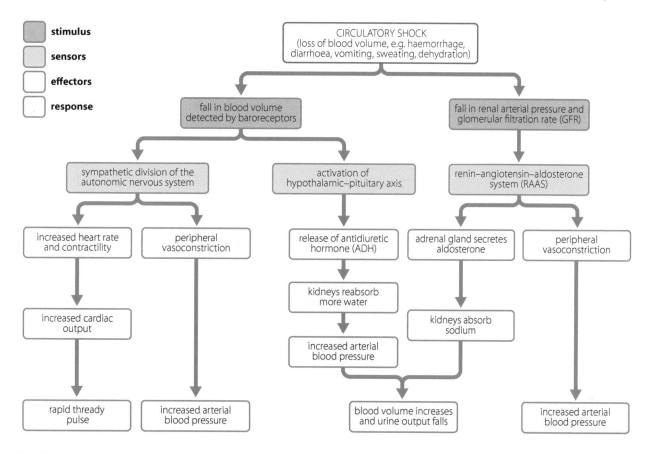

Fig. 16.1 Compensatory mechanisms that are activated in response to hypovolaemia (low circulating blood volume) to bring blood pressure back to normal.

Compensatory stage

The compensatory stage of shock follows the initial drop in blood pressure (→ Fig. 16.1). It describes the range of homeostatic responses that are activated to compensate for the hypoperfusion and hypoxia. Their role is to compensate for the initial disturbance and maintain an adequate blood pressure despite the reduction in circulating blood volume.

Progressive stage

The progressive stage of shock arises if compensatory mechanisms begin to fail. Cells shift to anaerobic respiration, leading to lactic acid production (metabolic acidosis) and inadequate ATP production for the body's needs (→ 6.6.6). These in turn lead to further cellular dysfunction and progressive decline in cardiac function with further loss of blood pressure.

16.5.1 Types of circulatory shock

The five main types of shock are linked with circulatory failure.

1. Hypovolaemic shock

Hypovolaemic shock is the result of a decrease in volume of circulating blood caused by severe haemorrhage, dehydration, severe vomiting or diarrhoea (→ Fig. 16.1). Compensatory mechanisms are triggered by the

Taking it Further
People who are diagnosed as being in circulatory shock are usually in an emergency setting. After checking for signs and symptoms of shock, a range of tests will be carried out to determine the person's physiological status.

You can find out more about the wide range of observations and measurements in online Chapter 17.

initial fall in blood pressure as the body attempts to maintain cardiac output. The sympathetic nervous system acts almost instantaneously to increase respiration, heart rate and cardiac contractility. This results in a rapid, thready pulse and shallow, rapid breathing.

2. Cardiogenic shock

Cardiogenic shock occurs when the heart muscle has been damaged to such an extent that it cannot function as an effective pump and it is unable to maintain the circulation of blood. This situation most commonly occurs during or after myocardial infarction (heart attack) or left ventricular failure.

3. Neurogenic shock

Neurogenic shock follows injury to the spinal cord and causes the walls of the blood vessels to relax (vasodilation) and impairs their ability to return blood flow from the periphery to the core circulation. The fall in venous return leads to reduced blood pressure. This makes the patient's skin warm and dry, leading to excessive heat loss and hypothermia.

4. Septic shock

Sepsis (septic shock; septicaemia; blood poisoning) occurs when the blood pressure drops to a dangerously low level due to systemic infection. Usually, the inflammatory response keeps an infection limited to one place as a localised infection. But if the immune system is suppressed or an infection is particularly severe, the pathogens, their toxins and immune cytokines (→ 14.1.1) can spread quickly through the bloodstream and cause a systemic inflammatory response, including a reduction in blood pressure (→ Box 16.19).

Any infection can cause sepsis but it is most commonly caused by pneumonia, kidney infections, abdominal infections, burns and pancreatitis.

Toxic shock syndrome (TSS) is a rare form of sepsis that occurs when the bacteria that normally live harmlessly on the skin, e.g. *Staphylococcus aureus* and *Streptococcus pyogenes*, invade the bloodstream and release toxins called **superantigens** which can directly activate up to half of all T cells. It is most notably caused when tampons are left in place too long.

5. Anaphylactic shock

Anaphylactic shock (anaphylaxis) is a severe life-threatening allergic reaction that can develop rapidly when a person is hypersensitive to a substance, one example being severe allergy to peanuts (→ 14.9.2). Large amounts of circulating inflammatory substances such as histamine cause widespread vasodilation, increase permeability of capillaries and consequently the blood pressure drops (→ Box 16.20).

16.6 Disorders of connective tissue

There are many known – and unknown – genetic variants that affect the function and type of connective tissue in a person's body. Some, including Ehlers–Danlos syndromes (→ 16.6.3), osteogenesis imperfecta and Marfan syndrome (→ 16.6.2), may offer distinct advantages, such as hypermobility, and are particularly prevalent amongst those who participate in flexibility sports including ballet, gymnastics and cricket.

Since connective tissue is present in all tissues and organs, disease that affects the connective tissue – the group of tissues that hold structures of the

Box 16.19 The symptoms of **sepsis** include fever, chills, shivering, and a rapid heart and breathing rate.

Recognition of the symptoms of sepsis in its earliest, most treatable phase is a public health issue and an essential aspect of the work of a health professional because, in some cases, severe sepsis can follow within hours. The Sepsis 6 is a bundle of six interventions, including oxygen therapy, intravenous fluids and antibiotics, that can be delivered by health professionals in the earliest stages.

Sepsis kills about 46,000 patients a year in the UK and causes millions of deaths worldwide.

Box 16.20 Signs of **anaphylactic shock:**
- swollen airways, making it difficult to breathe
- swollen eyes, lips, hands and feet
- itchy skin or a raised, red skin rash
- drop in blood pressure, causing dizziness, collapse and unconsciousness
- abdominal pain, nausea and vomiting.

body together (→ 2.5.2) – can affect any part of the body. The most common symptoms are joint pains, as experienced in arthritis (→ 4.5), skin rashes and tiredness, but other organs and systems are often affected.

16.6.1 Systemic lupus erythematosus

Systemic lupus erythematosus (SLE), commonly known as **lupus**, is an autoimmune disease (→ 14.9.3) of the connective tissue (→ 2.5.2). Like other more common autoimmune conditions, such as rheumatoid arthritis, it is thought that, in certain people, SLE is triggered by a combination of genetic and environmental factors.

Lupus is a disease which can present with many different symptoms. It is rare for two people to have exactly the same symptoms, which can vary from just one to many, be mild or severe, and change with time. The typical skin manifestations are 'butterfly rash' on the face and photosensitivity (sun allergy). The course of the disease is unpredictable with periods of illness (called flares) alternating with remissions (→ Box 16.21).

SLE occurs nine times more often in women than in men, especially in women aged 15–35, and is also more common in those of non-European descent. When SLE occurs in children, it generally presents between the ages of 3 and 15, with girls outnumbering boys 4:1.

Box 16.21 Lupus is a long-term, chronic and often disabling disorder that is sometimes known as 'the great imitator' because its symptoms are often confused with other diseases.

16.6.2 Marfan syndrome

Marfan syndrome is an inherited disorder caused by a defective gene that leads to abnormal production of a protein called fibrillin, which is essential for the formation of elastic fibres found in connective tissue. Typical characteristics of Marfan syndrome include:
- being tall
- abnormally long and slender limbs, fingers, and toes
- heart defects
- lens dislocation – the lens of the eye has an abnormal position.

The defective gene is an autosomal dominant allele (→ 13.6.2), which means there is a 50% chance that the child of a parent with Marfan syndrome will inherit the syndrome.

In some cases, neither parent has the syndrome, and the fibrillin gene changes (mutates) for the first time in the parent's egg or sperm.

16.6.3 Ehlers–Danlos syndromes

Collagen is a tough, fibrous protein that is a major architectural building block that provides both flexibility (e.g. cartilage) and strength (e.g. in bone) depending on where it is needed and located.

Ehlers–Danlos syndromes (EDS) are a group of disorders caused by different genetic alterations that affect collagen, with each subtype – of which there are at least thirteen – arising from distinct genetic change. People with EDS generally have problems involving skin, muscles, skeleton and blood vessels that predispose them to bruising, delayed wound healing, 'paper-thin' scars and hypermobile joints that are easily dislocated. People with each subtype will, however, have distinctive characteristics.

The disorder can be inherited as a dominant, recessive or spontaneous (*de novo*) genetic mutation.

Box 16.22 The effects on health make obesity one of the most important preventable health risks.

Box 16.23 Body Mass Index (BMI) is a simple index of weight-for-height that is commonly used to classify underweight, normal weight, overweight and obesity. It is defined as the weight of a person in kilograms divided by the square of their height in metres (kg/m²).

Box 16.24 Physical activity is important because it enables the energy in food (calories) to be used by the cells in the body and not stored as fat (→ Ch. 19).

Box 16.25 Age, gender, genetics and ethnicity are broad categories of factors that contribute to different patterns of adiposity (fat accumulation and distribution).

Taking it Further
Anthropometry is the measurement of body proportions.

Find out more about this kind of physiological observation in online Chapter 17.

Box 16.26 Excess adipose tissue packed within the abdominal cavity is strongly associated with cardiovascular risk in type 2 diabetes and **Alzheimer's disease**.

16.7 Obesity

Obesity is a term used to describe the physiological status of someone who is very overweight with a high degree of body fat (→ Boxes 16.22 and 16.23). It can be influenced by:

- a **sedentary lifestyle** and poor dietary habits learned during childhood (→ Box 16.24).
- certain **genetic traits** inherited from parents that exaggerate normal adiposity, disturb energy homeostasis and worsen metabolic syndrome (→ Box 16.25). These traits can make losing weight more difficult, but do not make it impossible.

16.7.1 Medical conditions and weight gain

Some medical conditions that can contribute to weight gain include:
- certain medicines, including some corticosteroids, antidepressants, antipsychotic medications and antidiabetic drugs
- Cushing's syndrome, a rare endocrine disorder that causes the over-production of steroid hormones by the adrenal glands
- an underactive thyroid gland (hypothyroidism)
- a side-effect of taking the combined contraceptive pill.

16.7.2 Psychological effects of obesity

People who are not happy with their weight may experience psychological difficulties such as low self-esteem and reluctance to mix with other people, which can lead to depression and affect relationships with family members and friends. The rising numbers of obese children and young people may be linked with the experience of bullying and isolation in schools.

16.7.3 The health risks associated with obesity

Obesity puts a strain on many of the body's systems, with wide-reaching effects on many body systems and aspects of long-term health:
- **impaired glucose tolerance** interferes with the ability to use insulin effectively
- **high cholesterol and lipid levels** in blood which can drive progression of atherosclerosis
- **osteoarthritis** due to excessive weight on the joints, causing pain which in turn prevents exercise and may lead to more weight gain
- **coronary heart disease** due to the higher risk of formation of plaques of fatty material which narrow the walls of arteries and increase the risk of heart attack or stroke
- **hypertension** – there is a close association between obesity and high blood pressure
- **Alzheimer's disease** (→ Box 16.26)
- **sleep apnoea** – a common disorder in people who have large fat stores around the neck; these narrow the airway and this leads to pauses in breathing while asleep
- increased risk of 13 different types of cancer including breast cancer and colon cancer.

16.8 Metabolic syndrome

Metabolic syndrome is the pathophysiological term for a combination of diabetes, hypertension (high blood pressure) and obesity, which increases the risk of heart disease and stroke (→ Box 16.27). This condition can develop in people who are within the normal weight range but the risk increases in:

- people with a sedentary lifestyle
- obese people with large amounts of visceral fat (→ Box 16.28)
- those with an inherited genetic tendency towards insulin resistance.

Signs of metabolic syndrome are:

- a waist circumference ≥94 cm (37 ins) for men and ≥80 cm (31.5 ins) for women
- high levels of LDL ('bad' cholesterol) and low levels of HDL ('good' cholesterol) in the blood, which can lead to atherosclerosis
- high blood pressure that is consistently ≥140/90 mmHg
- the inability to control blood glucose levels due to insulin resistance
- a tendency to develop inflammation (irritation and swelling of body tissue).

Box 16.27 Metabolic syndrome is estimated to affect one in four adults in the UK. It is especially prevalent in Asian and Afro-Caribbean people, and in women with polycystic ovary syndrome.

Box 16.28 Until recently adipose tissue was considered to be an inactive mass of stored fat but it is now known to produce physiologically active substances that directly influence insulin resistance and vascular injury. The development of blood clots such as deep vein thrombosis may be the first sign of metabolic syndrome in some people.

Key points

1. Multisystem disorders affect the physiological function of a number of body organs.
2. Diabetes is a metabolic disorder characterised by production of large volumes of urine, fatigue and excessive thirst, with the most common form being type 2 diabetes mellitus.
3. Stress is not a disease, but is characterised by an adverse reaction to perceived pressure when that pressure exceeds an individual's ability to cope; it can increase the risk of several major causes of premature mortality including hypertension, heart disease, respiratory disorders, cancer and suicide.
4. Circulatory shock is characterised by physical collapse and failure to maintain adequate blood pressure and oxygenation of organs.
5. Systemic lupus erythematosus (lupus) and Marfan syndrome are disorders of connective tissue and both affect all tissues and organs of the body.
6. The term metabolic syndrome refers to a trio of hypertension, diabetes and obesity that increase the risk of heart attack and stroke.

Test yourself! Go to *www.lanternpublishing.com/AandP* and try the questions to check your understanding.

GLOSSARY

100,000 Genome Project: the genomes of a large number of people are being sequenced to provide data for a new genomic medicine service

ABO system: universal system for classifying blood into four basic groups – A, B, AB and O

accessory muscles: not normally used for breathing but only when there is a high demand for gaseous exchange

accommodation: ability of the eye to change its focus

achondroplasia: a bone growth disorder that causes dwarfism

acid: in physiology, most often defined as a proton donor

acid–base balance: homeostatic regulation of the levels of acids and bases – and hence pH – of the body's extracellular fluid (ECF)

acidosis: occurs with either a rise in the amount of carbonic acid in extracellular fluid (ECF) or a decrease in the amount of bicarbonate (HCO_3^-) in ECF which, if uncompensated, would cause acidaemia

acinus: cluster of secretory cells at the terminal end of a duct of an exocrine gland (e.g. salivary gland or pancreas)

acne vulgaris: inflamed sebaceous glands, mostly on the face

acquired immunodeficiency syndrome (AIDS): progressive destruction of the immune system allowing life-threatening infections and cancers to thrive

actin: protein that forms the thin filaments in a sarcomere

action potential: change in electrical potential associated with the passage of an impulse along the plasma membrane of a neuron or muscle cell

active transport: uses energy to move substances across the plasma membrane against their concentration gradient

acute disease: short-term

acute respiratory distress syndrome (ARDS): type of respiratory failure characterised by trauma to the lungs caused by pneumonia, septic shock or breathing in noxious chemicals

adaptive (active) immunity: third line of defence against pathogens which is specific

addiction: compulsion to do something that can interfere with everyday life

Addison's disease: endocrine disorder characterised by adrenal damage

adenohypophysis: anterior pituitary gland

adenylate cyclase: enzyme in all cells that takes part in signal transduction

adipocytes: cells which store fat

adipose tissue: connective tissue packed with adipose (fat) cells

adrenal medulla: secretes adrenaline

adrenocorticotrophic hormone (ACTH): hormone from the anterior pituitary gland that controls the secretion of hormones from the adrenal cortex

aerobic bacteria: bacteria that require oxygen to survive

aerobic respiration: metabolic pathway that uses oxygen to release energy from glucose

afferent: neuron that conveys impulses to the central nervous system

afterload: pressure against which the heart must push to eject blood during systole

afterpains: pains after childbirth caused by contractions of the uterus

age-related macular degeneration (AMD): painless eye condition that leads to gradual loss of central vision due to changes in the macula of the retina

agglutination: a reaction in which red cells in the blood clump together

agnosia: difficulty in making sense of pictures, shapes and objects

agonist: a drug that triggers a response in the target cell

airway: path that air normally follows to get in and out of the lungs, with nose, mouth and trachea being normal entry points

albumin: plasma protein that helps to maintain osmotic pressure in the blood

alcohol dehydrogenase: an enzyme that breaks down alcohol to acetaldehyde (an even more toxic molecule)

aldosterone: corticosteroid hormone that stimulates the kidneys to absorb sodium

algor mortis: after-death change in body temperature to environmental temperature

alimentary canal (gastrointestinal tract; gut): tube about 9 m long in adults that extends from the mouth to the anus in which food is digested and absorbed

alkali: base

alkalosis: occurs when body fluids have too many bases; can be because of decreased blood levels of carbon dioxide or can be due to increased blood levels of HCO_3^-

alleles: alternative forms of a gene

allergy: immune reaction to a substance to which the body has become hypersensitive

alopecia: hair loss

alveolar sacs: air sacs in the lungs where gaseous exchange between air and blood takes place

Alzheimer's disease: progressive degenerative disease that affects brain function

amenorrhoea: absence of menstrual periods

amino acids: the building block of proteins; arranged in a variety of ways to form a vast number of different proteins

amnesia: profound disturbance of memory

amygdala: almond-shaped group of neurons on each side of the limbic cortex responsible for detecting fear and preparing for emergency events

amylase: digestive enzyme that splits up starch to maltose

amyotrophic lateral sclerosis (ALS): motor neurone disease

anabolic reactions: use ATP to synthesise (build up) macromolecules from smaller ones

anaemia: deficiency of haemoglobin, the red pigment in red cells that carries oxygen

anaerobic bacteria: bacteria that do not grow in the presence of oxygen

anaerobic respiration: a type of respiration that does not use oxygen

anaesthetic: drugs which make the body unable to feel pain

analgesia: loss of sensation of pain without loss of consciousness

analgesics: agents that produce diminished perception of pain without loss of consciousness

anaphylactic shock (anaphylaxis): severe allergic reaction that can develop rapidly

anatomical nomenclature: standard method of naming the position of anatomical structures

anatomy: structure of the human body

androgens: male sex hormones

angiogenesis: development of new blood vessels

angiotensin II: plasma that is a powerful vasoconstrictor and which promotes the secretion of aldosterone

angiotensin-converting enzyme: enzyme in the lung that converts angiotensin I to angiotensin II

angular gyrus: region of the brain involved in processes related to language, number processing, spatial cognition and memory retrieval

ankylosing spondylitis: chronic inflammation that mainly affects the lower part of the spine

annulus: strong outer ring of fibrocartilage of an intervertebral disc

anorexia nervosa: extreme self-induced undernutrition

antagonist: a drug that blocks a receptor response rather than activating it

anterior cavity of the eye: fluid-filled space between the cornea and the lens

antibiotics: chemicals that kill or inhibit the growth of bacteria

antibodies (Ab): immunoglobulins

antidiuretic hormone (ADH): prevents the production of dilute urine

antigen: substance that stimulates the production of antibodies

antigen-binding sites: site on an antibody molecule that binds to a specific antigen in a lock-and-key fashion

antigen presentation: link between innate and adaptive immunity as both macrophages and lymphocytes are involved

antigen-presenting cell: specialised cell that can 'present' an antigen to a T lymphocyte

anti-infective agents: protect against infection by microorganism

antiseptics: chemicals used on people to destroy or inhibit the growth of pathogens

antiserum: contains ready-made antibodies

anxiety: feeling fearful, tense or worried

APGAR score: assesses the physiological status of newborn babies

aphasia: disturbance in the production and/or expression of language

aphthous stomatitis (canker sores): mouth ulcers of unknown cause

apnoea: temporary cessation of breathing

apocrine sweat glands: secrete sweat containing sebum; characteristic odours are produced by bacterial action

apoptosis (programmed cell death): sequence of events that eliminates cells without releasing harmful substances that destroy surrounding tissue

appendicular skeleton: pectoral and pelvic girdles and the limbs attached to them

appetite: the physical desire for food, felt as hunger

aqueous humour: watery fluid in the space between the cornea and lens in the eyes

arachnoid mater: delicate cobweb-like middle layer of the meninges

areolar tissue: loose connective tissue that holds organs together

arteries: blood vessels that carry away from the heart

arterioles: small arteries with smooth muscle fibres in their wall

arthritis: inflammation of a joint which causes pain and limits movement

articular cartilage: covers the surfaces where a bone forms a synovial joint with another bone

ascending tracts (somatosensory pathways): bundles of afferent nerve fibres in the spinal cord that carry sensory impulses to the brain

asthma: inflammation of the airways that causes difficulty in breathing and wheezing

astigmatism: occurs when the cornea is unevenly curved and distorts vision

astrocytes (astroglia): star-shaped glial cells found throughout the central nervous system

atomic number: the number of protons in the nucleus of the atom

atom: the smallest particle of an element

ATP (adenosine triphosphate): high-energy molecule that supplies cells with energy

ATP–ADP cycle: a coupled process during which energy is stored in ATP and then released, leaving ADP and a phosphate group free to be re-used to make more ATP

ATP–PC system: process that provides energy during the first 5–8 seconds of exercise

atrioventricular bundle (AV bundle): bundle of fibres that carries impulses from the AV node through the atria to the septum separating the ventricles

atrioventricular node (AV node): a cluster of cells in the centre of the heart that delays the cardiac impulse before it is allowed to travel onwards from atria to ventricles

atrophy: waste away

attention deficit hyperactivity disorder (ADHD): condition characterised by short attention span, hyperactivity and impulsiveness

auditory cortex: processes auditory information (sounds)

autism: developmental disorder characterised by difficulty in social interaction and communication

autocrine signalling: occurs when a cell secretes a signalling molecule that may bind to receptors on the same cell

autolysis: when a cell dies the enzymes are released from lysosomes and break down the cell itself

autonomic nervous system: part of the nervous system responsible for involuntary control of functions such as breathing, heartbeat and digestion

autosomal recessive disorder: develops when an individual inherits two recessive alleles for that disorder

autosomes: chromosomes numbered 1–22 (excludes the sex chromosomes)

axon: nerve fibre that carries impulses away from the cell body

azoospermia: absence of sperm from semen

B cells: B lymphocytes

balanitis: inflammation of the glans (head of the penis)

baroreceptors: stretch receptors in blood vessels that respond to changes in blood pressure

baroreflex: homeostatic mechanisms for short-term regulation of blood pressure

Bartholin's glands: two glands beside the vaginal opening that secrete fluid during coitus

basal membrane: thin matrix that separates a layer of epithelium from underlying tissues

basal metabolic rate: the minimum amount of energy required to keep the body alive and functioning at rest

base (alkali): in physiology, base is most often described as a proton acceptor

base pair: the pairs of nucleotides that form the 'rungs' of the double helix

basophils: white cells involved in inflammation; they secrete histamine which promotes blood flow to tissues and heparin, which prevents blood from clotting too quickly

benign prostatic hyperplasia (BPH): enlarged prostate gland

benign tumour: non-malignant as it is not invading surrounding tissue or spreading to other sites

bicarbonate: neutralises acid and plays an essential role in acid–base homeostasis in the body

bile: yellow or greenish fluid which is secreted by the liver, stored in the gall bladder and aids the digestion of fat

bile duct: carries bile from the liver to the intestine

bilirubin: yellow pigment from the breakdown of red cells and excreted in bile, faeces and urine

binocular vision: when an object is viewed with both eyes

bioavailability: the portion of a drug that reaches the systemic circulation unchanged

biofilms: colonies of free-living bacteria that stick to each other and form slime

biotransformation: the way the intensity of a drug effect is determined by metabolic processes in the body

bipolar disorder: alternating periods of hypomania and severe depression

birth canal: channel formed by the uterus, cervix and vagina during parturition (labour)

bladder: hollow muscular sac that stores urine

blastocyst: fertilised egg about seven days after ovulation

blood bank: stores blood and blood components in sterile conditions

blood–brain barrier: membrane that separates blood in capillaries in the brain from the cerebrospinal fluid

blood pressure (BP): the force that blood exerts on the walls of blood vessels or the chambers of the heart. It is usually measured in the brachial artery

botulism: very severe form of food poisoning caused by the pathogen *Clostridium botulinum*

Bowman's capsule: cup-like structure at the beginning of a nephron

bradycardia: slower than normal heart rate (pulse)

brainstem: enlarged extension of the spinal cord in the brain responsible for control of the internal organs

brainstem death: occurs when a person no longer has any activity in the brainstem and therefore no potential for consciousness or independent breathing

Braxton Hicks contractions: sporadic tightening of the uterus

breathing (ventilation): regular and mainly automatic process in which air is alternately inhaled and exhaled

breech presentation: baby born bottom or leg first instead of head first

Broca's area: region of the brain involved in speech production situated in the frontal lobe of the cerebral hemisphere (usually the left)

bronchioles: narrower air tubes in which spirals of muscle tissue gradually replace cartilage

bronchitis: obstructive inflammation of the lining of the bronchi (the main airways of the lungs)

bronchus: large, branching air tube in the lungs

bruise: *see* haematoma

Brunner's glands: secrete an alkaline fluid that coats the duodenal wall and protects it from acid chyme

buffer: a solution that can resist a change of pH when a small amount of acid or of base is added to it

bulbo-urethral glands (Cowper's glands): pair of small glands that open into the urethra at the base of the penis

bulimia nervosa: a condition in which people have a persistent preoccupation with eating and a morbid dread of fatness

bundle of His: *see* atrioventricular bundle

bunion: swollen joint on the big toe

cachexia: weakness and weight loss as a result of severe illness

caesarean section (C section): delivery of a baby through a surgical incision in the mother's abdomen and uterus

calcitonin: hormone that lowers the level of calcium and phosphate in the blood

calcium: chemical element with symbol Ca and atomic number 20 which plays an essential role in physiological and biochemical processes

calluses: hard, rough areas of skin

cancer: one cell or a group of cells multiplies more rapidly than is necessary, typically forming a swelling called a tumour or growth

Candida albicans: a yeast (type of fungus) that normally lives harmlessly in the digestive tract and on skin but can sometimes cause thrush in the mouth, vulva or vagina

capillaries: network of tiny blood vessels with very thin walls that allow the exchange of substances between blood and tissues

capillary beds: interconnecting networks of capillaries between arterioles and venules

carbohydrate: compound containing atoms of carbon, hydrogen and oxygen

carbon: chemical element with atomic number 6 and symbol C which is the common element of all known life

carbon cycle: the pathway taken by carbon in various forms as it circulates continuously between the air, oceans, plants, animals and soil

carcinogens: substances capable of causing cancer

carcinoma: cancer arising from epithelial tissue of the skin or internal organs

cardiac cycle: sequence of events between one heartbeat and the next that ensure forward propulsion of blood

cardiac output: volume of blood ejected by the ventricles each minute

cardiac sphincter: ring of smooth muscle surrounding the opening between the oesophagus and stomach that prevents reflux into the oesophagus

cardiac tamponade: build-up of fluid or blood in the pericardial cavity

cardiogenic shock: heart muscle cannot function as an effective pump and it is unable to maintain circulation

cardiomyocytes: cardiac (heart) muscle cells that generate electrical impulses spontaneously and rhythmically

cardiovascular system: consists of heart, blood vessels and lymphatic system

carrier: person who harbours infectious pathogens without ill effect. Can also be a person who is not affected by a genetic disease but who is able to pass it on

carrier-assisted transport: uses carrier proteins in the plasma membrane to move molecules into or out of a cell

catabolic reactions: release ATP when macro-molecules are broken down into smaller ones

catalyst: substance that speeds up a chemical reaction without itself being changed

cataract: lens of the eye becomes progressively opaque, resulting in blurred vision

cauda equina: bundle of nerves from the lumbar, sacral and coccygeal regions of the spinal cord

cell: tiny unit of living matter

cell checkpoint: decision points in the cell cycle when the process can be halted until conditions are favourable for cell division

cell cycle: highly regulated sequence of events that occur when a cell divides to produce two new cells by the process of mitosis

cell division: the division of a cell into two daughter cells

cell lysis: cell destruction by rupture of the plasma membrane

cell membrane: *see* plasma membrane

cellular respiration: set of metabolic reactions that release of energy in the form of ATP in living cells that is required for all the cell's activities

central nervous system (CNS): composed of brain and spinal cord

centrioles: pair of organelles involved in cell division

cerebellum: part of the back of the brain that coordinates and regulates muscular activity

cerebral cortex: the outer layer of the cerebrum composed of folded grey matter that plays an important role in consciousness

cerebral haemorrhage (haemorrhagic stroke): occurs when blood vessels burst within the brain

cerebral hemispheres: two halves of the brain connected by the corpus callosum

cerebral palsy (CP): general term for a number of neurological conditions that affect movement and coordination

cerebrospinal fluid (CSF): colourless fluid that circulates through the brain and spinal cord

cerebrum: largest part of the brain, consisting of two cerebral hemispheres

cerumen (earwax): secreted by modified sebaceous glands in the auditory canal

cervical cancer: a form of cancer that is linked to infection with the human papillomavirus (HPV) that causes genital warts

cervical mucus (CM): produced by the epithelium that lines the cervix and undergoes changes in consistency during the menstrual cycle

cervix (neck of the womb): canal between the uterus and vagina

Chagas' disease: parasitic disease spread by insect vectors mainly in Latin America

chain of infection: sequence of events that happens for a pathogen to pass from one person to another

channel-mediated diffusion: occurs when protein molecules in membranes have a pore or channel that allows a specific substance to pass through

chemical bond: the force of attraction that holds atoms together in a molecule

chemical reaction: the rearrangement of atoms to form different substances

chemical signal molecule (first messenger): substance such as a hormone or cytokine which is released into body fluids that brings about a response inside a cell

chemoreceptor trigger zone: area of the medulla oblongata that is stimulated by drugs and other chemicals in the blood to communicate with the vomiting centre

chemotaxis: movement of white cells in response to the stimulus of a gradient of chemical concentration

chemotherapy: treatment that uses chemicals to destroy cancerous tissue

Cheyne–Stokes respiration: abnormal pattern of breathing that can be deep and rapid, interrupted by periods of apnoea

chiasma: point of contact at which exchange of genetic material takes place during the first meiotic division

chloride: negatively charged ion in extracellular fluids in association with sodium (sodium chloride NaCl)

cholecystokinin (CCK): hormone secreted by cells of the duodenal wall that stimulates the delivery of bile

cholestatic pruritus: intense sensation of itching that is associated with many forms of liver disease

cholesterol: fat-like substance present in the blood and most tissues throughout the body which is a precursor for steroid hormones, bile acids and vitamin D

chondrocytes: cells which secrete the cartilage matrix

chordae tendineae: thin, strong cords that anchor the tricuspid and mitral valves to the walls of the ventricles

choroid: thin, black, middle layer of the eyeball wall containing melanin and the main blood vessels

chromatin: substance in the nucleus, consisting of DNA, RNA and various proteins, that forms chromosomes during cell division

chromosome: long, thin, coiled macromolecule of DNA which contains part of the genetic material in a human cell

chromosome mutation: occurs when there is a change in the number of chromosomes or in the structure of one of the chromosomes

chronic disease: disease or condition that is long-term or frequently recurring

chronic fatigue syndrome (CFS) (myalgic encephalomyelitis): complex condition that typically occurs after infection and limits a person's ability to carry out ordinary daily activities

chronic obstructive pulmonary disease (COPD): collective term for lung disease that include chronic bronchitis and emphysema

chyme: semi-fluid mass of partly digested food and digestive juices

ciliary epithelium of the eye: produces aqueous humour

ciliary muscle of the eye: ring of smooth muscle that controls accommodation (focusing) of the lens

ciliary processes: suspend the lens

circle of Willis: system of arteries that encircles the base of the brain

circumcision: removal of the prepuce (foreskin) by surgery

cirrhosis: progressive disease in which healthy liver tissue is replaced by abnormal, lumpy, fibrous tissue

citric acid cycle (Krebs cycle): a series of chemical reactions to release energy from pyruvic acid

clavicles (collarbones): support the scapulae

clinical depression: feeling persistently and deeply sad for weeks or months, not just unhappy or fed-up for a few days

clitoris: small organ composed of erectile tissue; the female counterpart to the penis

clone: a group of identical cells that are derived from the same cell and hence share a common ancestry

coagulation: *see* haemostasis

coccyx: small bone at the end of the vertebral column formed from four fused sacral vertebrae

cochlea: sensory part of the inner ear concerned with hearing

co-dominant alleles: form of a gene that have equal dominance

codon: composed of three DNA or mRNA nucleotides arranged in a particular sequence that corresponds with a specific amino acid

coeliac disease: autoimmune disease that results in hypersensitivity to gluten

coenzymes: substances necessary to enhance and improve enzyme performance

cofactors: substances that must be present before certain enzymes can act

cognitive behavioural therapy (CBT): psychological therapy that helps people to change how they think ('cognition') and what they do ('behaviour')

coitus: sexual intercourse

colloid: mixture in which the particles are too small to ever settle out of the solvent, e.g. milk or jelly

colon: part of the large intestine that reabsorbs water back into the body

colostrum: early fluid produced by the breasts during lactation that is rich in antibodies

co-morbidity: two or more diseases existing together

compact bone: forms the hard outer shell of a bone

compartment syndrome: swelling within an enclosed bundle of muscles that can lead to ischaemia and necrosis in the affected area

complement proteins (complement): part of the innate immune system involved in inflammation, cell lysis (destruction) and opsonisation

compound: a molecule composed of two or more atoms

conception (fertilisation): fusion of male and female gametes

conduction velocity: speed at which nerve impulses travel

cones: photoreceptors in the retina responsible for colour vision and which work best in bright light

congenital heart disorders: range of birth defects that affect the normal workings of the heart

conjunctiva: mucous membrane that covers the cornea and lines the inner surface of the eyelid

conjunctivitis: infection and inflammation of the conjunctiva

connective tissue: tissue that provides physical support for other tissues and anchors them within the body

contagious disease: disease that is transmitted by contact

contraception: deliberate prevention of pregnancy

contraction cycle: series of events that results in contraction of a skeletal muscle

convalescence: time during which symptoms disappear and the patient regains strength

convergence: simultaneous movement of both eyes to focus on the same object

cord prolapse: when the umbilical cord drops through the open cervix into the vagina ahead of the baby

cornea: transparent layer of tissue at the front of the eye

corneal refraction: light rays enter the cornea and are refracted (bent) and brought into focus on the retina

corns: small circles of thick skin that develop on the toes

coronal plane: runs perpendicular to the sagittal plane and divides the body into front (anterior) and back (posterior) portions

corpus callosum: bundle of nerve fibres that connect the two cerebral hemispheres

corpus luteum: formed from an ovarian follicle and produces progesterone

corticospinal tract (pyramidal tract): column of nerve fibres that form a pathway from the cerebral cortex to the spinal cord

corticosteroids: steroid hormones secreted by the adrenal cortex

corticotrophin-releasing hormone (CRH): stimulates the release of adrenocorticotrophic hormone from the anterior pituitary

cortisol: steroid hormone from the adrenal gland that helps to control the use of glucose

costal cartilage: connects the ends of the ribs to the sternum

cough reflex: normal protective action to clear the airways

covalent bonds: atoms share electrons

Cowper's glands: *see* bulbo-urethral glands

cranial nerves: nerves that arise directly from the brainstem

cranium: skeletal structure of the skull

crenation: process due to osmosis that causes shrinkage of cells

cretinism: congenital disorder that is a result of hypothyroidism

Crohn's disease: inflammatory disease that can affect any part of the gastrointestinal tract

crossing over (recombination): occurs during meiosis when segments of chromosome are exchanged

crowning: baby's head emerges from the birth canal

cryoprecipitate: extract of blood clotting factors obtained from plasma

cryptorchidism: undescended testicles

crystallins: family of proteins that enable the lens to refract light whilst maintaining its transparency

cyanosis: bluish discolouration of the skin and mucous membranes

cyclo-oxygenases: family of enzymes involved in production of prostaglandins

cystic fibrosis: an autosomal recessive disease that causes build-up of sticky mucus

cytokines (signalling molecules): chemical signals involved in immunity and inflammation

cytoplasm: semifluid substance in the cell that contains the organelles

cytoskeleton: 3D structure consisting of protein tubules and fibres that support the cell and give it shape

deamination: the breakdown of amino acids to nitrogenous waste which can be excreted in urine

death: the end of a person's life on earth

deep vein thrombosis (DVT): blood clot that forms an obstruction in a vein

deglutition: swallowing

dementia: range of degenerative disorders characterised by death of neurons in the brain

dendrites: short, branching nerve fibres that carry impulses into the cell body

dendritic cells: cells that are specialised for presenting antigens to lymphocytes to initiate adaptive immunity

dental caries: tooth decay caused by softening of enamel and dentine due to acids made by bacteria

depolarisation: change in membrane potential of a cell when the inside becomes more positive (less negative) than at rest

dermis: middle layer of the skin

descending tracts: bundles of efferent nerve fibres in the spinal cord that carry motor impulses from the brain to the different parts of the body

detrusor muscle: contracts and expels urine from the bladder

developmental dysplasia of the hip (DDH): congenital condition in which the ball and socket joint of the hip is shallow, leading to dislocation

diabetes mellitus: chronic disorder resulting from defects in insulin production or its action on the body

diagnosis: process of determining the nature of the disease by clinical consideration of the patient's signs, symptoms and medical history

dialysis: artificial process of eliminating waste products and unwanted water from the blood by ultrafiltration

diapedesis: movement of white cells through the intact walls of capillaries

diaphysis: mid section of a long bone

diastole: the time of ventricular relaxation when the ventricles fill with blood from the veins

diencephalon: connects the cerebrum to the midbrain

dietary fibre: plant-based carbohydrate that cannot be digested in the small intestine and thus reaches the large intestine

diffusion: net movement of molecules from an area of higher concentration to an area of lower concentration along a concentration gradient

digestive system: comprises the alimentary canal and accessory organs of digestion

dihydrotestosterone: hormone from the testes that stimulates the development of male characteristics

diploid: two sets of chromosomes in a cell, one set from each parent

disaccharide: molecule that contains two simple sugar units linked by a glycosidic bond

disease: condition that impairs the normal functioning of the body

disinfectant: used to sterilise items that touch intact skin but do not penetrate the tissue

disorder: functional abnormality that may be used to distinguish physical disorders from infectious disease

disseminated disease: spreads to other parts of the body

DNA (deoxyribonucleic acid): material that carries genetic information

DNA repair genes: responsible for fixing and repairing DNA that has become damaged

DNA sequencing: laboratory process that identifies the order in which nucleotide bases of DNA are arranged

dominant alleles: form of a gene that masks the effect of recessive alleles

dopamine: neurotransmitter in the brain

double helix: the spiral shape of a double-stranded DNA molecule

Down syndrome: congenital disorder caused by the possession of an extra chromosome 21 (trisomy)

droplet infection: mode of transmission of infectious disease in minute droplets sprayed from an infected person in coughs and sneezes

drug: a medicine or other substance which has a physiological effect when introduced into the body

dry (atrophic) age-related macular degeneration (AMD): reduced blood supply to the macula with gradual loss of vision

ductus arteriosus: blood vessel in the foetal heart that connects the pulmonary artery to the descending aorta

ductus venosus: blood vessel in the foetus that connects the hepatic portal vein to the umbilical vein

duodenum: first part of the small intestine

dura mater: tough, strong outer layer of the meninges

dyslexia: difficulties in learning to read or interpret words, letters and other symbols

dyspepsia (indigestion; heartburn): pain or discomfort in the upper abdomen after eating

dysphagia: difficulty in swallowing

dysphoric milk ejection reflex (D-MER): abnormality of the milk ejection reflex that produces a state of unease just prior to milk ejection

dysplasia: cells lose the special features of the tissue in which they are growing and become abnormal

dyspnoea (shortness of breath; breathlessness): difficulty in breathing, sometimes accompanied by tightness in the chest; most commonly caused by exercise, being at high altitude, respiratory disease or anxiety

dyspraxia (clumsiness): developmental coordination disorder affecting planning of muscle movements and speech

eccrine sweat glands: secrete a colourless fluid to the skin surface

ectocervix (external os): the opening of the cervix into the vagina

ectoparasites: parasites that live on the skin

ectopic pregnancy: when a fertilised egg does not reach the uterus but remains in the fallopian tube

eczema (dermatitis): dry skin that is scaly, red and itchy

effacement: dilation of the cervix during birth

efferent: neurons that convey impulses away from the central nervous system

elastic cartilage: form of connective tissue that contains elastic fibres scattered throughout a solid but flexible matrix

electrocardiogram (ECG): records the heart's rhythm and electrical activity via electrodes on the skin

electroencephalogram (EEG): records brain wave activity via electrodes on the scalp

electrolytes: solutions that contain ions dissolved in water, blood or other body fluid

electron: a subatomic particle which carries one unit of negative electrical charge

electron transfer chain: chain of carrier molecules that transfer electrons from one carrier to the next to release energy

element: chemical substance consisting of atoms that have the same number of protons and cannot be broken down using chemical reactions

elephantiasis: disease caused by parasitic worms which become lodged in lymphatic vessels and block the flow of lymph

embolus: a thrombus, blood clot, air bubble, piece of fatty deposit or other object that travels in the bloodstream to lodge in a blood vessel and block it

emergency contraception: pill to prevent pregnancy following unprotected coitus

emesis (vomiting): reverse peristalsis

emphysema: disorder in which air sacs in the lungs become permanently damaged

endemic: disease that is always present in a particular population or in a certain area

endocarditis: inflammation of the endocardium

endocrine glands: ductless glands that manufacture one or more hormones and secrete them directly into the bloodstream

endocrine signalling: form of cell–cell communication that is carried out by hormones released into the bloodstream which bind with hormone receptors on the target cells

endocrine system: collection of glands that secrete hormones

endocrinology: study of hormones and the clinical practice related to hormones

endocytosis: process by which cells take in substances by engulfing them

endogenous: originating within the body

endogenous opioids (endorphins): produced by the central nervous system and pituitary gland that reduce the perception of pain

endometriosis: tissue similar to that in the uterus growing in other places in the abdomen

endometrium: the inner layer of the uterus wall that is shed during menstruation

endoplasmic reticulum (ER): network of membrane-bound canals in the cytoplasm

endothelium: tissue formed from a single layer of cells that line the heart, blood vessels and lymphatic vessels

energy balance: achieved by matching the intake of food with energy used by the body's activities

enosmia: permanent damage to the sense of smell

enteric division: division of the nervous system that governs gastrointestinal motility and secretions

Entonox: analgesic mixture of gas containing oxygen and nitrous oxide

enzyme: a protein made by a living cell that acts as a catalyst to increase the rate (speed) of chemical reactions

enzyme activators: bind to enzymes to increase their activity

eosinophils: white cells that destroy parasites

ependymal cells: columnar cells that line the cavities and canals in the brain and spinal cord through which cerebrospinal fluid flows

epidemic: disease that spreads rapidly and infects a large number of people

epidemiology: study and analysis of the distribution and determinants of health and disease

epidermis: outer layer of the skin

epididymal cyst: lump caused by a collection of fluid in the epididymis

epidural: injection of anaesthetic to block the sensation of pain below the waist

epiglottis: flap of cartilage located in the throat that stops food passing into the airway

epilepsy: a neurological disorder of the brain marked by sudden recurrent episodes of sensory disturbance, loss of consciousness, or seizures

epiphyseal plates: plates of tissue at each end of a long bone where growth in length takes place

episiotomy: surgical cut at the opening of the vagina to widen the birth canal

epistaxis: nosebleed

epithelium: tissue that covers the outside and inside surfaces of the body and forms many glands

erectile dysfunction (ED): inability to get or keep an erection firm enough to have coitus

erepsin: enzyme that splits up peptides to amino acids

erogenous zones: parts of the body that excite sexual feelings

erythema: heat and redness caused by dilation of the blood vessels and the increased blood flow to the area

erythrocytes: red cells in the blood

erythropoietin: hormone produced by the kidney that promotes the formation of red blood cells by the bone marrow

essential amino acids: cannot be synthesised in the body so it is vital that they are present in the diet

essential fatty acids: cannot be made in the body and must be obtained from foods

estimated date of delivery (EDD): the date on which a baby is most likely to be born

ethmoid bone: part of the skull which separates the nasal cavity from the brain

eumelanin: pigment that has two sub-types, black and brown – found in the skin of both light- and dark-complexioned people but in different amounts

Eustachian tube (pharyngotympanic tube): links the middle ear to the throat

excretion: removal of the waste products of metabolism to the external environment

exocrine glands: discharge their secretions through a duct into an external environment

exocytosis: transport of substances out of a cell in vesicles

exogenous: originating outside the body

expiration: the act of exhaling air out of the lungs

external respiration: exchange of oxygen and carbon dioxide between the air and the body which takes place in the lungs

extracellular fluid: all the fluid in the body that is not contained inside the cells

extraocular muscles: six muscles that control movement of the eyeball and one muscle that controls the eyelid

extrapyramidal effects: movement disturbances that can be experienced as side-effects of antipsychotic agents, e.g. restlessness, dystopia or parkinsonism

extrinsic sugar: all sugars added to foods by manufacturers, cooks or consumers and those in honey, syrups and unsweetened fruit juices

facets: flat surfaces that form joints with neighbouring vertebrae

facilitated diffusion: the passive movement of molecules across a membrane via specific integral proteins

factor VIII: a protein essential for blood clotting

facultative anaerobes: microorganisms that can live with or without oxygen

faecal–oral transmission: transmission of microorganisms from contaminated faeces to the mouth of another person

faeces: undigested food remains mixed with gut microbiota, mucus, bilirubin and water

fallopian tubes (oviducts): connect the ovaries to the uterus

fatty acid: a long hydrocarbon chain with a methyl group at one end and a carboxylic group at the other end

febrile response: fever

feedback system: homeostatic (self-correcting) process in which the input is used to control the output

female infertility: inability to conceive and bear children

fertilisation: fusion of the nuclei of male and female gametes (sperm and egg) to form a zygote

fever (pyrexia; febrile response): rise in body temperature above the normal range of 36.5–37.5°C

fibrinogens: plasma protein that help blood clots to form and stop bleeding

fibrocytes: cells in connective tissue that synthesise fibres and the gel-like matrix in which the fibres are embedded

fibroids: non-cancerous growths that develop in and around the uterus

fibrous tissue: consists mainly of bundles of collagen fibres

filum terminale: tapering end of the meninges

first messenger: hormone that binds to a protein receptor on the plasma membrane of the target cell in a lock-and-key manner

first pass effect: the amount of a drug that is lost on its journey from the mouth to the systemic circulation, generally related to liver activity

flare-up disease: refers to either the recurrence of symptoms or an onset of more severe symptoms

flatulence: excessive gas (flatus) in the digestive tract that is released through the anus

foetal alcohol syndrome (FAS): mental and physical defects associated with high alcohol consumption by the mother during pregnancy

foetal haemoglobin: has a greater affinity for oxygen than adult haemoglobin

foetus: developing baby from about 2 months after conception

follicle-stimulating hormone (FSH): anterior pituitary hormone that controls the production of eggs in the ovaries and sperm in the testes

follicular phase: phase in the menstrual cycle when a follicle in the ovary prepares for ovulation

fomites: non-living objects or substances capable of transmitting infection

fontanelles: flat triangular soft membranous gaps (soft spots) between cranial bones in a baby's skull

foramen ovale: small opening in the septum between the atria (upper chambers) of the foetal heart

fornix: band of nerve fibres linking the hypothalamus and hippocampus

fractionated blood: blood separated into its component parts

fragile X syndrome: inherited condition caused by the change to a gene on the X chromosome that results in a wide range of difficulties in learning, language and behaviour

G proteins: family of proteins that act as molecular switches inside cells

gallstones: small hard stones composed of cholesterol or bile salts that commonly form in the gall bladder

gametes: sperm and eggs, each with a haploid set of chromosomes

ganglion cells: cells in the retina sensitive to day length and which contain melanopsin

gangrene: death (necrosis) of soft tissue caused by loss of blood supply

gaseous exchange: movement of oxygen and carbon dioxide between air, blood and tissues across capillary membranes

gastrin: hormone that stimulates the secretion of gastric juices

gastroenteritis: inflammation of the lining of the stomach (gastritis) and intestines (enteritis)

gastrointestinal (GI) tract: alimentary canal

gated channels: proteins in cell membranes that provide a passageway for ions in response to stimulus

gene: sequence of nucleotide bases in DNA that contains the instructions for making a particular protein

gene expression: process by which a gene (sequence of DNA base pairs) is used to build a protein required by the cell

genetic profile (genetic fingerprinting): individual's unique pattern of DNA

genetics: study of heredity and the variation of inherited characteristics

genome: complete set of DNA in a cell

genome project: genomes of 100,000 people that were sequenced to provide data for a new genomic medicine service

genotype: defined as the complete set of genes inherited by an individual

germicides: chemicals used to destroy microbial pathogens

gestational diabetes: form of diabetes that occurs during pregnancy

ghrelin: hormone secreted by the stomach that stimulates the feeling of being hungry

gingivitis (gum disease): inflammation of the gums at the neck of teeth caused by bacteria, making them swollen and sore

gland: organ or group of cells that are specialised for synthesising and secreting a substance

Glasgow Coma Scale (GCS): system used to provide an initial assessment of a person's level of consciousness

glaucoma: increased pressure within the eyeball, causing gradual loss of sight

glia (microglia): specialised connective tissue in the nervous system

glomerulus: network of capillaries enclosed in Bowman's capsule of the nephron

glottis: V-shaped opening between the vocal cords

glucagon: pancreatic hormone that promotes the breakdown of glycogen to glucose

gluconeogenesis: conversion of amino acids or lipids into glucose during periods of fasting glucosuria: excess glucose sugar in the urine

glycogenolysis: breakdown of glycogen

glycolipids: fatty acids or lipids with a carbohydrate unit attached via a glycosidic bond

glycolysis: the process in which one glucose molecule is broken down to form two molecules of pyruvic acid

glycoprotein: a molecule with a carbohydrate chain attached to a protein

glycosidic bond: bonds between the sugar units

glymphatic system: waste clearance system in the central nervous system

goitre: benign enlargement of the thyroid gland

Golgi apparatus: processes materials made in the cell for secretion in vesicles

gonadotrophin-releasing hormone (GnRH): hormone from the hypothalamus that stimulates release of gonadotrophin hormones (LH and FSH) from the anterior pituitary

gonads: the organs that produce gametes – sperm or eggs

gout: type of arthritis in which small crystals of uric acid form inside a joint

G-protein (guanine nucleotide-binding protein): family of proteins whose function is to transmit a signal from a stimulus outside a cell to its interior

Gram stain: a dye used to distinguish between two groups of bacteria

granulomas: clusters of white cells that form in inflamed tissue

grey matter: nervous tissue that contains neuron cell bodies

growth hormones (GH; somatotrophin): hormone from the anterior pituitary that stimulates growth of the bones and muscles

gustation: act of tasting

gut flora: see gut microbiota

gut microbiota (gut flora): vast numbers of microorganisms that live in the colon

gyrus: raised area on the surface of the brain

haematology: the study of blood and blood disorders

haematoma (bruise): solid swelling of clotted blood in tissues

haematopoiesis (haemopoiesis): process of producing blood cells and platelets in the bone marrow

haemodialysis: uses a machine called an artificial kidney to filter blood

haemoglobinopathies: group of inherited diseases in which there is an abnormality in the production of haemoglobin

haemolytic disease of the newborn: see rhesus disease

haemolytic transfusion reaction: release of haemoglobin into the blood caused by the disintegration of red cells in the skin

haemophilia: disorder in which the blood's ability to clot is severely reduced

haemorrhage: bleeding or abnormal loss of blood

haemorrhagic stroke: see cerebral haemorrhage

haemostasis: process that causes bleeding to stop when blood vessels are injured

half-life: the time it takes for the effectiveness of a drug to be reduced by half

haploid: half the number of chromosome in the gamete

Hashimoto's disease (thyroiditis): chronic inflammation of the thyroid gland

haustra: small pouches that are repeated along the length of the colon

heart murmurs: abnormal sounds made by blood as it flows through the heart that can be detected with a stethoscope

heart rate: number of heartbeats per minute

heat exhaustion: loss of body fluid and salts after exposure to heat for a prolonged time

heat stroke: occurs when body temperature rises above 40°C and the body is no longer able to cool itself

Helicobacter pylori: bacterium that causes inflammation and ulcers in the stomach and duodenum

helminths: flatworms, tapeworms, thorny-headed worms and roundworms

hemiparesis: weakness or paralysis on one side of the body

hepatic artery: carries oxygenated blood from the aorta to the liver

hepatic portal vein: transports blood containing digested food materials from the gastrointestinal tract to the liver

hepatitis: inflammation of the liver

hepatocytes: cuboid epithelial cells that line the sinusoids and perform most of the liver's specialised functions

hernia: a part of the body that protrudes through the wall of the cavity containing it

herpes zoster: virus (varicella zoster) that reactivates to cause shingles

heterozygous: pair of alleles that have different effects, e.g. one gene encodes for blue eyes and the other encodes for brown eyes

hiatus hernia: part of the stomach that pushes up into the thorax through an opening in the diaphragm

hippocampus: curved ridge in the limbic cortex thought to be the centre for short-term memory

hirsutism: growth of coarse pigmented hair on face and body

histamine: chemical signal molecule that is released from mast cells in response to injury

histology: study of the microscopic structure of cells and tissues of living organisms

homeostasis: self-regulating process that enables the conditions inside the body to remain in a steady state for optimal health

homologous chromosomes: pair of chromosomes, one from each parent, that are similar in length and gene position

homozygous: pair of alleles that have the same effect, e.g. two genes encoding for blue eyes

horizontal plane: cross-section that divides the body into superior (upper) and inferior (lower) portions

hormone: chemical signal produced and secreted by an endocrine gland in one part of the body and transported in the bloodstream to affect tissues or organs in another part

host: individual that harbours a pathogen

human chorionic gonadotrophin (hCG): hormone secreted by the placenta during pregnancy which stimulates continued production of progesterone by the ovaries

Human Genome Project (HGP): an international scientific research project that determined the entire sequence of genes in the human chromosomes

human immunodeficiency virus (HIV): virus that infects and damages white cells and reduces the body's immunity

human papillomavirus (HPV): virus that causes genital warts

Huntington's disease: inherited neurodegenerative disorder with adult onset

hyaline tissue: bluish-white tissue that forms a smooth surface on bones at places where they meet a joint

hydrocele: swelling caused by fluid around the testicles

hydrogen: the most abundant element in the universe, with atomic number 1. It reacts with carbon to form a very wide range of combustible hydrocarbons, e.g. methane

hydrolysis: splitting of chemical bonds by water

hydrophobic: repelling water

hydrostatic pressure: pressure of circulating blood that forces fluid through the capillary walls into the interstitial spaces

hymen: membrane that covers the opening of the vagina

hyoid bone: small U-shaped bone in the neck

hyperbilirubinaemia: high levels of bilirubin in blood

hypercapnia (hypercarbia): elevated level of carbon dioxide in the bloodstream

hypercholesterolaemia: high levels of cholesterol in the blood

hypercoagulation: tendency for blood to form clots too easily

hyperglycaemia: glucose content in the blood is abnormally high

hypermetropia: being long-sighted; the image is formed too far behind the retina, causing a blurred image

hyperosmolar hyperglycaemic state (HHS): rare complication that occurs in people with diabetes mellitus or profound beta cell dysfunction

hyperoxia: excess oxygen in the body

hypertension (HTN): long-term condition characterised by high blood pressure

hyperthermia: when body temperature rises above the normal homeostatic range

hyperthyroidism: too much thyroid hormone is produced by an overactive thyroid gland

hyperventilation (overbreathing): unnaturally fast, deep breathing

hypoglycaemia: glucose content in the blood is abnormally low

hypomania: elation and hyperactivity

hypoperfusion: decreased blood flow through the organs

hypophysial portal system: system of blood vessels that connects the hypothalamus with the anterior pituitary via the pituitary stalk

hypotension: abnormally low blood pressure

hypothalamic–pituitary–adrenal axis: complex set of interactions and feedback loops between these three endocrine glands

hypothalamus: tiny region on the undersurface of the cerebrum that links the nervous system to the endocrine system via the pituitary gland

hypothermia: when body temperature drops and falls below the normal homeostatic range

hypothyroidism: disorder characterised by underactive thyroid gland

hypovolaemic shock: decrease in volume of circulating blood caused by haemorrhage, dehydration, severe vomiting or diarrhoea

hypoxaemia: abnormally low concentration of oxygen in blood

hypoxia: deficiency in the amount of oxygen reaching the tissues

identical twins: genetically identical individuals that come from the same fertilised egg

ileum: last part of the small intestine where most absorption of nutrients takes place

immune response: response of the immune system to antigens

immune tolerance: when the immune system does not respond to a specific antigen

immunisation (vaccination; inoculation): uses vaccines to protect against infectious disease

immunity: body's ability to resist infection by pathogens

immunoglobulins (Ig): a class of proteins that function as antibodies

immunosenescence: the gradual deterioration of the immune system that occurs as people get older

immunosuppressants: drugs that suppress the immune system

immunotherapy: monoclonal antibodies used as medication

implantation: embedding of a blastocyst in the uterus wall

in remission: disease that lessens in severity or temporarily disappears

incontinence: lack of voluntary control over urination or defecation

incretins: a group of hormones secreted by the gastrointestinal wall that stimulate the pancreas to secrete insulin

incubation stage of disease: time between entry of a pathogen and the appearance of signs and symptoms

induction: process of labour started artificially

infectious stage: time during which pathogens can be transmitted to others

infestation: the presence of unusually large numbers of parasite

inflammatory response: response by the body to injury or disease with symptoms of pain, localised heat, redness and swelling

influenza: highly contagious viral infection of the upper respiratory tract

inguinal hernia: part of the bowel that squeezes through the lower abdominal wall into the groin

inheritance: mechanism by which characteristics (traits) are transmitted from one generation to the next

innate: present at birth

innate response: response to 'non-self' particles that uses inflammation, phagocytes and natural killer cells (second line of defence)

inorganic compound: a compound in which two chemical elements other than carbon are combined

insertion: end of a skeletal muscle attached to a bone

insidious: develops gradually

inspiration: the act of inhaling air into the lungs

insula (insulary cortex): distinct part of the cerebral cortex; it is believed to have diverse functions linked to consciousness, memory, learning and emotional response

insulin: pancreatic hormone that regulates the amount of glucose in the blood

integral proteins: proteins that span across both phospholipid layers and are permanently attached to the plasma membrane

integrated healthcare: person-centred approach to health and illness that encompasses physical, emotional, mental and spiritual aspects

intercostal muscles: muscles between the ribs involved in facilitation of breathing

interferons: proteins produced in response to the presence of a virus to stop the disease process

internal respiration: exchange of oxygen and carbon dioxide between the blood and tissue cells

interneurons (association neurons): found only in the brain and spinal cord that enable communication between sensory and motor neuron

interstitial fluid: fluid that surrounds the cells and fills the spaces (interstices) between them

intertrigo: inflammation in folds of the skin

intracellular fluid: fluid inside the cell

intracranial pressure (ICP): pressure inside the skull

intrauterine device (IUD; coil): contraceptive device inserted into the uterus to prevent pregnancy

intravenous: administered into a vein

intravitreal: administered into the eyeball

intrinsic factor: substance secreted by the stomach that enables the absorption of vitamin B12

intrinsic sugars: part of the cellular structure of unprocessed food

invasive cancer: cancer that has spread beyond the layer of tissue in which it developed and is growing into surrounding, healthy tissues

ions: an atom or group of atoms that carries a positive or negative electric charge due to the loss or gain of electrons

iron: chemical element with symbol Fe and atomic number 26 that is essential for haemoglobin and myoglobin in the body

ischaemia: inadequate blood supply to part of the body

isotonic: relating to solutions with equal osmotic pressures

jaundice: high level of bilirubin in blood causing yellowing of the skin and eyes

jejunum: middle section of the small intestine where nutrients are absorbed

joint: place where two bones meet

juxtaglomerular cells: cells of the kidney that synthesise and secrete the enzyme renin

karyotyping: the process of photographing chromosomes from a cell when they become visible during cell division, and arranging them in order

keratin: tough, fibrous protein in the outermost epidermis

kernicterus: rare bilirubin-related injury to brain tissue in newborn babies

ketoacidosis: dangerously high levels of ketones in the blood that increase its acidity

ketones: waste product of fat metabolism

kidney stones: stones that form in the kidney from calcium deposits

kidneys: paired organs that regulate the composition and volume of all body fluids

kinesiology: study of body movement

Klinefelter syndrome: male born with an extra copy of the Y chromosome (XYY)

Kupffer cells: specialised macrophages break down worn-out red blood cells passing through the sinusoids of the liver

Kussmaul breathing: deep, laboured breathing

kyphosis: excessive outward curvature of the thoracic spinal curve

labia majora: two folds of skin that enclose the vulva

labia minora: two small folds on either side of the opening of the vagina

labyrinth: fluid-filled sensory organ of the inner ear concerned with balance

lachrymal glands: tear glands

lactase: enzyme that breaks down lactose to glucose and galactose

lactational amenorrhoea method (LAM): short-term family planning method based on sustained breastfeeding

lactic acid: produced continuously from pyruvate in the process of glycolysis (anaerobic respiration)

lactic acidosis: occurs when lactic acid accumulates in the bloodstream

lactose intolerance: occurs when the body does not produce enough lactase

Langerhans cells: specialised form of dendritic cells found in dermal layers of the skin, mucosal membranes and lymph nodes

lanugo: first hair to be produced by the foetal hair follicles

large intestine: last part of the gastrointestinal tract that consists of colon, rectum and anus

larynx: upper part of the trachea containing the vocal cords

latency period: time between infection and the ability of the disease to spread to another person

learned reflexes (conditioned reflexes): actions that have to be learnt before they become automatic

legionnaires' disease: atypical form of pneumonia caused by *Legionella* bacteria

lens: transparent, flexible structure suspended behind the iris of the eye

leptin: hormone from adipose tissue that reduces the desire and motivation to eat

leucocytes: white cells in the blood and body fluids that counteract foreign substances and disease

leukaemia: cancer that originates in bone marrow with the production of very large numbers of abnormal white cells

Lewy bodies: tiny deposits of an insoluble protein in nerve cells

Leydig cells: cells of the testis that secrete testosterone

ligament: band of tough fibrous tissue which limits the amount of movement at a joint

ligand: a molecule that binds to a receptor protein

ligand-gated ion channels: protein receptors that allow ions to pass through the plasma membrane when a ligand binds to it, e.g. neurotransmitter

limbic cortex: complex set of interconnected brain structures beneath the cerebrum responsible for emotions, memories and motivation

lipase: enzyme that splits up the molecules of fat into fatty acids and glycerol

lipids: organic substances that are insoluble in water and soluble in alcohol including fats, oils, waxes and steroids

liver: largest gland in the body which processes nutrients, produces bile and is involved in many metabolic processes

local anaesthetics: technique that induces temporary loss of sensation or pain using topically applied or injected agent without reducing the level of consciousness

localised disease: affects only one part of the body

loop of Henle: part of the nephron that forms a long loop in the medulla of the kidney

lordosis: excessive inward curve of the lumbar spine

lumbago: term (now rarely used) for pain in lower back

lung function: tests that assess how well the lung is functioning

lupus (systemic lupus erythematosus; SLE): autoimmune disease of the connective tissue affecting any part of the body

luteal phase: phase in the menstrual cycle when a follicle is developing and producing oestrogen

luteinising hormone (LH): controls the secretion of sex hormones

Lyme disease: illness caused by the bite of an infected tick

lymph: fluid that flows through the lymphatic system

lymph nodes (lymph glands): bean-shaped bodies containing lymphoid tissue that are situated along the course of lymph vessels

lymphatic filariasis: *see* elephantiasis

lymphocytes: a subtype of white cells that includes natural killer (NK) cells, B cells and T cells which are critical to immunity

lymphoid tissue: encompasses all of the various tissues and organs that contribute to the immune response

lymphoma: cancer of the lymphatic system

lysosomes: organelles in cytoplasm containing enzymes that engulf and break down unwanted matter

macrophages: phagocytic cells that patrol interstitial fluid and lymph and play a central role in immunity

macula: central area of the retina which provides sharp vision

magnesium: chemical element with the symbol Mg and atomic number 12 which is cofactor in many enzyme reactions

male infertility: low sperm count, or no sperm count at all

malignant disease: becomes life-threatening if not treated

maltase: enzyme that splits up maltose to glucose

mandible: lower jawbone

Marfan syndrome: inherited disorder of the body's connective tissue

mass: the amount of matter in an object; does not change with altitude, height and gravitational force applied to it

mast cells: help to initiate early events of the inflammatory response by releasing the signal molecule histamine

mastoiditis: infection in the mastoid bone behind the ear

maternal transfer of antibodies: antibodies from the mother's blood that reach the unborn baby via blood in the placenta, and the newborn through breast milk

matrix: ground substance in which the cells and fibres are embedded

mechanically-gated channels: channel proteins that open in response to distortion of the cell membrane, e.g. touch or pressure

median forebrain bundle: bundle of nerves that links the frontal lobes with the limbic system and hippocampus

medical history: record of the medical events and problems a person has previously experienced

medulla oblongata: part of the brainstem that contains the vital centres that control involuntary reflex actions

megaloblastic anaemia: bone marrow is producing abnormally large red cells

meiosis: type of cell division that occurs only in the production of gametes – sperm and eggs

Meissner's corpuscles: receptors that are sensitive to touch in the skin

melanocytes: cells that produce melanin

melanocytic naevi (moles): collections of naevus cells, which are variants of melanocytes; sometimes called a birthmark

melanoma: cancer that originates in melanocytes – the cells which are specialised to make the pigment melanin

melatonin: hormone from the pineal gland that is important in controlling circadian rhythms

membrane attack complex (MAC): circular structure typically formed on the surface of pathogen cell membranes as a result of the activation of the host's complement proteins

memory B cells: B cells that have 'learned' to make a particular type of antibody in response to specific antigens

menarche: first menstrual period

meningitis: inflammation of the meninges caused by infection by viruses or, less often, by bacteria

menopause (climacteric): cessation of menstrual periods

menorrhagia: excessive menstrual bleeding

mental health disorder: term that is commonly used in preference to mental illness or mental disease as it is considered more value-neutral and less stigmatising

Merkel's discs: touch receptors sensitive to pressure in the skin

messenger RNA (mRNA): conveys genetic information from the nucleus to the ribosomes

metabolic pathway: sequence of chemical reactions that is regulated by enzymes

metabolic rate: rate at which metabolism occurs

metabolic syndrome: combination of diabetes, high blood pressure and obesity which increases the risk of stroke and heart disease

metabolise: change a substance by chemical reactions

metabolism: the sum of all the chemical processes that occur in the body in order to maintain life

metastasis: development of secondary malignant growths at a distance from a primary cancer

methicillin-resistant *Staphylococcus aureus* (MRSA): bacteria which have multiple resistance to antibiotics

microbial signature: an individual's unique collection of microorganisms colonising the gut

microglia: function as macrophages (scavengers) in the central nervous system

micronutrients: essential elements, including vitamins and minerals, that are required in small amounts every day

microvilli: hair-like structures that project from some intestinal cells, increasing their surface area

midbrain: part of the brainstem that connects the pons and the cerebellum

migraine: severe, recurrent and disabling headache

milk ejection reflex (let-down reflex): release of oxytocin in response to suckling that causes milk to flow freely from the breasts

minerals: elements obtained from food and used to build and maintain the body's tissues

miscarriage: spontaneous abortion

mitochondria: organelles in cytoplasm that generate most of the ATP needed for the cell's activities

mitochondrial DNA: DNA that is only found in mitochondria

mitosis: type of cell division that results in two daughter cells each having the identical DNA as the parent cell

mitral regurgitation: leakage of the mitral valve so some blood flows backwards into the atria during every heartbeat

mixture: a combination of two or more substances which keep their original properties

molecule: two or more atoms linked together by chemical bonds

monoclonal: clone derived from a single cell

monoclonal antibodies (MAB): ready-made antibodies

monocytes: circulating phagocytic white cells capable of migrating from blood into tissues where they enlarge and develop into macrophages

mononuclear phagocytic system: part of the immune system that consists of phagocytic cells located in reticular (fibrous) connective tissue of lymph nodes and spleen, and also scattered through tissues including liver, lung and skin

monosaccharide: a simple single sugar unit

mons pubis: pad of fat lying over the pubic symphysis

Montgomery tubercles: small glands in the areola producing an oily fluid that lubricates the nipple

mood disorders: mental or behavioural pattern that causes either suffering or the inability to function normally in ordinary life

morbid: 'sick' or 'unhealthy' and indicates the presence of disease

morula: an early-stage embryo consisting of a ball of cells

motor cortex: region in cerebral cortex that transmits impulses to skeletal muscles to initiate movement

motor (efferent) nerves: convey impulses from the CNS to muscles or glands

motor end plate: the flattened end of a motor neuron that connects to a muscle fibre; also called a neuromuscular junction

motor neurone disease (MND) (amyotrophic lateral sclerosis): degeneration of motor neurons with progressive weakness and wasting of skeletal muscles

motor neurons: nerve cells that transmit impulses away from the CNS to the muscles and glands

motor unit: all the muscle fibres that are innervated by a single motor neuron

mucosa (mucous membrane): mucus-secreting tissue lining the cavities and canals in the body that are linked to the external environment

mucus: clear, thin viscous fluid produced by the goblet cells in the mucosa

Müllerian duct: embryonic tissue that develops into fallopian tubes, uterus and vagina

multifactorial inheritance: polygenic inheritance that also includes interactions with the environment

multiple melanoma: cancer that originates in plasma cells which can form tumours all through the body

multiple sclerosis (MS): progressive autoimmune disease of the peripheral nervous system that destroys myelin sheaths

multipotent: stem cells that can develop into more than one type of cell

muscle tone: state of slight tension in which contraction of muscle is maintained that helps to maintain posture and keeps muscles ready for action

muscular dystrophy: rare inherited disease in which muscles progressively waste away

musculoskeletal system: gives shape and support to the body and enables it to move

mutation: change in the genetic material

myalgic encephalomyelitis (ME): chronic fatigue syndrome (CFS)

mycoses: fungal infections

mydriasis: dilation of the pupils

myelin sheath: surrounds and insulates some nerve fibres; its white colour is due to the presence of the fatty substance myelin

myeloid tissue: red bone marrow

myocardium: cardiac (heart) muscle

myocytes: muscle cells

myofibril: elongated contractile fibres in skeletal muscle

myogenic: the ability of cardiac or smooth muscle to contract in response to stretch

myometrium: thick layer of smooth muscle in the uterus wall

myopathies: diseases of skeletal muscles marked by degeneration and weakness

myopia: near-sightedness; results from images being focused in front of the retina

myosin: protein that forms the thick filaments in a sarcomere

naive B cells: B cells that have not yet been exposed to an antigen

natural killer cells (NK cells): cytoxic cells that secrete substances that rapidly induce apoptosis (cell death) in tumour- and virus-infected cells

necrosis: death of most or all cells in a tissue or organ

negative feedback: self-correcting process to restore homeostasis

neonatal hypoglycaemia: low glucose levels in newborn babies

neonatal non-haemolytic jaundice: *see* hyperbilirubinaemia

neonatal period: time between birth and 28 days of age

nephrons (renal tubules): microscopic functional units of the kidneys

nephropathy: disease or damage of the kidney, that can eventually lead to kidney failure

nerve impulse (action potential): short burst of electrochemical change that travels along an axon

nerves: bundles of parallel nerve fibres

nervous system: vast network of neurons specialised to carry impulses to, and from, all parts of the body

neurocrine signalling: occurs when neurons release chemical signals into the bloodstream that affect distant cells

neurodevelopmental disorders: disorders resulting from atypical changes in the processes of brain and skills development

neuroendocrine system: complex ways in which the nervous and endocrine systems communicate and act together

neurogenic shock: injury to the spinal cord that causes systemic vasodilation

neuroglia: *see* glia

neuroleptic drugs: class of drugs, also known as antipsychotics, that may help control symptoms of schizophrenia, bipolar disorder and other psychotic disorders

neuromuscular junction: the flattened end of a motor neuron that connects to a muscle fibre; also called a motor end plate

neurons: cells that specialise in transmitting electrical impulses

neuropathic pain: form of pain associated with dysfunction of sensory nerves

neuropathy: damage to peripheral nerves causing numbness or weakness and pain, usually in hands and feet

neuroreceptors: postsynaptic receptor proteins that are activated by a neurotransmitter at the synapse

neurotransmitter: signal molecule that is released from a presynaptic neuron and diffuses across the synaptic cleft to either excite or inhibit the target cell

neutron: a subatomic particle in the nucleus of an atom with no electrical charge and one unit of atomic mass

neutrophils: most abundant phagocytes in the bloodstream

nitrogen: chemical element with symbol N and atomic number 7 which exists in air in the form of N_2 gas and in all organisms in amino acids, proteins, nucleus acids and ATP

nociceptive pain: form of pain associated with physical damage to tissues and organs

nociceptors: sensory neurons that respond to painful stimuli

non-coding DNA: parts of the chromosomes that do not code for proteins but have other functions

non-gated channel: a channel that spans a membrane and is always open, allowing particles to diffuse along a concentration gradient from high to low

non-polar bond: a bond between two atoms where there is equal sharing of the electrons

non-specific immune system: physical and chemical barriers that defend the body against pathogens (first line of defence)

non-steroidal anti-inflammatory drugs: class of drugs used to relieve pain, reduce inflammation, reduce fever and prevent blood clots

nuclear membrane: membrane that encloses the nucleus of a cell

nuclear receptors: receptor proteins in the nucleus

nucleic acid: substances present in living cells, e.g. DNA and RNA, that consist of nucleotides linked together in a long chain

nucleolus: plays an important part in the synthesis of ribonucleic acids (RNA) and ribosomes

nucleotide: organic molecules formed from a sugar, nitrogenous base and phosphate group which are basic units for nucleic acids

nucleus: contains chromosomes that direct the activities of the cell

nucleus pulposus: soft jelly-like centre of an intervertebral disc

nutrition: the science of food and the dietary needs of the body

obesity: state of being very overweight with a high degree of body fat

obsessive–compulsive disorder (OCD): anxiety disorder that is characterised by recurrent, intrusive thoughts or images

occiput: back of the head

occult blood loss: slow and unnoticed bleeding from the gastrointestinal tract

oculomotor dysfunction (OMD): when the movements in one or both eyes do not move smoothly, accurately and quickly across a line when reading

oedema: retention of fluid in the interstitial spaces

oestrogens: female sex hormones

olfaction: the sense of smell

olfactory bulb: receives information relating to smell from the olfactory epithelium of the nose

olfactory epithelium: small (2.5 cm) patch of highly specialised tissue sensitive to odours situated on the roof of the nasal cavity

olfactory glomerulus: where synapses form between the olfactory receptors and sensory neurons

oligodendroglia: support and insulate axons (nerve fibres) by creating the myelin sheath

oligosaccharides: polymers that contain 3–10 sugar units

oncogenes: genes that have the potential to cause cancer

oncology: branch of medicine that deals with the prevention, diagnosis and treatment of cancer

oncotic pressure: form of osmotic pressure created by proteins in plasma that tends to draw water from the interstitial spaces back into the capillaries

oogenesis: development of an ovum in the ovary

opiates: drugs derived from opium poppy that are used to treat pain or induce sleep, e.g. morphine

opsonisation: process in which complement proteins and/or antibodies tag pathogens to attract phagocytes which will eliminate them

optic chiasma: X-shaped structure formed by the two optic nerves as they partly cross over in the base of the cerebrum

organ: part of the body with a special function or functions

organelle: membrane-bound structures in the cytoplasm, with each type having its own particular function

organic compound: any chemical substance that contains carbon

origin: end of a skeletal muscle attached to a bone that does not move

osmoreceptors: sensory neurons that respond to changes in the composition of blood and body fluids

osmoregulation: homeostasis of water content

osmosis: movement of water from a high to a low concentration through a semipermeable membrane

ossicles: three tiny bones in the inner ear

ossification: the processes of laying down new bone tissue

osteoarthritis: degenerative disease of the joints caused by wear and tear of the cartilage

osteocytes: bone cells

osteons (Haversian systems): basic units of compact bone

otitis media (glue ear): infection in the middle ear producing thick, sticky fluid which causes temporary deafness

ovarian reserve: estimate of the number of eggs that could be fertilised during a woman's reproductive life

ovulation: rupture of a follicle to release an ovum from the ovary

ovum (egg): female sex cell

oxygen: the chemical element with symbol O and atomic number 8 which exists in air as a colourless and odourless gas with the chemical formula O_2

oxygen debt: the amount of oxygen needed to oxidise lactic acid to carbon dioxide and water after exertion has stopped

oxytocin: stimulates the uterus to contract at the end of pregnancy and triggers the milk let-down reflex

Pacinian corpuscles: detect changes in pressure and vibration in the skin

pain: unpleasant sensory and emotional experience

pain pathway: route taken by nerve impulses from sensory receptors via the spinal cord to the brain, where pain is perceived

pallor mortis: after-death paleness that occurs in those with light skin

palpation: using the hands to feel or check a part of the body

pancreas: functions as both a digestive gland and an endocrine gland

pancreatitis: inflammation of the pancreas that can be acute or chronic

pandemic: outbreak of an infectious disease that crosses international boundaries

panic disorder: disorder characterised by recurring but unpredictable panic attacks

papilla: small, rounded protuberance on a part of the body

paracrine signalling: cell–cell communication in which cells produce signals that induce a quick response in nearby cells

parasympathetic division: part of the autonomic nervous system that prepares the body for rest, excretion and reproduction

parathyroid hormone (PTH): hormone from the parathyroid glands that regulates calcium and phosphate levels in blood and bone

Parkinson's disease: progressive disease of the nervous system marked by tremor, muscular rigidity and slow, imprecise movement

partial pressure: pressure exerted by each constituent gas in a gas mixture

particle: very tiny portion of matter such as an atom or molecule

parturition (labour; delivery): action of giving birth

passive immunity: short-term protection from ready-made antibodies

passive transport: movement of substances without using energy

pathogens: microorganisms (microbes) that cause infectious disease – mainly bacteria, viruses, fungi, protozoa and prions

pathology: study of nature and causes of disease

pathophysiology: study of the disordered physiological processes that are typically associated with, or lead to, disease

peak flow: maximum speed of expiration as measured by a peak flow meter

pectoral girdle: composed of two clavicles and two scapulae

pelvic girdle: consists of the right pelvis, left pelvis and sacrum

pelvic inflammatory disease (PID): infection of the upper female genital tract

pepsin: digestive enzyme in gastric juice that breaks down proteins into peptides

peptic ulcers: open sores that develop on the lining of the stomach or small intestine

periaqueductal grey (PAG): primary control centre for the modulation and adjustment of pain

pericarditis: inflammation of the pericardial sac

pericardium: sac of connective tissue that surrounds and encloses the heart and roots of the attached blood vessels

perimetrium: thin layer of serosa that surrounds the uterus

perineum: the diamond-shaped skin region between the anus and the scrotum or vulva

periodontitis: chronic inflammatory disease which affects the periodontal membrane that holds teeth in place

periosteum: connective tissue membrane that covers the outer surface of a bone

peripheral nervous system (PNS): part of the nervous system that is outside the brain and spinal cord

peripheral proteins: proteins that adhere to the outer surface of the phospholipid bilayer of a plasma membrane

peristalsis: rhythmic wave-like movements of the gut wall that push (squeeze) the contents forward in one direction only

peritoneal dialysis: process that uses the peritoneum as a filter for removing waste substances from the blood

peritoneum: connective tissue that lines the abdominopelvic cavity and covers the viscera

pernicious anaemia: deficiency of vitamin B12 in the body that prevents the bone marrow from making enough red cells

pertussis (whooping cough): highly contagious bacterial infection of the lungs and airways

pethidine: synthetic opiate pain-relieving drug

Peyer's patches: patches of lymphoid tissue in the digestive tract

pH scale: the scale that is used to express acidity or alkalinity

phagocytes: white cells that engulf and destroy bacteria and other small particles

phagocytosis: process by which white cells engulf and destroy bacteria and other small particles

phagosome: vesicle in which pathogenic microorganisms or worn-out parts of the cell are broken down by phagocytes

pharmacodynamics: the study of the physiological, biochemical and molecular effects of drugs and molecular effects of drugs and their side-effects

pharmacogenomics: the study of how genes affect an individual's response to drugs

pharmacokinetics: the study of the way a drug is absorbed and processed by the body

pharmacology: study of the science of drugs and their actions on the human body

pharynx (throat): muscular cavity that links the mouth and nasal passage to the oesophagus and trachea

phenotype: individual's observable characteristics determined by the interaction between genotype and environmental factors

pheomelanin: reddish-yellow form of the pigment melanin that occurs in the lips, nipples and glans of the penis

pheromones: chemical signals that elicit responses from members of the opposite sex

phlegm: thick mucus secreted in the respiratory tract during inflammation and disease

phobia: extreme and debilitating fear of a particular object, place or situation

phospholipid bilayer: two-layered arrangement of phospholipid molecules that form the basic structure of the plasma membrane

phosphorus: chemical element with symbol P and atomic number 15 that is essential for life

phosphorylation: biochemical process that involves the addition of a phosphate group to a molecule

photoreceptors: light-sensitive rods and cones

photosynthesis: a series of chemical reactions that use light energy to produce glucose and sugars from carbon dioxide and water

physiology: study of the logic of life

physiotherapy: professional practice that aims to improve flexibility, mobility and quality of life for people affected by injury or illness

pia mater: innermost layer of the meninges

pineal gland: tiny gland in the centre of the brain which produces melatonin

pinna: outer part of the ear

pituitary gland: major endocrine gland at the base of the brain

plasma: fluid part of blood

plasma cell: B lymphocyte that produces a single type of antibody

plasma membrane (cell membrane): thin semi-permeable layer around the outside of the cell which separates it from its surroundings

pleura: a two-layered sac that reduces friction between lungs and chest wall

pleural fluid: fluid in the pleural sac

pleurisy: inflammation of the pleura – the double layer covering the lungs

pluripotent: the potential to differentiate into different types of specialised stem cells

pneumothorax (collapsed lung): a build-up of air in the pleural cavity

point mutation (single gene mutation): mutation that produces a different form (allele) of the gene

polar bond: a covalent bond between two atoms where the electrons forming the bond are unequally placed

polycystic ovary syndrome (PCOS): hormone-related disorder caused by small cysts growing on the ovaries

polygenic inheritance: characteristics that are controlled by many different genes, e.g. height or hair colour

polypeptides: chains of amino acid

polyuria: production of abnormally large volumes of dilute urine

pons: part of the brainstem responsible for many of the automatic functions in the body such as breathing, swallowing, bladder and bowel control

portal circulation: special network of blood vessels that connects two organs by veins

positive feedback: homeostatic feed-forward mechanism that occurs when the input of a system is used to increase the output and amplify the response

posterior cavity of the eye: space behind the lens filled with vitreous humour

posterior pituitary (neurohypophysis): endocrine gland that releases the neurohormones, oxytocin and antidiuretic hormone (ADH)

post-herpetic neuralgia: persistent pain that occurs at the site of a previous attack of shingles

post-natal depression: severe form of depression in the early years following childbirth

post-partum (post-natal) period: first six weeks following childbirth

post-partum haemorrhage (PPH): loss of more than 500 cm³ blood following childbirth

post-traumatic stress disorder (PTSD): anxiety disorder that persists after a life-threatening event

potassium: chemical element with symbol K and atomic number 19 which is vital for the function of all living cells

Prader–Willi syndrome: rare genetic defect on chromosome number 15 causing restricted growth, short stature and compulsive behaviours

pre-ejaculate: fluid released from the bulbo-urethral glands

prefrontal cortex: region of the brain responsible for executive functions

preload: the volume of blood in the ventricles at the end of diastole

premature ovarian failure (POF): ovaries stop working before the age of natural menopause

premenstrual dysphoric disorder (PMDD): intense type of premenstrual syndrome

premenstrual syndrome (PMS): physical, psychological and behavioural symptoms that can occur in the days before menstruation

prepuce (foreskin): retractable fold of skin that covers the end of the penis

presbyopia: gradual changes in the structure of the lens as people grow older, reducing the ability to focus on close objects

pressure ulcers (bed sores): injury to soft tissues in response to prolonged pressure

priapism: abnormally prolonged, often painful erection of the penis

prions: defective proteins that damage neurons in the brain

professional antigen-presenting cell: immune cells that specialise in presenting antigens to T lymphocytes

progesterone: steroid hormone secreted by the corpus luteum and placenta

prognosis: assessment of the future course and outcome of a patient's disease

progressive disease: ailment or disorder whose course leads to degeneration over time

prolactin: hormone from the anterior pituitary gland that stimulates breast development and milk production in women

prolapsed disc (herniated disc; slipped disc): occurs when pressure on the disc causes a portion of the nucleus pulposus to push through a crack in the annulus

proprioception: conscious awareness of the position of the parts of the body and the strength required for rapid movement

proprioceptors: nerve endings in muscle spindles in tendons, joints and ligaments that detect changes in the position of the parts of the body

prosopagnosia: difficulty in making sense of faces

prostaglandins (PG): group of substances synthesised from fatty acids that have a wide range of functions

prostate gland: gland that lies just below the bladder in men

prostatitis: inflammation of the prostate gland

protease: protein-digesting enzyme

protein: molecule composed of one or more long chains of amino acids joined together by peptide bonds

prothrombin time (PT): blood test that measures how long it takes blood to coagulate

proton: a subatomic particle in the nucleus of an atom with one unit of positive electric charge

proto-oncogenes: genes which, when altered by mutation, become oncogenes

protozoa: single-celled organisms; a few can live and multiply inside the body and cause disease, e.g. *Plasmodium* causes malaria

proximal convoluted tubule: part of the nephron between Bowman's capsule and the loop of Henle

proximal epiphysis: enlarged terminal part of a bone

psoriasis: autoimmune condition that results in scaly patches of skin that itch

pubic symphysis: cartilaginous joint between the right and left pelvic bones

pulse: rhythmic expansion and contraction of arteries as blood is ejected from the ventricles during systole with each heartbeat

pulse oximeter: device that measures the oxygen saturation (%) of a person's blood

Purkinje fibres: conducting fibres embedded in the ventricles that transmit impulses to all parts of the muscular walls

pustules: blisters containing pus

pyloric sphincter: ring of smooth muscle at the junction between the stomach and duodenum that opens to allow the passage of chyme

pyrexia: fever

pyrogens: fever-inducing agents

radiotherapy: uses radiation to destroy cancerous tissue

rash: outbreak of red spots or patches on the skin

reaction: a chemical process in which substances, the reactants, are converted to one or more different substances

receptor proteins: proteins that bind specifically to signal molecules and relay the signals between the cell's external and internal environments

recessive alleles: only expressed when two recessive alleles for the same characteristic are in the genome

reciprocal innervation: describes the dual supply of autonomic nerves to organs

recombinant chromosomes: containing a unique combination of genes that increase genetic diversity

red bone marrow: contains stem cells which produce three blood components – red cells, white cells and platelets

red nucleus: group of cells in the midbrain involved in posture and balance

reflex action: rapid involuntary response to a stimulus that follows a specific nerve pathway

refractory disease: disorder or ailment that resists treatment

releasing hormones: hormones produced by the hypothalamus that control the release of the anterior pituitary hormones

renin: an enzyme made by the juxtaglomerular cells of the kidney that catalyses the production of the peptide angiotensin

renin–angiotensin–aldosterone system (RAAS): group of hormones that work together to regulate blood pressure and fluid balance

rennin: an enzyme made by the stomach that assists the digestion of milk in infancy

repetitive strain injury (RSI): refers to overuse injuries involving muscles, tendons, ligaments and nerves

reservoir of infection: the site where a pathogen lives and multiplies

respiration rate: number of breaths taken in one minute

respiratory acidosis: impaired ability to excrete carbon dioxide, making body fluids acidic and causing pH of blood to decrease

respiratory pump: expansion and contraction of the thorax that facilitates venous return

respiratory system: organ system concerned with ventilation (breathing) and gaseous exchange

respiratory tract: pathway along which air flows in and out of the body

resting potential: potential difference between the two sides of the plasma membrane of a neuron when it is not conducting an impulse

reticular activating system: bundles of neurons in the brainstem responsible for regulating level of consciousness

retina: thin lining of the eyeball containing the light-sensitive cells

retinal detachment: retina at the back of the eye begins to pull away from the blood vessels that supply it with oxygen and nutrients

retinopathy: damage to the blood vessels in the eye, leading to haemorrhage into the retina and a major cause of blindness

retrovirus: virus containing RNA

rhabdomyolysis: breakdown of skeletal muscle resulting in the release of myocyte contents into the circulation

rhesus disease (haemolytic disease of the newborn): destruction of red cells in the foetus by antibodies from the mother's blood

rhesus factor system (RhD): blood group system based on the presence or absence of the RhD antigen

rheumatoid arthritis: autoimmune disease of the synovium that usually starts in the wrists, hands or feet

rhinitis: inflammation of the nasal mucosa causing excess mucus

rhodopsin (visual purple): pigment in rods of the retina that bleaches to visual yellow in bright light and re-forms when the light becomes dim

ribosomal RNA (rRNA): found only in ribosomes where it links amino acids together to form a protein

ribosomes: organelles in cytoplasm that manufacture proteins

rigor mortis: after-death stiffening of the body

ringworm: fungal infection that feeds on keratin in skin

risk factor: condition that increases the likelihood of developing a disease or injury

RNA (ribonucleic acid): single strand of nucleotides essential for making proteins

rods: photoreceptors in the retina that function in dim light

root abscess: pus-filled swelling in the root of the tooth

rubrospinal tracts: bundle of motor nerve fibres responsible for large muscle movements of the upper limbs

saccadic eye movements: tiny, unconscious movements of the eyes as they move rapidly from one point to another

sacrum: triangular bone at the base of the vertebral column formed from five fused vertebrae

sagittal plane: runs vertically through the centre of the body, dividing it into left and right portions

salivary amylase: enzyme that begins the digestion of starch by breaking it down into disaccharides called maltose

salivary glands: three pairs of glands that secrete saliva into the mouth

salt: yields both positive ions and negative ions

saltatory conduction: movement of an action potential along a myelinated nerve fibre as it jumps from one node of Ranvier to the next

sarcomere: basic contractile unit of a myofibril

saturated fats: fatty acids with only single bonds between the carbon atoms in the chain

scapula: shoulder blade

schistosomiasis: tropical disease caused by parasitic flatworms

schizophrenia: chronic mental health disorder of the mind characterised by confused thinking and odd perceptions

Schwann cells: form the myelin sheath around axons in the peripheral nervous system

sciatica: irritation or compression of a sciatic nerve that causes pain

sclera (white of the eye): opaque, fibrous, protective outer layer of the eyeball that is continuous with the transparent bulging in front of the eye

sebaceous glands: glands in skin that produce a greasy liquid called sebum

second messenger: intracellular signalling molecule that makes the hormone effective inside the cell by causing biochemical reactions

secretin: a gastrointestinal hormone that inhibits intestinal motility and the release of gastric acid while stimulating secretion of alkaline pancreatic juice and bile

seizure: sudden surge of electrical activity in the brain

semen (seminal fluid): fluid secreted by the seminal vesicles, prostate gland and bulbo-urethral glands that may contain sperm

semicircular canals: part of the inner ear concerned with balance

seminiferous tubules: tubules within the testes in which sperm are produced

sensory (afferent) nerves: convey impulses from sense organs to the CNS

sensory cortex: region of the cerebral cortex that receives and processes information received from the sensory organs

sensory nerves: transmit impulses from the sense organs towards the central nervous system

sensory receptors: specialised nerve endings that respond to stimuli by converting them into nerve impulses

sensory system: part of the nervous system responsible for processing sensory information

sensory threshold: minimum amount of a given stimulus that gives rise to a sensation

sepsis (septic shock; septicaemia; blood poisoning): form of circulatory shock that occurs when the blood pressure drops to a dangerously low level due to an infection

serosa (serous membrane): thin layer of epithelium that covers the walls and organs within the thoracic and abdominal cavities

serous fluid: thin watery fluid found in many body cavities

serum: plasma with the fibrinogen removed

set point: level at which a homeostatic process is maintained (set) for optimum health

sex-determining region Y (SRY): gene that promotes development of the testes in the embryo

sex-linked inheritance: gene inherited on either the X or Y chromosome

shock (circulatory shock): extreme physical collapse that occurs when there is not enough pressure to maintain the blood flow to the tissues

shunt: process or anatomical structure that diverts fluid from one place to another

sickle cell anaemia: inherited disorder that is characterised by sickle-shaped red cells

signal molecules: substances whose physiological function is communication from one cell to another

signal transduction: cascade of chemical reactions in a cell that occurs when a hormone binds to a receptor on the plasma membrane

signs: objective evidence of disease that can be observed by a health professional

sinoatrial (SA) node: located in the upper wall of the right atrium and contains pacemaker cells that generate the cardiac impulse

sinusoids: blood-filled channels surrounded by hepatocytes (liver cells)

situs inversus: heart and other organs lie on the opposite side of the body from what is normal

skeletal-muscle pump: skeletal muscle contraction compresses veins and forces blood towards the heart

skin: sensory organ that covers the body's surface and forms a barrier

skin biota (commensal bacteria): microbes that live on or near the epidermis of the skin

skin integrity: the skin is healthy, undamaged and able to perform its basic function

snoring: vibration of the soft tissue at the back of the mouth, nose or throat when a person breathes in or out during sleep

sodium: chemical element with symbol Na and atomic number 11 which is the major cation in extracellular fluids and helps in maintaining fluid balance

solutes: substances in solution

solution: liquid mixture in which one or more chemical substances are dissolved

somatosensory pathways: ascending tracts of nerve fibres from the body to the brain

sperm (spermatozoa): male gametes (sex cells)

spermatic cord: connects the testicles to the abdominal cavity

spermatids: transform into mature sperm

spermatocytes: divide by meiosis to produce spermatids

spermatogenesis: development of mature sperm from spermatogonia in seminiferous tubules of the testes

spermatogonia: cells that line the walls of the seminiferous tubules and divide by mitosis to produce spermatocytes

sphincter: ring of muscle that can close an opening or tube

spinal canal: passage that runs through the vertebral column containing the spinal cord and cerebrospinal fluid

spinal nerves: nerves that connect to the spinal cord

spinous processes: bony projections from vertebrae

spiral arteries: small arteries that supply blood to the endometrium

spirometer: instrument for measuring the air entering and leaving the lungs

spleen: organ involved in the production and removal of blood cells

spongy bone: consists of a meshwork of trabeculae (bony bars) with many interconnecting spaces filled with marrow

spontaneous abortion (miscarriage): when the embryo/foetus leaves the uterus too early to survive on its own

spores: dormant forms of bacteria that are highly resistant to destruction

stable disease: disease that is neither increasing nor decreasing in extent or severity

statins: class of lipid-lowering medications that can lower levels of cholesterol

status epilepticus: emergency situation when a seizure lasts for more than 30 minutes

stem cell: unspecialised cell that can give rise to one or more different types of specialised cell

stereocilia: hair cells in the inner ear that respond to motion

sterile: free from microorganisms

steroid hormones: family of signal molecules made from lipid molecules based on cholesterol

strabismus (squint): condition in which the eyes look in different directions

stratum basale (basal layer): continuously produces new epidermal cells by mitosis

stratum corneum: outermost layer of the skin consisting of keratinised cells

stress: adverse reaction to perceived pressure when that pressure exceeds the individual's ability to cope

stridor: noisy breathing caused by obstruction of airway or larynx

stroke volume: the volume of blood ejected from each ventricle with each contraction

structural protein: protein that builds a part of the cell

subacute sclerosing panencephalitis (SSPE): type of encephalitis that can follow an attack of measles if the virus remains passively in the brain

subatomic particle: protons, neutrons and electrons

sublingual: applied under the tongue

substrate: substance upon which an enzyme acts

sucrase: enzyme that splits up sucrose to glucose and fructose

sulcus: groove or furrow on the surface of the cerebral cortex

sulphur: an essential element for living organisms with the symbol S and atomic number 16

suppository: solid block of medication applied to the rectum or vagina

suspension: a mixture in which the particles settle out of the solvent phase after a period of time, e.g. sand in water

suspensory ligament: connective tissue that holds the lens in place

sutures: form of immovable joint that forms the junction between bones

swelling: result of vascular leakage (oedema)

sympathetic division: division of the autonomic nervous system that prepares the body for action

symptoms: evidence of disease noticed by the affected individual, e.g. inflammation, pain, rash or fever

synapse: junction between two neurons

synaptic signalling: when neurons secrete chemical signals that cross a synapse

syndrome: combination of several signs and symptoms that are characteristic of a particular disease or disorder, e.g. Down syndrome

synovial joint: freely movable joint with a capsule that contains synovial fluid

synovium: lines the inner surface of a synovial joint and secretes synovial fluid

synthesis: process of uniting simpler chemical substances to form a complex chemical compound

system: group of organs working together to carry out one or more functions

systemic disease: disorder or condition that affects the entire body

systole: the time when muscular chambers of the heart contract and eject blood

T cells: T lymphocytes

tachycardia: fast heart rate that exceeds the normal resting rate for age and gender

tachypnoea: rapid breathing rate

taeniae coli: ribbon-like smooth muscles of the colon

target cells: cells with the specific receptors to receive signalling molecules

taste buds: sensory receptors situated in the sides of papillae on the tongue and in the lining of the mouth

telomere: section of DNA found at the end of a chromosome

temperature set point: homeostatic level at which the body attempts to maintain its temperature

tendonitis: inflammation of a tendon

tendons: tough cords of connective tissues that attach muscles to bones

TENS: transcutaneoous electrical nerve stimulation for pain relief

teratogenic: drugs taken in pregnancy which are harmful to the foetus

testes (testicles): male reproductive glands that produce sperm

testicular torsion: painful swelling when a spermatic cord becomes twisted

thalamus: two egg-shaped groups of neurons – one on each side of the limbic system – that act as relay centres

thalassaemia: inherited anaemia caused by mutations in the gene for haemoglobin

therapeutic: healing of disease

therapeutic index: the relationship between the dose of a drug that has a therapeutic effect and the dosage that could be lethal

therapeutic window (safety window): the range of dosages of a drug that produces a therapeutic response without causing significant adverse effects in the person

thermoreceptors: sensory endings that respond to temperature changes

thermoregulation: homeostatic process that maintains core body temperature

thoracic cage: body cavity formed by the thoracic vertebrae, ribs and sternum

'thready' pulse: pulse that feels like a mobile thread under a finger

thrombocytopenia: reduced number of platelets in the blood that increases the potential for haemorrhage

thrombosis: formation of a blood clot (thrombus) in a blood vessel, obstructing flow

thymus: organ in the neck where T lymphocytes mature and which reduces in size at puberty

thyroid: butterfly-shaped endocrine gland situated at the base of the neck in front of the trachea

thyroid-stimulating hormone: anterior pituitary hormone that regulates the secretion of thyroxine by the thyroid gland

thyrotropin-releasing hormone (TRH): hypothalamic hormone that stimulates the release of thyroid-stimulating hormone and prolactin

thyroxine: main hormone from the thyroid gland

tinnitus (ringing in the ears): condition that is characterised by the sensation of hearing sound(s) in the absence of any external sound

tissue: group of cells specialised to perform a particular function

tissue fluid: interstitial fluid

tissue-typing (HLA typing): diagnostic tests before an organ transplant to determine whether the tissues of a donor and recipient are compatible

tongue: muscular organ in the mouth that manipulates food and is the primary organ for taste sensation

tonsils and adenoids: patches of lymphoid tissue in the pharynx (throat)

topical route: applied directly to body surfaces

TORCH complex: vertically transmitted infection passed from mother to foetus

toxic effects: adverse effects of drugs that are induced by an exaggerated response compared to the therapeutic one

toxic shock syndrome (TSS): rare form of sepsis

toxicology: the branch of pharmacology which deals with poisons (toxins)

toxocariasis: infection caused by larvae of the roundworm *Toxocara*

trachea (windpipe): the airway tube that connects the larynx with the bronchi of the lungs

trachoma: infectious disease caused by infection with the bacterium *Chlamydia trachomatis*

transamination: the process of converting non-essential amino acids to essential ones

transcellular fluids: fluids derived from plasma, e.g. saliva, sweat, urine and breast milk

transcription: the process of copying a section of DNA (a gene) to make a strand of mRNA

transduction: process that converts energy from one form to another

transfer RNA (tRNA): form of nucleic acid that helps to decode mRNA to enable ribosomes to build a protein

transferrin: plasma protein that binds to iron and acts as a carrier in the bloodstream

translation: the information in mRNA is decoded to build a protein

transport proteins: proteins that transport substances across cell membranes

trauma: serious injuries to the body

trigeminal neuralgia: severe facial pain associated with the trigeminal nerve (cranial nerve V)

triglyceride: molecule that contains one glycerol molecule and three fatty acids

trigone: triangular sensory region on the floor of the bladder

trophoblast: outer layer of cells of a blastocyst which gives rise to stem cells that form the placenta

trypsin: enzyme that splits up protein to peptides in the small intestine

tuberculosis (TB): bacterial infection caused by *Mycobacterium tuberculosis* (MTB)

tumour suppressor genes: genes that inhibit cell proliferation and act as 'brakes' to slow the process of cell division

type 1 diabetes: autoimmune disorder caused by destruction of beta cells in the islets of Langerhans in the pancreas, resulting in little or no secretion of insulin

type 2 diabetes: condition characterised by cells of the body becoming resistant to insulin, or the pancreas cannot produce enough insulin for the body's needs

typhoid fever: infectious disease caused by *Salmonella typhi* that spreads through the faecal–oral route

ulcer: inflamed break in a surface inside or outside the body that fails to heal

ultrafiltration: high pressure filtration of plasma through the semipermeable structure of the glomerulus

unsaturated fats: fatty acids with at least one double bond within the fatty acid chain

urea: a waste product of protein metabolism

urethritis: inflammation of the urethra

uric acid: a waste product of nucleotide metabolism

urinary system (renal system): regulates the composition of the blood and body fluids and removes waste substances from them

urinary tract: system of ducts and channels that conduct urine from the kidneys to the exterior

urine: fluid produced by the kidneys

uterus (womb): hollow muscular organ in the female abdomen

vaccine: special preparation of antigenic material that is used to produce active immunity to a specific disease

varicocele: swelling caused by dilated (enlarged) veins within the scrotum

varicose vein: swollen veins, usually seen on the legs

vas deferens (plural vasa deferentia): duct that connects the epididymis to the urethra

vascular dementia: degenerative disorder caused by problems in the blood supply to the brain

vascular resistance: resistance that must be overcome to push blood through the circulatory system

vasectomy: surgical procedure in which the vasa deferentia are cut and sealed off

vasoconstriction: narrowing of arterioles by contraction of the smooth muscle reducing blood flow through tissue

vasodilation: widening of arterioles that results from relaxation of the muscle tissue, increasing blood flow to capillaries

vasospasm: sudden constriction of a blood vessel

vectors: organisms that transmit parasitic diseases to humans

veins: thin-walled vessels that convey blood towards the heart

ventilation: the movement of air between the atmosphere and the lungs by means of inhalation and exhalation (breathing)

ventouse: vacuum extraction using a suction cap on the baby's head

venules: tiny veins that collect blood from capillaries

vertebral column (spine): column of 33 small bones called vertebrae separated by intervertebral discs

vesicle: small membrane-bound sac that can store or transport substances inside the cell

vesicle-mediated transport: vesicles are used to move substances in or out of cells

vestibular apparatus: sensory nerve that transmits sound and balance information from inner ear to the brain

vestibulocochlear nerve (8th cranial nerve): to the auditory cortex of the brain where they are interpreted as sounds we hear

villi (singular villus): tiny finger-like projections that increase the surface area of the small intestine

Virchow's triad: three major factors that contribute to the risk of thrombosis

virulent: having a rapid, harmful effect

virus: non-living particles consisting of a strand of either DNA or RNA surrounded by a protein coat

viscera: the soft internal organs of the body, especially those contained within the abdominal, pelvic and thoracic cavities

vision (sight): ability to see

visual impairment: sight loss that cannot be fully corrected by spectacles or contact lenses

visual neglect: seeing only one side of objects

vitamin D: plays an essential role in calcium homeostasis

vitamins: substances required by the body for growth and health

vitreous humour: clear gel in the space behind the lens of the eye

vocal cords (voice box): two folds of tissue that project across the larynx

voiding: discharge of urine from the body

voltage-gated channels: protein channels embedded in cell membranes that respond to changes in the electrical properties of the membrane, e.g. depolarisation

warts: small lumps of keratin that develop in the epidermis

weight: the heaviness of a person or thing; the force of gravity on an object

Wernicke's area: located in the left side of the brain and responsible for the comprehension of speech

wet age-related macular degeneration (AMD): leakage of fluid and blood from blood vessels under the retina and the gradual loss of vision

white matter: tissue of the brain and spinal cord, consisting of nerve fibres with their white myelin sheaths

Williams syndrome: rare developmental disorder that occurs when a region of chromosome 7 containing 25 genes is deleted

Wolffian duct: embryonic tissue that develops into the male genitalia

wound: breakdown in the continuity of the skin's integrity

zymogen: inactive form of an enzyme

APPENDIX: FIGURE ACKNOWLEDGEMENTS

Figs. 2.5–2.8, 2.17 (adapted), 5.11
Science Photo Library.

Fig. 3.2
Adapted from image by Kilbad. Public domain.

Fig. 3.6
Reproduced with permission from DermNetNZ.

Fig. 5.31
Reproduced from www.footiq.com

Fig. 6.8a
Image provided by Midmark Corporation, Miamisburg, OH.

Fig. 6.9
By Mikael Häggström, used with permission. – Nunn, A. J., and I. Gregg. 1989. New regression equations for predicting peak expiratory flow in adults. *Br. Med. J.* **298**: 1068–1070. Adapted by Clement Clarke for use in EU scale.

Fig. 7.14a
Reproduced from www.calgarygi.com

Fig. 8.10
Reproduced from Wikimedia under the Creative Commons Attribution-Share Alike 4.0 International licence. Author: Jakupica.

Fig. 9.23
Reproduced from *Clinical Skills for OSCEs*, 5th ed. © Neel Burton, 2015.

Fig. 9.24
Illustration by Hilary Strickland.

Fig. 10.9
Reproduced under a Creative Commons Attribution-Share Alike 4.0 International Licence. Attribution: Diaconu Paul.

Fig. 10.10
Häggström, Mikael. "Medical gallery of Mikael Häggström 2014". Wikiversity Journal of Medicine 1 (2). doi: 10.15347/wjm/2014.008. ISSN 20018762. – Own work.

Fig. 13.7
Reproduced from *New Clinical Genetics*, 3e, by Andrew Read and Dian Donnai. © Scion Publishing Ltd.

Fig. 15.10
Centers for Disease Control and Prevention/Dr Mae Melvin.

Fig. 15.11
Reproduced under a Creative Commons Attribution-Share Alike 3.0 Unported licence. Attribution: Joel Mills.

Fig. 15.12
Reproduced under a Creative Commons Attribution-Share Alike 4.0 International Licence from *A New View on Lyme Disease: Rodents Hold the Key to Annual Risk*. Gross L, PLoS Biology Vol. 4/6/2006, e182. doi:10.1371/journal.pbio.0040182

The following figures were supplied by the author: 17.1, 17.3b, 17.4, 17.19, 17.20.

Fig. 17.2
Reproduced under the Creative Commons CC 1.0 Universal Public Domain Dedication. Author: UusiAjaja. https://commons.wikimedia.org/wiki/File:Wrist-oximeter.jpg

Fig. 17.3a
Reproduced under a Creative Commons Attribution-Share Alike 4.0 International Licence. Author: Tiia Monto. https://commons.wikimedia.org/wiki/File:Erka_sphygmomanometer.jpg

Fig. 17.5
Adapted from Thim, T., Krarup, N.H., Grove, E.L. et al. (2012) Initial assessment and treatment with the Airway, Breathing, Circulation, Disability, Exposure (ABCDE) approach. *Int. J. Gen. Med.* **5**: 117–121.

Fig. 17.7
Reproduced from Wikimedia Commons. Author: Wolfgang Moroder. https://commons.wikimedia.org/wiki/File:CRL_Crown_rump_length_12_weeks_ecografia_Dr._Wolfgang_Moroder.jpg

Fig. 17.9
Adapted from image at http://grhfad.cias.rit.edu/pligGH/ribXrays.html

Fig. 17.10
Science Photo Library (adapted).

INDEX

Bold indicates main entry; f indicates a Figure; t a Table and b a Box. Blue entries relate to online chapters 17–20. → means see/see also.